THE
Clinician's Guide to
Pediatric Nutrition

NATALIE D. MUTH
MD, MPH, RDN, FACSM, FAAP

MARY TANAKA
MD, MS, FAAP

Enjoy!
DrNatalieMuth

Happy Eating!
MaryTanaka

American Academy of Pediatrics
DEDICATED TO THE HEALTH OF ALL CHILDREN®

American Academy of Pediatrics Publishing Staff

Mary Lou White, *Chief Product and Services Officer/SVP, Membership, Marketing, and Publishing*

Mark Grimes, *Vice President, Publishing*

Sara Weissenborn, *Editor, Professional/Clinical Publishing*

Theresa Wiener, *Production Manager, Clinical and Professional Publications*

Amanda Helmholz, *Medical Copy Editor*

Mary Louise Carr, MBA, *Marketing Manager, Clinical Publications*

Published by the American Academy of Pediatrics
345 Park Blvd
Itasca, IL 60143
Telephone: 630/626-6000
Facsimile: 847/434-8000
www.aap.org

The American Academy of Pediatrics is an organization of 67,000 primary care pediatricians, pediatric medical subspecialists, and pediatric surgical specialists dedicated to the health, safety, and well-being of all infants, children, adolescents, and young adults.

While every effort has been made to ensure the accuracy of this publication, the American Academy of Pediatrics does not guarantee that it is accurate, complete, or without error.

The recommendations in this publication do not indicate an exclusive course of treatment or serve as a standard of medical care. Variations, taking into account individual circumstances, may be appropriate.

Statements and opinions expressed are those of the authors and not necessarily those of the American Academy of Pediatrics.

Any websites, brand names, products, or manufacturers are mentioned for informational and identification purposes only and do not imply an endorsement by the American Academy of Pediatrics (AAP). The AAP is not responsible for the content of external resources. Information was current at the time of publication.

The persons whose photographs are depicted in this publication are professional models. They have no relation to the issues discussed. Any characters they are portraying are fictional.

The publishers have made every effort to trace the copyright holders for borrowed materials. If they have inadvertently overlooked any, they will be pleased to make the necessary arrangements at the first opportunity.

This publication has been developed by the American Academy of Pediatrics. The contributors are expert authorities in the field of pediatrics. No commercial involvement of any kind has been solicited or accepted in the development of the content of this publication.

Every effort has been made to ensure that the drug selection and dosages set forth in this publication are in accordance with the current recommendations and practice at the time of publication. It is the responsibility of the health care professional to check the package insert of each drug for any change in indications or dosage and for added warnings and precautions.

Every effort is made to keep *The Clinician's Guide to Pediatric Nutrition* consistent with the most recent advice and information available from the American Academy of Pediatrics.

Please visit www.aap.org/errata for an up-to-date list of any applicable errata for this publication. Special discounts are available for bulk purchases of this publication. Email Special Sales at nationalaccounts@aap.org for more information.

Printed in the United States of America

9-490/1222   1 2 3 4 5 6 7 8 9 10
MA1081
ISBN: 978-1-61002-661-1
eBook: 978-1-61002-662-8

Cover and publication design by Peg Mulcahy

Library of Congress Control Number: 2022905483

American Academy of Pediatrics Reviewers

Authors

Natalie D. Muth, MD, MPH, RDN, FACSM, FAAP
W.E.L.L. Clinic Director and Pediatrician
Children's Primary Care Medical Group
Carlsbad, CA
Adjunct Assistant Professor
Community Health Sciences
UCLA Fielding School of Public Health
Los Angeles, CA

Mary Tanaka, MD, MS, FAAP
Pediatrician
Children's Primary Care Medical Group
Carlsbad, CA

To the pediatricians at Children's Primary Care Medical Group

Equity, Diversity, and Inclusion Statement

The American Academy of Pediatrics is committed to principles of equity, diversity, and inclusion in its publishing program. Editorial boards, author selections, and author transitions (publication succession plans) are designed to include diverse voices that reflect society as a whole. Editor and author teams are encouraged to actively seek out diverse authors and reviewers at all stages of the editorial process. Publishing staff are committed to promoting equity, diversity, and inclusion in all aspects of publication writing, review, and production.

Contents

Acknowledgments

Thank you to our patients and families at Children's Primary Care Medical Group (CPCMG), where both of us practice as primary care pediatricians and dedicate 1 day per week to the CPCMG W.E.L.L. Clinic, a primary care–based healthy living, nutrition, and obesity clinic. Our patients have given us a hands-on opportunity to not only deepen our understanding of a large breadth of nutritional concerns but also hone our approach to communicating what we have learned and how to best provide tailored guidance and recommendations to optimize their nutrition, across a variety of concerns and health conditions. We also want to thank the other 150 pediatricians and the leadership at CPCMG for the referrals and support of our nutrition clinic. We dedicate this resource to them, because they have trusted us with their patients and helped us deepen our expertise in pediatric nutrition. We are thrilled to have the opportunity to share this information with other pediatricians and clinicians who care for infants, children, and adolescents.

The idea for this guide came after attending a session with the publishing team of the American Academy of Pediatrics (AAP) at the AAP National Conference and Exhibition in New Orleans. We want to thank the AAP publishing team, in particular Jeff Mahony, Barrett Winston, and Sara Weissenborn, for believing in our idea and helping us turn our vision of creating a practical pediatric nutrition resource for clinicians into this book. It is a privilege to publish with the AAP. We give an extra-special heartfelt thank-you to our editor extraordinaire, Sara Weissenborn, whose attention to detail and quality of editing is unmatched. We also want to thank our copy editor, Amanda Helmholz, for ensuring the quality and consistency of the book. We cannot thank enough the expert volunteer reviewers from the many committees, councils, and sections of the AAP who provided invaluable feedback and input on each of the chapters. We especially want to thank the Section on Breastfeeding and the Section on Allergy and Immunology, who went above and beyond to help ensure the highest quality and utility of the information provided in the book. Thank you also to University of California San Diego undergraduate student Sarah Lobo for her help with preliminary research.

Thank you to our families—Bob, Thomas, and Mariella Muth and Leo, Everett, and Walden Tanaka—for their support and patience and for the hands-on opportunities they have given us to deploy much of our nutrition information and advice over the years.

Finally, thank you to pediatricians Drs Alice Kuo, Wendy Slusser, and Kate Perkins and to the UCLA Pediatrics Residency Training program that brought us together as interns more than 10 years ago, supported our interests in nutrition, and provided the opportunity for us to grow our friendship, leading us to many fun nutrition and cooking adventures together, including this latest one, *The Clinician's Guide to Pediatric Nutrition*.

Introduction

Whether through anticipatory guidance or recommendations for the management of many acute or chronic health concerns, pediatric clinicians are trusted by families to provide nutrition information and advice to support and optimize a child's health. However, even though physicians report that they are willing to provide nutritional counseling to patients and families, and patients deem them a credible source of nutrition information, few provide this nutritional counseling. Most physicians cite lack of knowledge and lack of training as key barriers.[1]

Although the National Academy of Sciences recommends that all medical students receive at least 25 hours of nutrition education, only 29% of medical schools meet this recommendation.[1] The reality is that most physicians receive very little nutrition training during medical school and residency.[2] Without sufficient training, medical students are unlikely to develop the knowledge, attitudes, skills, and confidence to provide nutritional coaching or counseling to patients and their families when they become attending physicians, yet patients and their families have many nutritional concerns and questions. Most pediatricians have limited access to a nutrition specialist, such as a registered dietitian nutritionist, to refer patients to. Given the time demands and limited training, clinicians need an easy-to-use, credible, evidence-based resource to optimize nutritional management.

The Clinician's Guide to Pediatric Nutrition is a resource written for primary care clinicians who work with infants, children, and adolescents. It includes the most up-to-date evidence-based and evidence-informed nutrition recommendations across the variety of topics that clinicians routinely encounter. With this resource, clinicians can feel confident that they are providing their patients the best nutritional advice.

An Overview

The Clinician's Guide to Pediatric Nutrition features many of the most common nutrition topics encountered in the primary care setting and provides guidance, resources, and recipes to help families translate guidance into nutritional changes. This guide helps pediatricians effectively apply nutrition information to the unique nutritional concerns their patients experience in the context of a busy primary care practice.

This book shows clinicians how to

- Evaluate growth and development, weight and adiposity, and signs of nutritional deficiency or excess.
- Complete a nutritional assessment, including a nutritional history, and provide a patient-specific nutritional treatment plan.
- Recognize whether a child has an unhealthy nutritional profile, such as malnutrition or nutritional deficiencies, and develop a plan to improve nutritional health.

- Determine macronutrient, micronutrient, and fluid needs for infants, children, and adolescents based on the Dietary Reference Intakes, a set of reference values used to plan and assess nutrient intakes of apparently healthy people who have typical growth and plasma nutrient levels.
- Select and interpret findings from screening and laboratory tests and diagnostic procedures to assess and manage a patient's nutrition.
- Use behavior change strategies and coaching techniques matched to a patient and family's readiness for change, including motivational interviewing, SMART goal setting, problem-solving, self-monitoring, stimulus control, and the 5 A's (ask, assess, advise, assist/agree, and arrange).
- Provide age-specific nutritional guidance for newborns or infants, toddlers, pre-schoolers, school-aged children, and adolescents on the basis of the most up-to-date information, including the *2020–2025 Dietary Guidelines for Americans.*
- Most effectively incorporate scientifically sound nutritional guidance into the treatment of many common pediatric concerns, such as anemia, reflux, constipation, underweight, childhood overweight and obesity, dyslipidemia, prediabetes, fatty liver disease, hypertension, disordered eating, attention-deficit/hyperactivity disorder, and autism.
- Consult or refer to a registered dietitian and other health care professionals and community resources as appropriate.
- Screen for food insecurity, and connect with public health resources.
- Confidently answer the most common nutrition questions that parents and patients ask their pediatrician.
- Integrate nutrition principles into everyday life through application of culinary medicine and recipes.

Target Audience

The primary audience for this book is the pediatric primary care clinician who cares for children and adolescents in the outpatient setting, routinely providing nutrition-related anticipatory guidance during health supervision visits and addressing nutrition-related concerns, from the newborn stage to young adulthood. This includes primary care pediatricians, family physicians, pediatric and family nurse practitioners, and pediatric and family physician assistants. The secondary audience for this book includes pediatric residents, clinicians from other specialties who commonly work with children and adolescents, registered dietitians, and other allied health professionals.

Key Themes

The Clinician's Guide to Pediatric Nutrition emphasizes several key themes that are discussed and elaborated on throughout the text.

- Nutrition recommendations are best tailored to a child's age and developmental stage.
- A healthy, balanced eating pattern consistent with federal MyPlate recommendations provides a simple framework for nutritional guidance and applies to most children

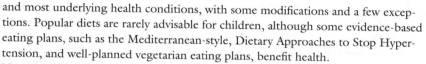

and most underlying health conditions, with some modifications and a few exceptions. Popular diets are rarely advisable for children, although some evidence-based eating plans, such as the Mediterranean-style, Dietary Approaches to Stop Hypertension, and well-planned vegetarian eating plans, benefit health.

- Nutrition plays an important role in and influences many common health conditions that infants, children, and adolescents experience, across all major organ systems and pediatric specialties.
- The knowledge of how to eat and the psychology of food and nutrition are as important as the understanding of what to eat when providing nutrition recommendations. This point is especially true in pediatrics, in which pediatricians offer nutritional advice most often to a parent or another caregiver who is then responsible for implementing the guidance with a child who may or may not be on board with the recommendations.
- Effective communication, an understanding of social determinants of health, and tailoring of guidance to a patient and family's current understanding, access to resources, and readiness to change are essential to support translation of nutrition information into patient-level behavior changes.

Features

The Clinician's Guide to Pediatric Nutrition includes several features that help clinicians translate knowledge gained into action to provide better and more efficient nutritional care to children, adolescents, and their families.

- **Clinical Practice Tips.** These boxes include easy-to-use and easy-to-access tools, resources, and information to help streamline nutritional assessment and counseling for busy clinicians.
- **In Greater Depth.** The evidence behind commonly discussed nutrition topics and controversies is explored in these boxes.
- **Frequently Asked Questions.** Quick answers to parents' and patients' most common questions are featured in this chapter of Part 5, Frequently Asked Questions, Case Studies, and Recipes.
- **Case Studies.** Patient examples bring key principles to life in this chapter of Part 5, Frequently Asked Questions, Case Studies, and Recipes.
- **Recipes and culinary tips.** Included in the book are recipes and culinary tips that clinicians can share with patients and families to make it fun and easy to translate information into real-world, actionable change leading to improved nutrition. Recipes and culinary tips related to chapter content can be found in Part 5, Frequently Asked Questions, Case Studies, and Recipes. Culinary tips are also included in Chapter 13, Culinary Medicine and Strategies for Healthy Eating.

Ultimately, *The Clinician's Guide to Pediatric Nutrition* will help pediatric clinicians develop a strong foundation and skills in nutritional assessment and counseling to help patients and their families thrive.

References

1. Aspry KE, Van Horn L, Carson JAS, et al; American Heart Association Nutrition Committee of the Council on Lifestyle and Cardiometabolic Health, Council on Cardiovascular and Stroke Nursing, Council on Cardiovascular Radiology and Intervention, and Stroke Council. Medical nutrition education, training, and competencies to advance guideline-based diet counseling by physicians: a science advisory from the American Heart Association. *Circulation.* 2018;137(23):e821–e841 PMID: 29712711 doi: 10.1161/CIR.0000000000000563

2. Crowley J, Ball L, Hiddink GJ. Nutrition in medical education: a systematic review. *Lancet Planet Health.* 2019;3(9):e379–e389 PMID: 31538623 doi: 10.1016/S2542-5196(19)30171-8

PART 1

Nutrition Essentials

A varied and healthy eating plan is essential for children to obtain adequate energy and the necessary nutrients for physiological function, growth, and maturation and to fuel physical activity and exercise. When children optimize nutrition intake, including meeting recommendations for macronutrients (carbohydrates, protein, and fat), micronutrients (vitamins and minerals), and fluids (water), they are poised for good health during childhood, adolescence, and adulthood.

Chapter 1, Dietary Reference Intakes (DRIs), outlines the types of DRIs and details how to determine a child's recommended caloric intake. Chapters 2 through 4, Carbohydrates, Protein, and Fats, apply the DRIs in discussion of macronutrients, and Chapters 5 through 7, Vitamins, Minerals, and Water and Hydration, apply the DRIs in discussion of micronutrients and water. For pediatric clinicians, this information serves as the foundation for applying nutritional assessment and guidance throughout infancy, childhood, and adolescence and in addressing the role of nutrition in the prevention and management of chronic disease.

CHAPTER 1

Dietary Reference Intakes

Children have unique nutritional needs to support optimal growth, optimal development, and overall health. The Dietary Reference Intakes (DRIs) provide a bench-
mark to help ensure that children obtain appropriate intakes of calories, macronutrients
(carbohydrates, protein, and fat), micronutrients (vitamins and minerals), and fluids.
Familiarity with the DRIs is important for pediatric clinicians to apply when advising
patients and their families about what and how much to eat to optimize pediatric health
and nutrition.

The DRIs include a set of 6 nutrient-based reference values used to assess nutrient
intake and plan healthy diets for people across age, sex, and 22 life stages: the estimated
average requirement (EAR), recommended dietary allowance (RDA), adequate intake (AI),
tolerable upper intake level (UL), estimated energy requirement (EER), and acceptable
macronutrient distribution range (AMDR).[1] The DRIs form the basis for nutritional
assessment and counseling described in parts 2, Nutritional Assessment, and 3, Nutritional
Counseling.

The EAR, RDA, and AI are used as follows to define nutritional adequacy:

- The EAR is the median usual intake needed to meet nutrient requirements of
  half the population for age and sex.
- The RDA is the level needed to meet nutrient requirements of nearly all healthy
  individuals (97%–98%). The RDA is set at 2 SDs above the EAR. When available,
  the RDA is the target intake for age and sex.
- The AI is the approximate intake that healthy individuals need to meet nutrient
  requirements. This value is used when there are insufficient data available to determine the EAR and RDA. The AI is the target intake for age and sex for nutrients
  for which there are not enough data to establish an RDA. This is often the case
  in infancy.

Tables A-1 through A-3 in the Appendix detail the RDA for the macronutrients,
micronutrients, and water by age and sex.

The UL is used as follows to define potential risk of toxicity:

- The UL is the highest level of daily intake of a nutrient to pose no risk of toxicity in
  almost all individuals.

Tables A-4 and A-5 in the Appendix detail the UL for vitamins and minerals.

Estimated Energy Requirement

The EER is an equation used to approximate caloric needs for a child based on age,
sex, weight, height, and physical activity level. It takes into account the energy necessary for basic physiological functions such as metabolism, circulation, respiration,
and protein synthesis; the thermic effect of food (energy required for consumption,

3

digestion, transport, metabolism, and storage of food); thermoregulation; growth and development; and physical activity. Most other commonly used predictive equations do not account for all these factors.[1] The EER is the preferred predictive equation for estimating a child's caloric needs. Refer to **tables A-6 and A-7** in the Appendix for the formulas needed to calculate the EER.

A General Estimate of Energy Needs

For clinicians who may not be inclined to use the EER equation to estimate a child's caloric needs, **Table 1-1** provides a general estimate of daily calories needed to support typical growth and development, based on a child's age. This estimate is adapted from the US Department of Agriculture and US Department of Health and Human Services *Dietary Guidelines for Americans* and based on the EER, using reference (average) heights and reference (healthy) weights by age and sex. Calories are supplied by the macronutrients as follows: carbohydrates (4 kcal/g), protein (4 kcal/g), and fat (9 kcal/g). Because these values are estimates, clinicians should monitor and adjust intakes based on a child's individual growth trajectory.

Acceptable Macronutrient Distribution Range

The AMDR is the DRI that describes the proportion of daily caloric intake derived from carbohydrates, protein, and fat that not only provides the AI of essential nutrients but also helps reduce risk of chronic diseases such as heart disease, diabetes, obesity, and cancer.[1] Refer to **Table A-8** in the Appendix for AMDR by age.

The AMDR advises that children 3 years and older obtain 45% to 65% of their daily calories from carbohydrates such as whole grains, vegetables, and fruits; 25% to 35%, from fats such as nuts, seeds, and oils; and 10% to 30%, from proteins such as fish, poultry, meat, and beans. Children aged 1 to 3 years need slightly more calories from fat (30%–40%) and slightly less calories from protein (5%–20%). Note that most foods may be predominantly one type of macronutrient but generally contain smaller amounts of one or more of the other macronutrients. For example, black beans are 71% carbohydrate, 27% protein, and 3% fat. As discussed in Chapter 5, Vitamins, clinicians can help families meet these recommendations through encouraging consumption of a varied diet of whole foods.

The DRI Calculator for Health Care Professionals discussed in **Box 1-1** provides clinicians with a convenient tool to easily determine the DRIs for any individual patient.

Interpreting Dietary Reference Intakes on the Nutrition Facts Label

Federal law requires that packaged foods and beverages include a Nutrition Facts label. The nutrition label helps translate the DRIs into practical nutrition information that families can use to make healthier choices to meet nutritional needs. Clinicians can help families use the label to compare products, make healthier choices, and meet nutritional

Table 1-1. Approximate Caloric Needs Based on Age, Sex, and Physical Activity Level

Age	Caloric needs for males[a]			Caloric needs for females[a]		
12 mo	800			800		
15 mo	900			800		
18 mo	1,000			900		
21–23 mo	1,000			1,000		
	Activity level					
	Sedentary	Moderately active	Active	Sedentary	Moderately active	Active
2 y	1,000	1,000	1,000	1,000	1,000	1,000
3 y	1,000	1,400	1,400	1,000	1,200	1,400
4 y	1,200	1,400	1,600	1,200	1,400	1,400
5 y	1,200	1,400	1,600	1,200	1,400	1,600
6 y	1,400	1,600	1,800	1,200	1,400	1,600
7 y	1,400	1,600	1,800	1,200	1,600	1,800
8 y	1,400	1,600	2,000	1,400	1,600	1,800
9 y	1,600	1,800	2,000	1,400	1,600	1,800
10 y	1,600	1,800	2,200	1,400	1,800	2,000
11 y	1,800	2,000	2,200	1,600	1,800	2,000
12 y	1,800	2,200	2,400	1,600	2,000	2,200
13 y	2,000	2,200	2,400	1,600	2,000	2,200
14 y	2,000	2,400	2,800	1,800	2,000	2,400
15 y	2,200	2,600	3,000	1,800	2,000	2,400
16 y	2,400	2,800	3,200	1,800	2,000	2,400
17 y	2,400	2,800	3,200	1,800	2,000	2,400
18 y	2,400	2,800	3,200	1,800	2,000	2,400

Adapted from US Department of Agriculture, US Department of Health and Human Services. *Dietary Guidelines for Americans, 2020–2025.* 9th ed. 2020. Accessed September 14, 2022. https://www.dietaryguidelines.gov.

[a] Caloric needs are approximate. They may vary for individual children and adolescents, especially for children aged < 3 y, and older children on the basis of other factors such as height. Patients can find individualized plans at MyPlate (www.myplate.gov/myplate-plan).

needs (**Box 1-2**). An overview of the components of the nutrition label is included in **Figure 1-1**. Note that the nutrition label is based on a standard 2,000-Cal diet, so the actual "% Daily Value" may be a greater percentage of the daily RDA for children and adolescents who need less than 2,000 Cal/d.

CLINICAL PRACTICE TIP

Box 1-1. Dietary Reference Intake Calculator for Health Care Professionals

The DRI Calculator for Health Care Professionals, available at the National Agriculture Library website (www.nal.usda.gov/human-nutrition-and-food-safety/dri-calculator), is a free tool from the National Academy of Sciences that calculates a patient's nutrient needs based on their age, sex, height, weight, and activity level. After inputting this patient demographic information, the clinician receives a report of the child's body mass index, estimated daily caloric needs, and recommended intake of macronutrients (including carbohydrate, total fiber, protein, fat, saturated fat, alpha-linolenic acid, and linoleic acid), dietary cholesterol, total water, and micronutrients, including all water- and fat-soluble vitamins and essential and nonessential minerals.

CLINICAL PRACTICE TIP

Box 1-2. Continuing Medical Education Program for Pediatricians and Labels Unwrapped

Clinicians can learn more about how to best teach patients and families to read the Nutrition Facts label, access patient resources, and obtain continuing medical education credit at the Continuing Medical Education Program for Pediatricians website developed by the US Food and Drug Administration and the American Academy of Pediatrics (www.fda.gov/food/healthcare-professionals/nutrition-facts-label-continuing-medical-education-program-pediatricians). Additionally, clinicians can encourage families interested in learning more about nutrition labels to visit Labels Unwrapped (https://labelsunwrapped.org), a website from the Vermont Law School Center for Agriculture and Food Systems that details information about the nuances of the nutrition label and, in issue briefs, highlights up-to-date information on nutrition label hot topics.

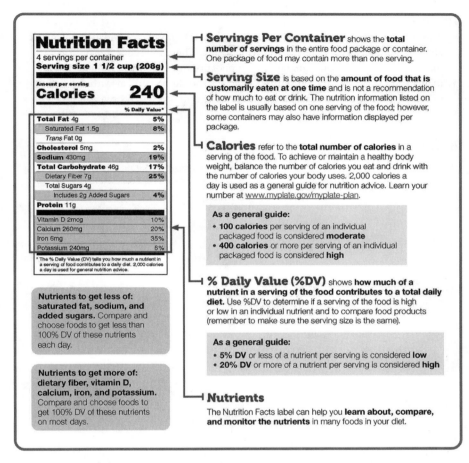

Figure 1-1. Understanding and using the Nutrition Facts label.

Reproduced from US Food and Drug Administration. https://www.accessdata.fda.gov/scripts/interactivenutritionfactslabel/assets/InteractiveNFL_UnderstandingTheNFL_October2021.pdf. Accessed September 14, 2022.

In Sum

- The 6 DRIs (EAR, RDA, AI, UL, EER, and AMDR) provide guidance on caloric and nutrient needs for children and adolescents. These reference intakes form the foundation for nutritional guidance to support optimal growth, optimal development, and overall nutritional status. Clinicians should be familiar with the definition of each DRI and how to calculate recommended intakes based on a child's age, sex, height, weight, and activity level.

Reference

1. Institute of Medicine. *Dietary Reference Intakes for Energy, Carbohydrate, Fiber, Fat, Fatty Acids, Cholesterol, Protein, and Amino Acids.* National Academies Press; 2005

CHAPTER 2

Carbohydrates

Children and adolescents need about half their total daily calories from carbohydrates, which are found primarily in grains, vegetables, and fruits. Carbohydrates serve as the body's preferred energy source. The brain and red blood cells rely almost exclusively on carbohydrates for fuel, whereas other cells prefer carbohydrates but can also use protein or fat. Carbohydrates facilitate cardiovascular and digestive health, help regulate glucose and insulin metabolism, support cholesterol and triglyceride metabolism, and provide a sweet taste to foods, which helps increase palatability. They also serve as a gut microbial energy source, playing an important role in supporting a healthy microbiome.

Carbohydrate Needs

The acceptable macronutrient distribution range for carbohydrates in children and adolescents is 45% to 65% of total daily calories, most of which should be derived from whole grains (refer to **Table A-8** in the Appendix). The recommended dietary allowance for carbohydrates is 130 g for children 1 year and older, adolescents, and most adults (refer to **Table A-1** in the Appendix).[1] When carbohydrates are consumed in excess or when consumption of highly processed or refined carbohydrates (eg, sugary drinks, candies, baked goods) is high, children may experience atypical weight gain, tooth decay, and other health risks. When intake is very low, such as during fasting, starvation, or carbohydrate restriction, protein and fat are used for energy. This produces a state of ketosis, and long-term effects may include bone mineral loss, hypercholesterolemia, kidney stones, and decreased mental functioning.[1]

Carbohydrate Structure and Types

Carbohydrates are named for their chemical composition of carbon, hydrogen, and oxygen atoms. They are made of short or long chains of monosaccharides, or sugars. Monosaccharides contain the general chemical structure of $C_6H_{12}O_6$.

Monosaccharides are found in nature in primarily 5 forms, as follows:

- Glucose is the body's primary energy source.
- Fructose is fruit sugar that is also found in honey, agave nectar, some vegetables, and many processed foods with added sugars (eg, sucrose, high-fructose corn syrup).
- Galactose is about as sweet as glucose, usually found as disaccharide (lactose).
- Xylose is sugar derived from plant cell walls. Its derivative, xylitol, is often used as a low-calorie sugar substitute and sweetener in food products. In contrast to other sugars, which can cause tooth decay, xylitol can help prevent tooth decay. It contains fewer calories than glucose because it can be only partially metabolized in the human gut.
- Ribose is a sugar produced by the body. It is an important component of adenosine triphosphate, which provides energy to the body's cells.

Disaccharides are sugars that include 2 monosaccharides joined together, and in this process, 2 hydrogen molecules and 1 oxygen molecule are eliminated in the form of water. The general chemical structure is $C_{12}H_{22}O_{11}$. Disaccharides include the following combinations:

- Glucose + fructose = sucrose (table sugar).
- Glucose + galactose = lactose (milk sugar; the major carbohydrate in human milk, which increases in content as colostrum progresses to mature milk).[2]
- Glucose + glucose = maltose (less sweet than sucrose and lactose, often used in hard candies and frozen desserts because of its high tolerance to heat and cold).

Short-chain carbohydrates (monosaccharides and disaccharides) are referred to as *sugars* or *simple sugars* and include fruit juice and the many variations of sugar (**Box 2-1**). Simple sugars are digested quickly, causing a rapid rise in blood glucose and subsequent insulin secretion from the pancreas. This can be beneficial in providing a quick energy source; however, excess sugar consumption is detrimental to health, contributing to atypical weight gain, worsened cardiovascular health, and tooth decay.[4]

Sugars are often added to foods and beverages to sweeten, preserve, or add viscosity, texture, body, or browning capacity to them.[1] Food manufacturers are continually searching for ways to sweeten foods while responding to consumer demand for less added sugars and sweeteners. Most recently, some manufacturers have begun to sweeten foods with allulose, a relatively rare sugar that has 70% of the sweetness of sugar—with 0.4 Cal/g, compared to 4 Cal/g of sugar. Although present naturally in a few foods such as jackfruit and raisins, allulose used in the food supply is manufactured by converting fructose from corn into allulose via microbial enzymes. The US Food and Drug Administration allows for allulose to be excluded from the total and added sugars declarations on the nutrition and supplement facts labels because it has a low-calorie level and minimal effect on blood glucose and insulin levels and does not promote tooth decay.

The *Dietary Guidelines for Americans, 2020–2025,* and the American Heart Association advise that infants and children younger than 2 years consume no added sugars from food or beverages.[5,6] Children older than 2 years and adolescents should limit added sugar intake to no more than 6% of total calories, as recommended by the Scientific Report of the 2020 Dietary Guidelines Advisory Committee,[5] or 25 g, as recommended by the American Heart Association,[4] whichever is lower. Actual intake is typically much higher. Data from the National Health and Nutrition Examination Survey suggest that 84% of children younger than 2 years consume added sugars,[7] and average daily intake for children, adolescents, and young adults aged 2 to 19 years is 17 tsp (68 g) of added sugars per day.[8] Although children consume added sugars from obvious sources such as soda and cookies, added sugars are also hidden in seemingly healthy foods (**Box 2-2**). Refer to Part 5, Frequently Asked Questions, Case Studies, and Recipes, for recipes that are low in added sugars and can satisfy children's desire for sweet food and drinks while promoting good nutrition.

Complex carbohydrates are made up of 3 or more monosaccharides joined together and include oligosaccharides (3–10 monosaccharides) and polysaccharides (>10 monosaccharides). There are more than 100 different oligosaccharides in human milk, which are important nutrition sources and play an important role as prebiotics, or food

Box 2-1. The Various Forms of Sugar in the Food Supply

Sugars that occur naturally in foods, such as fructose in fruits and lactose in dairy products, are usually present alongside other nutrients (eg, fiber, vitamins, and minerals) that support optimal health. An exception is honey, which is a natural sugar that contains only trace amounts of other nutrients. Added sugars, which some food and beverage manufacturers use in excess to promote a sweet taste and improve palatability, typically provide no nutritional value and contribute to excess caloric intake and increased risk of many health concerns, such as obesity, type 2 diabetes, cardiovascular disease, some cancers, and tooth decay. Sugar shows up on the ingredient list in packaged foods in at least 61 ways,[3] as noted in the following list, and many food products targeted toward children contain multiple forms of added sugars:

- Agave nectar
- Barbados sugar
- Barley malt
- Barley malt syrup
- Beet sugar
- Brown sugar
- Buttered syrup
- Cane juice
- Cane sugar
- Caramel
- Carob syrup
- Caster sugar
- Coconut palm sugar
- Coconut sugar
- Confectioners' sugar
- Corn sweetener
- Corn syrup
- Corn syrup solids
- Date sugar
- Dehydrated cane juice
- Demerara sugar
- Dextrin
- Dextrose
- Evaporated cane juice
- Free-flowing brown sugars
- Fructose
- Fruit juice
- Fruit juice concentrate
- Glucose
- Glucose solids
- Golden sugar
- Golden syrup
- Grape sugar
- High-fructose corn syrup
- Honey
- Icing sugar
- Invert sugar
- Malt syrup
- Maltodextrin
- Maltol
- Maltose
- Mannose
- Maple syrup
- Molasses
- Muscovado
- Palm sugar
- Panocha
- Powdered sugar
- Raw sugar
- Refiners' sirup
- Rice syrup
- Saccharose
- Sorghum syrup
- Sucrose
- Sugar (granulated)
- Sweet sorghum
- Syrup
- Treacle
- Turbinado sugar
- Yellow sugar

CLINICAL PRACTICE TIP

Box 2-2. Teaching Patients to Look for Added Sugars

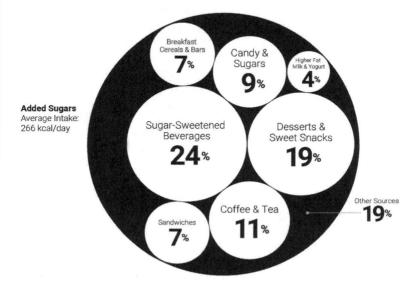

Added Sugars
Average Intake:
266 kcal/day

Breakfast Cereals & Bars **7%**

Candy & Sugars **9%**

Higher Fat Milk & Yogurt **4%**

Sugar-Sweetened Beverages **24%**

Desserts & Sweet Snacks **19%**

Sandwiches **7%**

Coffee & Tea **11%**

Other Sources **19%**

Top sources and average intakes of added sugars: US population ages 1 and older.

Reproduced from US Department of Agriculture, US Department of Health and Human Services. *Dietary Guidelines for Americans, 2020–2025.* 9th ed. 2020. Accessed September 14, 2022. https://www.dietaryguidelines.gov.

Added sugars are present in larger than expected amounts in known sugary items such as soda and suspected "healthy" foods such as yogurt and granola bars. Clinicians can help school-aged and adolescent patients and the families of children of all ages limit sugar intake by teaching them how to read a Nutrition Facts label and, specifically, how to identify the number of grams of added sugars per serving.[a]

This can be an easy and effective hands-on activity done in the clinic with just a few props: a 20-fl oz (0.6-L) bottle of soda, an empty 6-fl oz (0.2-L) cup of yogurt, 1 granola bar, a set of measuring cups and spoons, and a paper towel or clear bag. Clinicians or other clinical team members first review a nutrition label with patients and identify the number of grams of added sugars stated. Then, they measure 1 tsp of sugar for every 4 g of

CLINICAL PRACTICE TIP

Box 2-2 (*continued*)

added sugars and place it onto a paper towel or clear bag. Then, they show the patient and/or family the amount of sugar on the paper towel or bag, compare that to the total recommended amount for the day, and ask whether the amount is more or less than the patient and/or family expected.

Additionally, per the US Food and Drug Administration, sugars included in a product must be included on the ingredient list and can be listed by the various names included in **Box 2-1**. Clinicians may show interested patients and their families how to use the ingredient list to identify obvious and added sugars.

[a] 4 g = 1 tsp.

sources for healthy gut bacteria.[2] Maltodextrin and raffinose are examples of oligosaccharides in the food supply. Manufacturers add maltodextrin to foods such as pastries, candies, and sugary drinks to improve flavor, thickness, or shelf life. Raffinose is a glucose-galactose-fructose chain found in vegetables such as beans, cabbage, brussels sprouts, broccoli, and asparagus. The human digestive tract does not contain the enzyme needed to digest raffinose, which is one reason why these foods tend to cause flatulence. Raffinose may serve as an important prebiotic. Prebiotics are detailed more in **Box 2-3**.

Starch, the plant storage form of carbohydrate, is a polysaccharide comprised of long chains of amylase (long, linear glucose chains) and amylopectin (highly branched glucose chains). Starchy foods include many grains, potatoes, and other root vegetables. On the whole, polysaccharides take longer to digest than simple sugars, causing a slower and more steady increase in blood glucose and insulin levels than that of simple sugars.

Glycemic Index

Glycemic index (GI) is a measure of blood glucose response after a person consumes a carbohydrate. This scale ranks carbohydrates from 0 to 100 on the basis of how quickly blood glucose level rises after consumption. Starchy foods that are less processed and more slowly absorbed have a lower GI and are generally healthier than highly processed or rapidly absorbed starches and sugar. However, this health benefit may be caused more by their fiber content than GI.[9]

- Low-glycemic foods (≤55) include steel-cut oatmeal, oat bran, muesli, sweet potatoes, peas, legumes, most fruits, and non-starchy vegetables.
- Medium-glycemic foods (56–69) include quick oats, brown rice, and whole wheat bread.
- High-glycemic foods (70–100) include white bread, cornflakes, white potatoes, pretzels, rice cakes, and popcorn.

Glycemic load (GL) is a measure of the GI and the total amount of carbohydrate in a serving. It is calculated by multiplying the GI by the grams of carbohydrate per serving divided by 100. In general, a GL of 20 or higher is high; 11 to 19, intermediate; and 10 or lower, low. Following are examples of how GL may be of more utility than GI:

- White rice has a GI of about 67, with 53 g of carbohydrate per 1-c (150-g) serving. The GL is calculated as $67 \times 53/100 = 35$. Although white rice is a medium-GI food, a 1-c serving has a high GL.
- White bread has a GI of 71, with 14 g of carbohydrate per 1 slice (30 g). The GL of a sandwich with 2 slices of white bread is calculated as $71 \times 28/100 = 20$. This is in contrast to 2 slices of whole grain bread. Whole wheat bread has a GI of 51 and 13 g of carbohydrate per 1 slice. The GL is calculated as $51 \times 26/100 = 13$.
- Watermelon has a GI of about 76, with 11 g of carbohydrate per 1-c (150-g) serving. The GL for a 1-c serving of watermelon is calculated as $76 \times 11/100 = 8$. In contrast to white bread, which is a high-GI food and has high GL, watermelon is a high-GI food, but a 1-c serving has a low GL.

Values of GI and GL for foods are available at The University of Sydney website (https://glycemicindex.com).

Fiber

Fiber refers to all parts of plant-based foods that cannot be fully digested or metabolized by the body, such as cellulose, hemicellulose, and pectin. *Dietary fiber* refers to insoluble and soluble fiber obtained through consumption of foods such as fruits, vegetables, whole grains, and legumes (**Table 2-1**).

Insoluble fiber passes through the gastrointestinal tract undigested, where it absorbs water in the large intestine, softening and bulking stool. It also serves as a prebiotic to support healthy gut bacterial growth. Foods high in insoluble fiber include brans, seeds, vegetables, brown rice, and potato skins.

Soluble fiber is partially digested in the gastrointestinal tract, forming a gel-like substance in the intestines. Soluble fiber helps decrease levels of blood cholesterol and low-density lipoprotein, decrease straining with bowel movements, and blunt postprandial glucose levels. Fleshy fruits, oats, broccoli, and dried beans are high in soluble fiber.

Functional fiber is isolated, extracted, or synthetically manufactured fiber that serves a beneficial physiological purpose. Functional fibers include plant-derived pectin and gums, animal-derived chitin and chitosan, and commercially produced resistant starch and polydextrose. Functional fibers are common components in fiber supplements.

Most children do not consume the recommended daily intake of fiber (refer to **Table A-1** in the Appendix).

Carbohydrate Digestion, Absorption, and Storage

Carbohydrate digestion starts in the mouth when the salivary enzyme amylase breaks down starches into smaller polysaccharide chains and maltose. Stomach acids inactivate amylase, essentially halting carbohydrate digestion in the stomach. The presence of

Table 2-1. Sources of Dietary Fiber

Food	Fiber content (g)
Fruits	
Raspberries (1 c)	8.0
Blackberries (1 c)	7.6
Pear (1 medium)	5.5
Apple with skin (1 medium)	4.4
Blueberries (1 c)	3.6
Orange (1 medium)	3.4
Banana (1 medium)	3.1
Strawberries (1 c)	2.9
Yellow peach with skin (1 medium)	2.6
Fig (1 large)	1.9
Medjool date (1 pitted)	1.5
Vegetables	
Artichoke hearts (1 c)	9.6
Green peas (1 c)	8.3
Edamame (1 c)	8.1
Tomatoes, red, ripe, canned in tomato juice (1 c)	4.6
Sweet potato with skin (1 medium)	3.8
Sweet corn (1 c)	3.5
Brussels sprouts (1 c)	3.3
Broccoli (1 c)	2.3
White potato with skin (1 medium)	2.1
Carrot (1 medium)	1.7
Whole grains and legumes	
Lentils, cooked (1 c)	15.6
Chickpeas (garbanzo beans), cooked (1 c)	12.5
Barley, cooked (1 c)	6.0

Continued

Table 2-1 (*continued*)

Food	Fiber content (g)
Whole grains and legumes (*continued*)	
Whole wheat pasta, cooked (1 c)	5.5
Quinoa, cooked (1 c)	5.2
Oatmeal, cooked (1 c)	4.0
Popcorn, air-popped (3 c)	3.5
Brown rice (1 c)	3.2
Peanuts (1 oz, 35 peanuts)	2.5
Whole wheat bread (1 slice)	2.0
Nuts and seeds	
Chia seeds (1 oz)	9.8
Flaxseeds (1 oz)	5.7
Almonds (1 oz, 23 nuts)	3.5
Pecans (1 oz, 19 halves)	2.7
Walnuts (1 oz, 14 halves)	1.9

Data from US Department of Agriculture FoodData Central. Accessed September 14, 2022. https://fdc.nal.usda.gov.

fiber in the stomach delays the passage of carbohydrates from the stomach to the small intestine (gastric emptying), contributing to a feeling of fullness and satiety. Delaying gastric emptying may also reduce postprandial glucose concentrations and improve insulin sensitivity.[1]

Carbohydrate digestion resumes in the small intestine, where pancreatic and intestinal enzymes break down polysaccharides, oligosaccharides, and disaccharides into monosaccharides. For example, pancreatic lactase digests lactose into galactose and glucose, whereas intestinal sucrase digests sucrose into glucose and fructose. Any carbohydrates not digested in the small intestine (primarily fibers) pass to the large intestine, where they serve as prebiotics (**Box 2-3**) and produce short-chain fatty acids (propionate, butyrate, and acetate) and methane (responsible for flatulence) as by-products. Short-chain fatty acids serve as a nutrient source for colonocytes, but in excess, they contribute to diarrhea and abdominal cramping.

Once carbohydrates are digested, the small intestine absorbs the monosaccharide glucose, fructose, and galactose and transports the nutrients to the portal bloodstream and the liver. As glucose passes to the liver, it may then be stored as glycogen (through glycogenesis), transported to the systemic circulation, or delivered to the cells as a source of energy or to the muscles as a means of storage. The body can store glucose at a capacity of approximately 90 g in the liver and 150 g in the muscle.

> ### Box 2-3. A Primer on Prebiotics
>
> Prebiotics are nondigestible fibers that serve as food for healthy gut bacteria and probiotics. Prebiotics also help increase calcium absorption, decrease pathogenic bacteria populations, decrease allergy risk, improve immune system defenses, and improve gastrointestinal barrier integrity.[10] Excellent sources of prebiotics include beans, asparagus, cabbage, brussels sprouts, broccoli, bananas, soybeans, artichoke hearts, whole wheat, and other high-fiber fruits, vegetables, and whole grains. Refer to Part 5, Frequently Asked Questions, Case Studies, and Recipes, for several recipes high in prebiotics.

The presence of absorbed glucose in the bloodstream prompts the pancreas to release insulin. Insulin signals the body's cells to absorb glucose for energy. When blood glucose levels are low, the pancreas releases glucagon, which releases stored glycogen from the liver (through glycogenolysis). Additionally, if needed, glucose can be produced from noncarbohydrate sources such as amino acids from protein or glycerol from triglycerides. Note that fatty acids cannot be converted into glucose.

Any carbohydrates consumed in excess of what the body can use or store as glycogen are converted into fat. Carbohydrates provide 4 Cal/g, except for fiber, dextrose, and xylitol. Although fiber passes through the body largely unabsorbed, it indirectly provides 1.5 to 2.5 Cal/g by way of the energy produced by colonic bacteria from short-chain fatty acids, which is then used by the colonocytes. Dextrose, which is a rapidly digested processed corn sugar used in baked products as a sweetener and in intravenous fluids, provides 3.4 Cal/g. Xylitol is derived from xylose, a monosaccharide in plant cell walls that is often used as a low-calorie sugar substitute and sweetener in food products. It contains 2.4 Cal/g.

Carbohydrate Metabolism Disorders

Pediatricians encounter patients with many types of carbohydrate-related metabolic disorders. Several of the most common are detailed herein.

Lactose intolerance, the inability to break down lactose because of lactase deficiency, affects many children. Almost all babies are born with high lactase production, although a small amount of lactose in human milk is not absorbed, helping support a softer stool consistency, decreased fecal flora, and improved mineral absorption.[2] After weaning, there is a genetically programmed decrease in lactase levels (referred to as *lactase non-persistence*) in about two-thirds of the world's population. Lactase persistence, in which lactase production continues at infantile levels, occurs primarily in Northern European descendants of populations that traditionally practiced cattle domestication and in pastoralist populations from Africa. This frequency in some populations is thought to be caused by natural selection because lactase persistence has a complex but clear genetic basis and seems to be inherited in a dominant fashion.

Lactase persistence is less common in Southern European and Middle Eastern populations and is uncommon in non-pastoral Asian, African, and American Indian communities.[11,12] Lactase non-persistence often results in lactose intolerance, which manifests with bloating, diarrhea, and abdominal cramps after ingesting lactose-containing foods or drinks because of the bacterial fermentation of undigested lactose in the colon. The presence and extent of clinical symptoms depend on many factors, including the amount of lactose ingested, lactase activity, other foods ingested with lactose, the extent of colonic fermentation of lactose, and individual sensitivity to the by-products of fermentation.[11]

Often lactose intolerance is diagnosed clinically, but diagnosis can be confirmed with a hydrogen breath test (also known as a *lactose breath test*) or with a blood glucose level test performed before lactose ingestion and repeated after. An increase in breath hydrogen level of 20 ppm or more from baseline after digestion of lactose-containing product indicates lactose intolerance or small intestinal bacterial overgrowth (SIBO), depending on clinical symptoms. SIBO is described later in this section. A rise in glucose by 30 mg/dL (1.7 mmol/L) or more is considered within reference range, indicating typical digestion of lactose into glucose and galactose, whereas a rise by less than 30 mg/dL is suggestive of lactose intolerance.

It is important to ensure that children and adolescents with lactose intolerance still consume recommended amounts of calcium and vitamin D. To help them do so, clinicians should consider the following findings[11]:

● Children and adolescents with lactose intolerance can generally tolerate at least 12 g of lactose in a single dose (approximately 1 c of milk or yogurt; most types of cheese are low in lactose). This amount may vary by person; some people may tolerate a lactose intake of more than 12 g without clinical symptoms, whereas others may experience symptoms with an intake of less than 12 g of lactose.

● Most children and adolescents are better able to tolerate lactose in larger amounts if lactose-containing products are consumed in small portions with other foods throughout the day.

● Consuming lactase enzyme–containing products such as Lactaid or taking a lactase enzyme supplement with dairy products may help prevent symptoms.

● Regularly consuming lactose-containing products increases lactose tolerance over time.

● Nondairy (ie, lactose-free) sources of calcium and vitamin D such as fortified plant-based milk alternatives may be acceptable, although they may have less bioavailability of calcium and vitamin D than that of dairy sources.

Hereditary fructose intolerance occurs because of congenital absence of the enzyme fructose-biphosphate aldolase, which is necessary to break down fructose. Children with fructose intolerance experience vomiting and liver dysfunction after fructose or sucrose ingestion. They tend to strongly dislike sweet foods. Treatment includes avoiding all foods containing fructose or sucrose, which includes all fruits and most sweets.

Fructose malabsorption, also known as *dietary fructose intolerance,* occurs when digestive enzymes are unable to fully metabolize fructose, causing symptoms of abdominal pain, diarrhea, gassiness, and bloating after consumption of fructose-rich foods such as table sugar, many fruits, and some vegetables. In some cases, fructose malabsorption is caused by fructan intolerance. Fructans are fermentable carbohydrates with small chains of fructose and a single attached glucose molecule. They are detailed more in relation to the low fermentable oligosaccharide, disaccharide, monosaccharide, and polyol (FODMAP) diet in Chapter 21, Nutrition for Common Gastrointestinal, Autoimmune, and Inflammatory Conditions.

Galactosemia results from the inability to break down galactose because of an inherited enzyme deficiency (typically, galactose-1-phosphate uridyltransferase). For infants with classic galactosemia, consuming lactose-based formula or human milk (glucose-galactose chains) causes an accumulation of metabolites galactitol and galactose-1-phosphate, rapidly leading to feeding difficulties, excessive vomiting, metabolic decompensation, liver dysfunction, jaundice, coagulopathy, cataracts, and sepsis. Treatment includes dietary elimination of galactose, including human milk and all formulas that contain galactose, and feeding with an elemental formula. However, protein hydrolysate and soy formulas, which are lactose-free formulas that are less expensive and more palatable than elemental formula, have been found to be generally well tolerated in infants with galactosemia, although they contain very small amounts of galactose.[13] Galactosemia is detected on the newborn screening.

Non-classic galactosemia causes different symptoms than the more severe classic galactosemia. Children with galactosemia type II (also called *galactokinase deficiency*) often develop cataracts if a lactose-free diet is not maintained but usually do not have other complications. Children with type III galactosemia (also called *galactose epimerase deficiency*) may have mild to severe symptoms, which can include cataracts, delayed growth and development, intellectual disability, liver disease, and/or kidney problems. Because of the genetic variation, children with type III galactosemia depend on exogenous galactose and require a galactose-restricted but not galactose-free diet.[14]

Glycogen storage diseases describe a group of diseases that result from the inability to break down stored liver or muscle glycogen into glucose because of an enzyme deficiency. Liver glycogen is an important source of glucose during periods of fasting. Hepatic glycogen storage diseases (eg, glycogen storage disease type I, also known as *von Gierke disease*) lead to fasting hypoglycemia and to elevated lactic and uric acid and triglyceride levels. These diseases are usually first identified in late infancy as time between feedings is increased. Treatment includes continuous gastrostomy tube feedings or very frequent glucose-containing feedings. Muscular glycogen storage diseases (eg, glycogen storage disease type V, also known as *McArdle disease*) result from the absence of myophosphory-lase, leading to exercise-induced muscle pain, fatigue, and rhabdomyolysis.

Lysosomal storage disorders occur when one or more lysosomal enzymes are deficient. Lysosomes are cell organelles full of enzymes that digest large molecules such as fats and sugars. Lysosomal storage disorders result in accumulation of a large, bulky mole-cule in the cells, causing cellular dysfunction and clinical features such as enlarged liver, coarse facial features, bony deformity, and developmental regression. Named lysosomal storage disorders affecting carbohydrate metabolism include Hurler syndrome, Hunter syndrome, Fabry disease, Gaucher disease type I, Krabbe disease, and glycogen storage disease type II (also known as *Pompe disease*).

Small intestinal bacterial overgrowth occurs when gut bacteria overpopulate the intestines. This usually occurs because of dysmotility, infection, or medications. The excess bacteria cause increased sugar fermentation, which results in symptoms of bloating and flatulence, diarrhea or constipation, abdominal pain, nausea, and fatigue. SIBO is diagnosed through a positive result on a lactulose breath test: A quick rise in hydrogen and methane levels (≥ 20 ppm from baseline) resulting from bacterial fermentation of the nondigestible lactulose indicates SIBO. SIBO is often treated with the antibiotic rifaximin.

Pancreatic insufficiency resulting from cystic fibrosis, chronic pancreatitis, or a pancreatic tumor leads to decreased release of pancreatic enzymes necessary for carbohydrate digestion. Only 10% of pancreatic amylase is necessary to prevent carbohydrate malabsorption. People with pancreatic insufficiency usually take pancreatic enzyme capsules before each meal.

Celiac disease decreases carbohydrate absorption caused by villous atrophy. A gluten-free diet results in mucosal healing and improved carbohydrate absorption. Celiac disease is detailed more in Chapter 21, Nutrition for Common Gastrointestinal, Autoimmune, and Inflammatory Conditions.

Nutritional Impact

High consumption of whole grain carbohydrates is associated with reduced obesity, insulin resistance, and cardiovascular disease risk.[15] This may be in large part caused by the high fiber content of whole grains. However, overconsumption of refined grains and added sugars, particularly from drinks, is associated with obesity, dyslipidemia, insulin resistance, cardiovascular disease risk, and dental caries.[6]

In Sum

- Carbohydrates play important roles in pediatric health. Although all carbohydrates are ultimately digested into glucose and then further broken down to serve as an energy source, they do not have equivalent health impacts. Whole grains, fruits, and vegetables contain fibers that are important for cardiovascular and gut health.
- Carbohydrates contain 4 Cal/g. Calories from carbohydrates should comprise 45% to 65% of pediatric caloric intake, according to the acceptable macronutrient distribution range. The recommended dietary allowance for carbohydrates for children and adults 1 year and older is 130 g/d.
- Added sugars are ubiquitous in the food supply and contribute to negative health effects such as excess weight gain and worsened cardiovascular health. Added sugars are ideally limited to less than 6% of total calories or 25 g/d for children and adolescents. The average 2- to 19-year-old consumes approximately 17 tsp (68 g) of added sugars per day.

- There are several types of carbohydrate metabolism disorders. The most common is lactose intolerance, which results from low activity of the enzyme lactase. Children with lactose intolerance can generally tolerate about 1 c of dairy (12 g of lactose) in a single dose. Regular consumption of small portions of lactose-containing products throughout the day can help increase lactose tolerance over time. Consuming lactase enzyme–containing products or a lactase enzyme supplement with dairy products may help prevent symptoms.

References

1. Institute of Medicine. *Dietary Reference Intakes for Energy, Carbohydrate, Fiber, Fat, Fatty Acids, Cholesterol, Protein, and Amino Acids.* National Academies Press; 2005
2. Schanler RJ, Krebs NF, Mass SB, eds. *Breastfeeding Handbook for Physicians.* 2nd ed. American Academy of Pediatrics, American College of Obstetricians and Gynecologists; 2014
3. University of California San Francisco. Hidden in plain sight: added sugar is hiding in 74% of packaged foods. SugarScience. Accessed September 14, 2022. https://sugarscience.ucsf. edu/hidden-in-plain-sight/#.YVThB5rMI2w
4. Johnson RK, Appel LJ, Brands M, et al; American Heart Association Nutrition Committee of the Council on Nutrition, Physical Activity, and Metabolism and Council on Epidemiology and Prevention. Dietary sugars intake and cardiovascular health: a scientific statement from the American Heart Association. *Circulation.* 2009;120(11):1011–1020 PMID: 19704096 doi: 10.1161/CIRCULATIONAHA.109.192627
5. Dietary Guidelines Advisory Committee; Scientific Report of the 2020 Dietary Guidelines Advisory Committee. *Advisory Report to the Secretary of Agriculture and the Secretary of Health and Human Services.* Agricultural Research Service, US Dept of Agriculture; 2020
6. Vos MB, Kaar JL, Welsh JA, et al; American Heart Association Nutrition Committee of the Council on Lifestyle and Cardiometabolic Health, Council on Clinical Cardiology, Council on Cardiovascular Disease in the Young, Council on Cardiovascular and Stroke Nursing, Council on Epidemiology and Prevention, Council on Functional Genomics and Translational Biology, and Council on Hypertension. Added sugars and cardiovascular disease risk in children: a scientific statement from the American Heart Association. *Circulation.* 2017;135(19):e1017–e1034 PMID: 27550974 doi: 10.1161/CIR. 0000000000000439
7. Herrick KA, Fryar CD, Hamner HC, Park S, Ogden CL. Added sugars intake among US infants and toddlers. *J Acad Nutr Diet.* 2020;120(1):23–32 PMID: 31735600 doi: 10.1016/j.jand.2019.09.007
8. Food patterns equivalents intakes from food: mean amounts consumed per individual. In: *What We Eat in America, NHANES 2017–2018.* Agricultural Research Service, US Dept of Agriculture; 2020
9. Vega-López S, Venn BJ, Slavin JL. Relevance of the glycemic index and glycemic load for body weight, diabetes, and cardiovascular disease. *Nutrients.* 2018;10(10):1361 PMID: 30249012 doi: 10.3390/nu10101361
10. Carlson JL, Erickson JM, Lloyd BB, Slavin JL. Health effects and sources of prebiotic dietary fiber. *Curr Dev Nutr.* 2018;2(3):nzy005 PMID: 30019028 doi: 10.1093/cdn/nzy005
11. Suchy FJ, Brannon PM, Carpenter TO, et al. NIH consensus development conference statement: lactose intolerance and health. *NIH Consens State Sci Statements.* 2010;27(2):1–27 PMID: 20186234

12. Anguita-Ruiz A, Aguilera CM, Gil Á. Genetics of lactose intolerance: an updated review and online interactive world maps of phenotype and genotype frequencies. *Nutrients.* 2020;12(9):2689 PMID: 32899182 doi: 10.3390/nu12092689

13. Bosch AM. Classic galactosemia: dietary dilemmas. *J Inherit Metab Dis.* 2011;34(2):257–260 PMID: 20625932 doi: 10.1007/s10545-010-9157-8

14. US National Library of Medicine, National Institutes of Health, Department of Health & Human Services. Galactosemia. MedlinePlus. Updated August 1, 2015. Accessed October 5, 2022. https://medlineplus.gov/genetics/condition/galactosemia/#resources

15. Zong G, Gao A, Hu FB, Sun Q. Whole grain intake and mortality from all causes, cardiovascular disease, and cancer: a meta-analysis of prospective cohort studies. *Circulation.* 2016;133(24): 2370–2380 PMID: 27297341 doi: 10.1161/CIRCULATIONAHA.115.021101

CHAPTER 3

Protein

When guidelines for healthy, balanced eating are followed, protein comprises about one-tenth to one-third of a child's or an adolescent's total daily caloric intake. Proteins are found primarily in meat, poultry, fish, legumes, nuts, seeds, and dairy products. They are also found in some whole grains and vegetables. Proteins serve a critical role in infant and pediatric growth. From 6 months to 13 years of age, 58% of dietary protein is used to support growth; from 14 to 18 years, 43%.[1] Proteins provide structure to all cells of the body, including major organs and muscle tissue. They also function as enzymes, transport carriers, antibodies, hormones, and precursors for DNA, vitamins, and other molecules. Lactoferrin, lysozyme, and secretory immunoglobulin A are whey proteins found only in human milk that line the gastrointestinal tract and serve a critical role in host defense.[2] Proteins also serve a critical role in maintenance of acid-base and fluid balances. When energy is deprived or carbohydrates are restricted, the body can metabolize proteins to produce energy.

Protein Needs

For children 4 years and older and adolescents, the acceptable macronutrient distribution range for protein is 10% to 30% of total daily calories from protein; for children aged 1 to 3 years, 5% to 20% (refer to **Table A-8** in the Appendix). An acceptable macronutrient distribution range is not established for infancy; however, human milk contains about 5% of calories from protein. Like carbohydrate, protein contains 4 Cal/g. Although adults require protein of about 0.8 g/kg of body weight per day, children and adolescents require larger amounts to support growth and development. The recommended dietary allowance (RDA) is 13 g/d for children aged 1 to 3 years, 19 g/d for children aged 4 to 8 years, 34 g/d for children and adolescents aged 9 to 13 years, 52 g/d for males aged 14 to 18 years, and 46 g/d for females aged 14 to 18 years (refer to **Table A-1** in the Appendix). An RDA is not established for infancy. However, for newborns and infants aged 0 to 6 months, the adequate intake of protein is 9.1 g/d on average or can be determined for an individual infant as 1.52 g/kg/d; for infants aged 7 to 12 months, it is 11 g/d on average or can be determined for an individual infant as 1.0 g/kg/d.[1]

Protein Structure

Proteins are folded, 3-dimensional molecules made of amino acids (nitrogen, carbon, hydrogen, and oxygen, plus a variable side chain) joined together by peptide bonds. There are 20 amino acids, 9 of which are essential because they cannot be made by the human body and must be consumed in the diet. The 9 essential amino acids are histidine, isoleucine, leucine, lysine, methionine, phenylalanine, threonine, tryptophan, and valine.

Several amino acids are considered "conditionally essential" because the body cannot produce them in certain stressful situations, such as preterm birth (in an infant), severe catabolic stress, and cancer. These amino acids include arginine, cysteine, glutamine, glycine, proline, and tyrosine. The amino acids alanine, aspartic acid, asparagine, glutamic acid, and serine are nonessential because they can be produced by the human body.

Protein Quality

Protein quality is generally based on a food's essential amino acid composition, digestibility, and bioavailability. Beef, pork, poultry, fish, egg, dairy, soy, and quinoa proteins are high-quality proteins because they contain sufficient levels of the essential amino acids, are easily digested, and are bioavailable. Despite being a high-quality protein, protein in cow milk has been found to be only 70% as efficiently used as protein in human milk in studies of 1-year-old infants. Human milk is 70% whey protein and 30% casein, whereas cow milk is 18% whey protein and 82% casein.[1] Whey protein is generally more easily digested than casein. Additionally, the whey fraction of human milk is predominately α-lactalbumin compared to β-lactoglobulin, the predominant whey fraction of cow milk. α-Lactalbumin provides many benefits to the growing infant, including increased calcium and zinc absorption, balanced supply of essential amino acids, and immuno-protective proteins such as lactoferrin, lysozyme, and secretory immunoglobulin A.[2]

Although plant proteins contain the essential amino acids, they contain very low amounts of certain rate-limiting amino acids, usually lysine or methionine. For example, grains are low in lysine and high in methionine; legumes are low in methionine and high in lysine. Combining plant proteins such as grains and legumes (as in a peanut butter sandwich or rice and beans) or those such as legumes and seeds (as in falafel) to ensure adequate intake of all essential amino acids provides a complete, high-quality protein. Note that the complementary proteins need not be consumed at the same meal. Most children and adolescents obtain sufficient intake of the essential amino acids without much effort, although those who follow a vegan diet may need to partner with their clinician in more careful planning to ensure optimal intake. Part 5, Frequently Asked Questions, Case Studies, and Recipes, includes several recipes that can help children who follow a vegan or vegetarian eating plan ensure sufficient and high-quality protein intake. Ultimately, even though plant protein quality is somewhat lower than animal protein quality, the clinical significance is minimal most of the time.[3]

Protein Digestion, Absorption, and Storage

Dietary proteins are digested into amino acids in the stomach and small intestine. Hydrochloric acid in the stomach begins the digestive process by denaturing the protein and making the amino acid chain more accessible to enzymatic action. Pepsin then cleaves the protein into smaller oligopeptide chains. As these chains pass into the small intestine, pancreatic enzymes further cleave oligopeptides into tripeptides, dipeptides, and individual amino acids. These products can all be taken up by intestinal cells, where dipeptides and tripeptides are broken down into amino acids. Some amino acids are part of the process of synthesizing intestinal enzymes and new cells. Most enter the bloodstream and are transported to other parts of the body.

Nitrogen Balance

Proteins undergo constant turnover, by being digested into amino acids that are then reconfigured to create new protein structures. The amino acids are continuously recycled through the addition and removal of nitrogen groups. Amino acids cannot be stored; they are incorporated into protein, converted into fat or glucose, or excreted as nitrogen-containing products such as urea and ammonia. A person who consumes more nitrogen from protein than they excrete in urine from amino acid breakdown is in positive nitrogen balance. In other words, they are incorporating nitrogen into newly formed protein such as muscle. A person who excretes more nitrogen than they consume is in negative nitrogen balance. When energy availability is low, because of either rapidly increased demands (eg, critical illness) or low intake (eg, starvation), the body breaks down proteins from muscle and tissue stores to provide amino acids for energy. Although nitrogen balance is often assessed in hospital settings, it is rarely evaluated in pediatric outpatient settings.

Protein Metabolism Disorders

Protein metabolism is a complex process with many opportunities for dysfunction. Protein metabolism disorders generally fall into 1 of 3 categories: aminoacidopathies, organic acidemias, and urea cycle disorders. Most are detected on the newborn screening.

Aminoacidopathies include phenylketonuria, maple syrup urine disease, homocystinuria, and tyrosinemia. These are autosomal recessive conditions resulting from an enzyme deficiency that impairs the digestion of specific amino acids. The amino acids then accumulate in the blood and urine, causing various toxicities. Treatment is complete avoidance of foods containing the amino acid that cannot be metabolized, which in most cases includes high-protein foods such as meat, fish, dairy products, eggs, legumes, and nuts. Thus,

- People who have phenylketonuria must avoid phenylalanine. Phenylalanine is present in most protein-containing foods and in some protein-free products such as soda. Infants with phenylketonuria are fed a phenylalanine-free formula. Once they begin solid foods, a metabolic dietitian can help provide a specialized meal plan that includes specialized formulas.
- Those who have maple syrup urine disorder must avoid the 3 branched-chain amino acids: leucine, isoleucine, and valine. The branched-chain amino acids are present in most protein-containing foods. Children with maple syrup urine disorder require a specialized diet that is strictly monitored and controlled. Even then, metabolic crises can occur with fasting, infection, or metabolic, physical, or psychological stress.
- Those who have homocystinuria must avoid methionine, which accumulates alongside homocysteine because of the body's inability to convert methionine to cysteine.

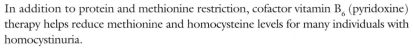

In addition to protein and methionine restriction, cofactor vitamin B_6 (pyridoxine) therapy helps reduce methionine and homocysteine levels for many individuals with homocystinuria.

- Those who have tyrosinemia must avoid tyrosine and phenylalanine, the precursor to tyrosine. Treatment includes a specialized diet and a specialized therapeutic nitisinone, a tyrosine metabolism inhibitor.

Organic acidemias include propionic acidemia, methylmalonic acidemia, glutar-icaciduria, isovaleric acidemia, and biotinidase deficiency and result from an inability to digest amino acids after the removal of the nitrogen group. These acidic amino acid fragments accumulate in the blood and urine, leading to metabolic acidosis. All these disorders are autosomal recessive and detected on newborn screening. Long-term treatment includes restricted intake of the affected amino acids, carnitine (because there is usually secondary carnitine deficiency), cofactor (eg, biotin for biotinidase deficiency and vitamin B_{12} [cyanocobalamin] for methylmalonic acidemia), and metabolic formula supplementation.

Urea cycle disorders include ornithine transcarbamylase deficiency, citrullinemia, argininosuccinicaciduria, and carbamyl phosphate synthetase I deficiency. The urea cycle rids the body of toxic ammonia, the product of the deamination of amino acids, by converting ammonia into urea. When the urea cycle malfunctions, because of a specific urea cycle enzyme deficiency, ammonia accumulates in the blood, causing serious toxicity, which can result in altered mental status, lethargy, vomiting, cerebral edema, coma, and death. Long-term treatment of urea cycle disorders includes protein restriction, arginine or citrulline supplementation, sodium or glycerol phenylbutyrate, and sick-day management.

Nutritional Impact

Sufficient protein intake is critical to support typical growth and development. Proteins from plant sources such as beans, legumes, nuts, and seeds and from fish are associated with reduced risk of cardiovascular disease. Protein cannot be stored in the body, and any protein consumed in excess of dietary needs is converted in the body to glucose or fat. Excessive protein intake may place additional metabolic burden on the kidneys, bones, and liver and can be especially detrimental for certain populations, such as those with chronic kidney disease. However, most of the time, the risk of excess protein intake is primarily excess weight gain from caloric overconsumption. Additionally, proteins from processed meats such as deli meats, bacon, sausage, and hot dogs are associated with increased risk of cardiovascular disease, likely because of their higher saturated fat, sodium, and nitrate or nitrite content.[4]

In Sum

- Proteins serve many important roles for pediatric growth and development. Over half of dietary protein intake is used to support growth from ages 6 months to 13 years, and just under half of dietary protein intake is used to support growth from ages 14 to 18 years. Proteins also provide structure to all cells of the body; form enzymes, transport carriers, antibodies, hormones, and precursors for DNA, vitamins, and other molecules; and maintain acid-base and fluid balance. Human milk includes a unique composition of whey proteins that offer superior digestibility and bioavailability and provide immuno-protection. When energy is deprived or carbohydrates are restricted, body proteins can be broken down to provide energy.

- Proteins from plant sources (eg, beans, legumes, nuts, seeds) and from fish are associated with reduced risk of cardiovascular disease. Proteins from processed meats such as deli meats, bacon, sausage, and hot dogs are associated with increased risk of cardiovascular disease.
- Protein contains 4 Cal/g. Children 4 years and older and adolescents should obtain 10% to 30% of their total daily calories from protein. Children aged 1 to 3 years need 5% to 20% of their total daily calories from protein. The RDA is 13 g/d for children aged 1 to 3 years, 19 g/d for children aged 4 to 8 years, 34 g/d for children aged 9 to 13 years, 52 g/d for males aged 14 to 18 years, and 46 g/d for females aged 14 to 18 years. An RDA is not established for infancy. However, for newborns and infants aged 0 to 6 months, the adequate intake of protein is 9.1 g/d on average or can be determined for an individual infant as 1.52 g/kg/d; for infants aged 7 to 12 months, it is 11 g/d on average or can be determined for an individual infant as 1.0 g/kg/d.[1]
- Protein consumed in excess cannot be stored in the body. Rather, it is converted into fat for storage, and the nitrogen group is excreted in the urine.
- There are several types of protein metabolism disorders. Most are detectable on the newborn screening.

References

1. Institute of Medicine. *Dietary Reference Intakes for Energy, Carbohydrate, Fiber, Fat, Fatty Acids, Cholesterol, Protein, and Amino Acids.* National Academies Press; 2005
2. Schanler RJ, Krebs NF, Mass SB, eds. *Breastfeeding Handbook for Physicians.* 2nd ed. American Academy of Pediatrics, American College of Obstetricians and Gynecologists; 2014
3. Gardner CD, Hartle JC, Garrett RD, Offringa LC, Wasserman AS. Maximizing the intersection of human health and the health of the environment with regard to the amount and type of protein produced and consumed in the United States. *Nutr Rev.* 2019;77(4):197–215 PMID: 30726996 doi: 10.1093/nutrit/nuy073
4. LaPelusa A, Kaushik R. *Physiology, Proteins.* StatPearls Publishing; 2020

CHAPTER 4

Fats

Children and adolescents require approximately one-third of total calories from dietary fats. Dietary fats are found in oils, nuts, seeds, fatty fish, meats, dairy products, and certain fruits, such as avocado and olives. Dietary fats serve as a source of energy and aid in absorption of the fat-soluble vitamins A, D, E, and K. They also serve as structural components of cell membranes and signaling molecules and have an especially important role in typical brain development during infancy and early childhood.

Dietary Fat Needs

The acceptable macronutrient distribution range for dietary fat for children aged 1 to 3 years is 30% to 40% of total daily calories from fat, whereas the range for children and adolescents aged 4 to 18 years is 25% to 35%. An acceptable macronutrient distribution range is not established for infancy; however, fat is the major source of energy for exclusively breastfed infants aged 0 to 6 months. The adequate intake (AI) for infants aged 0 to 6 months is 31 g/d and approximately 55% of total caloric intake. This value is based on the average intake of infants exclusively fed human milk. The AI for infants aged 7 to 12 months is 30 g/d and approximately 40% of total caloric intake. The AI is lower for these infants because the proportion of total calories from fat decreases from ages 7 to 12 months, when complementary foods are introduced. There is no established recommended dietary allowance for total fat intake. However, inadequate fat intake can stunt growth and increase the risk of chronic disease. Unlike carbohydrates and protein, which contain 4 Cal/g, dietary fat is a more concentrated source of energy, containing 9 Cal/g.

Dietary Fat Structure

Dietary fats consist of chains of triacylglycerols (also referred to as *triglycerides*), which are 3 fatty acids linked to a glycerol (carbon and hydrogen) backbone. Each fatty acid contains an even number of carbons and varying degrees of saturation with hydrogen. The human body requires fatty acids of differing chain lengths and saturations to meet structural and metabolic needs. The major categories of fatty acids are saturated, monounsaturated, polyunsaturated, and trans fatty acids. Linoleic acid (omega-6) and linolenic acid (omega-3) polyunsaturated fatty acids are the only *essential fatty acids,* meaning they cannot be synthesized by the human body and must be consumed in the diet. Saturated and trans fats are solid at room temperature, whereas unsaturated fats are liquid at room temperature.

Saturated Fats

Saturated fats are solid at room temperature. Medium-chain fatty acids contain 7 to 12 saturated carbons, whereas long-chain fatty acids contain 13 or more. Saturated fats consist of primarily 4 forms in the food supply.

- **Lauric acid** (12:0; medium-chain fatty acid) raises both low-density lipoprotein (LDL) and high-density lipoprotein (HDL) but decreases the total cholesterol to HDL ratio. Sources include coconut oil, palm kernel oil, and dairy products.
- **Myristic acid** (14:0; long-chain fatty acid) raises both LDL and HDL but minimally affects the total cholesterol to HDL ratio. Sources include palm kernel oil, coconut oil, and butter.
- **Palmitic acid** (16:0; long-chain fatty acid) raises both LDL and HDL but minimally affects the total cholesterol to HDL ratio. Sources include palm kernel oil, dairy fat, meats, cocoa butter, soybean oil, and sunflower oil. Palmitic acid is present in human milk and serves an important role in helping increase fat and mineral absorption.
- **Stearic acid** (18:0; long-chain fatty acid) lowers LDL. It has a neutral effect on cardiovascular disease risk. Sources include fatty meats, dairy, and chocolate.[1,2]

Monounsaturated Fats

Monounsaturated fats have 1 unsaturated carbon. They are liquid at room temperature. Oleic acid is the most commonly consumed monounsaturated fat in the United States. Most plant oils (eg, olive, canola, sesame, peanut) and nuts, seeds, and avocado are excellent sources of monounsaturated fat. Monounsaturated fats lower the level of LDL cholesterol. Chapter 20, Obesity and Related Health Conditions, includes further discussion of the role of cholesterol lipoproteins in cardiovascular disease.

Polyunsaturated Fats

Polyunsaturated fats include 2 or more unsaturated carbons. Like monounsaturated fats, they are liquid at room temperature. The essential omega-6 fatty acid linoleic acid, the essential omega-3 fatty acid alpha-linolenic acid (ALA), and the omega-3 fatty acids eicosapentaenoic acid (EPA) and docosahexaenoic acid (DHA) are all types of polyunsaturated fats.

Linoleic acid cannot be produced by the body and must be consumed in the diet. It is important for the production of eicosanoids, such as prostaglandins, thromboxanes, leukotrienes, and arachidonic acid. Foods rich in linoleic acid include nuts, seeds, and vegetable oils (eg, sunflower, safflower, corn, soybean). Human milk contains an abundance of linoleic acid and its derivative, arachidonic acid, which is found only in human milk and not in cow milk. Arachidonic acid helps improve retinal and neurodevelopmental outcomes.[3]

Alpha-linolenic acid is found primarily in plant foods such as walnuts, seeds such as chia seeds and flaxseeds, soybeans, and spinach. Human milk is also a rich source of ALA for infants. Alpha-linolenic acid must be converted into EPA and DHA to benefit health. This conversion is inefficient, with about only 10% of ALA converted into EPA and DHA. Many products include front-of-package nutrition claims that they are fortified with omega-3 fatty acids. Most of the time, this fortification is from ALA, which has few health benefits.

The omega-3 fatty acids EPA and DHA are particularly important for human health because they reduce blood clotting, dilate blood vessels, reduce inflammation, and act to reduce cholesterol and triglyceride levels. Additionally, DHA is important for neurogenesis, neurotransmitter metabolism, learning, and visual function.[4] Eicosapentaenoic acid and DHA are naturally found in egg yolk (amounts vary depending on the chicken feed) and in cold water fish and shellfish such as tuna, salmon, mackerel, cod, crab, shrimp, and oyster. In addition, human milk is a rich source of DHA.

Understanding the potential benefit of DHA supplementation on child health outcomes is an area of active research. A systematic review on the effects of algal DHA or DHA-enriched fish oil supplementation on maternal and child health showed that supplementation may be associated with a small but positive effect on pregnancy duration and a positive effect on birth weight in healthy full-term infants. It did not show any association between supplementation and the risk of preterm birth, peripartum depression, gestational hypertension or preeclampsia, postnatal growth outcomes, visual acuity, neurological and cognitive development (other than a possible small effect from fortification of preterm infant formula with DHA plus arachidonic acid), autism spectrum disorder, attention-deficit/hyperactivity disorder, learning disorders, or atopic conditions such as asthma, eczema, or allergies. Other than mild gastrointestinal symptoms, omega-3 fatty acid supplementation was not associated with any adverse events.[5]

Linoleic acid and ALA are the only essential fats, although small amounts of EPA or DHA can contribute toward reversing an omega-3 fatty acid deficiency. Adequate intake by age is shown in **Table A-1** in the Appendix. Deficiency is rare; however, during total parenteral nutrition with dextrose solutions, insulin concentrations are elevated, impairing mobilization of fat tissue. This impairment results in signs of essential fatty acid deficiency, including rough, scaly skin; dermatitis; and an elevated eicosatrienoic acid to arachidonic acid (triene to tetraene) ratio.[6]

Trans Fats

Artificial trans fats are manufactured by converting an unsaturated fat to a saturated fat to improve shelf life. This process is known as *hydrogenation*. Trans fats are now banned from the food supply because of their serious harmful effects on health, including increased level of LDL cholesterol and increased risk of heart disease. However, in some cases, small amounts of trans fats may still be present in the food supply. Consumers can identify whether trans fats are present in packaged foods by looking for "partially hydrogenated" oils on the ingredient list. Naturally occurring trans fats that are produced by bacteria in the stomach of cattle, sheep, and goats are present in small amounts in some meat and dairy products. Their health impact is not well understood.

Phospholipids

Phospholipids such as lecithin and sphingomyelin are structurally like triglycerides, but the glycerol backbone is modified so the molecule is water soluble at one end and water insoluble at the other end. Phospholipids play a critical role in maintaining cell-membrane structure and function. Lecithin is a major component of HDL. Common food sources of lecithin include liver, egg yolks, soybeans, and legumes.

Sterols

Sterols are a class of lipids that share a ringlike carbon structure. The most abundant sterol is cholesterol, which provides cells with structure and integrity. Cholesterol also serves as the precursor to vitamin D. When the skin is exposed to sun, cholesterol in the epidermal layer of the skin is converted into cholecalciferol. Cholecalciferol is then converted in the body to calcitriol, the active form of vitamin D. Other sterols form the building blocks of the steroid hormones such as cortisol, aldosterone, androgens, estrogens, and bile acids.

Sterols are not only produced by the body but can also be consumed through food sources. Cholesterol is present in animal products, whereas soy, vegetables and fruits, grains and cereals, legumes, vegetable oils, nuts, and seeds contain plant sterols.

The Milk Fat Globule

The milk fat globule found in human milk is a complex fat structure that functions to support optimal growth and nutrition during infancy. The milk fat globule is a spherical structure that is secreted by human mammary epithelial cells, that consists of a milk fat globule membrane comprised of membrane phospholipids and sphingolipids, and that surrounds triacylglycerols of primarily palmitic acid (18%–23%), oleic acid (20%–35%), linoleic acid (8%–18%), and smaller quantities of linolenic acid, arachidonic acid, EPA, and DHA. The milk fat globule also contains gangliosides and cholesterol. The composition of milk fat varies over the course of lactation on the basis of several factors, including the lactation duration, genetic factors, maternal diet, gestational age and sex of the infant, and length of a specific feeding, with more fat composition in hind milk than foremilk. In addition to the milk fat globule's important role in optimizing infant nutrition, there is emerging evidence suggesting that the globule may play an important role in developing the infant gut microbiome and immune function.[7]

Fat Digestion, Absorption, and Storage

Dietary fat is both consumed and stored as triglyceride. Fat digestion begins in the mouth when triglycerides are cleaved into short- and medium-chain fatty acids. The fatty acids are further digested in the stomach before passing into the small intestine. In the small intestine, cholecystokinin stimulates the release of gastric inhibitory peptide, which decreases gut movement and slows digestion, leading to increased satiety. Enzymes further digest the short- and medium-chain fatty acids into fatty acids, cholesterol, and lysolecithin. Micelles carry these fats and fat-soluble vitamins to the absorptive surface of the intestinal cells, where they diffuse across the luminal membrane and are converted back into triglycerides, cholesterol, and phospholipids. Whereas medium-chain triglycerides can pass directly into the portal circulation, long-chain triglycerides join an apoprotein to form a chylomicron. In the liver, chylomicrons are degraded and the lipids can be repackaged into lipoproteins, the vehicle by which they are transported to cells for supply of energy via beta oxidation or to adipose tissue for storage.

To obtain energy from fat, the enzyme hormone-sensitive lipase cleaves triglycerides into glycerol and omega-3 fatty acids. In the case of the milk fat globule, palmitic acid remains bound to the glycerol backbone of the triglyceride following hydrolysis with the bile salt–stimulated lipase contained within human milk. This process prevents the glycerol from forming micelles and facilitates enhanced fat and mineral absorption. This may also have implications for formation of the breastfed infant gut microbiome. Hormone-sensitive lipase is activated by low insulin and high glucagon levels, such as in hypoglycemia caused by starvation (eg, anorexia nervosa), severely restricted carbohydrate intake (eg, ketogenic diet), or insulin deficiency (eg, type 1 diabetes). Albumin transports the fatty acids through the bloodstream to the working cells. With the help of carnitine, fatty acids enter the mitochondria, where they undergo beta oxidation, ultimately forming acetyl coenzyme A (CoA) and hydrogen. Note that in the case of very long-chain fatty acids, this process occurs in the peroxisome organelle rather than the mitochondria. In muscle and cardiac cells, the acetyl CoA enters the citric acid cycle to form carbon dioxide and adenosine triphosphate and to generate the energy-containing compounds reduced nicotinamide adenine dinucleotide and flavin adenine dinucleotide. In liver cells, the acetyl CoA generated from fatty acid oxidation is broken down into the ketone bodies acetone, acetoacetate, and β-hydroxybutyrate. The ketone bodies can be readily used by the body's cells for energy. Refer to Chapter 19, Mental Health, Behavioral, and Developmental Conditions, for further discussion of ketosis in the context of the ketogenic diet.

Fatty Acid Metabolism Disorders

Fatty acid metabolism disorders come in primarily 3 forms: fatty acid oxidation disorders, peroxisomal disorders, and lysosomal storage disorders.

Fatty acid oxidation disorders are autosomal recessive disorders that result from a deficiency of an enzyme necessary for the breakdown of fatty acids into energy. They include medium-chain acyl CoA dehydrogenase deficiency, long-chain fatty acid oxidation disorders, primary carnitine deficiency, palmitoyltransferase II deficiency, and glutaricaciduria type II. The inability to metabolize fatty acids results in decreased production of acetyl CoA, which is required for production of ketone bodies, a necessary energy supply for the brain during periods of low glucose availability. This results in hypoketotic hypoglycemia during periods of relative fasting or low carbohydrate intake. Clinically, patients experience vomiting, lethargy, and, in the most severe cases, brain injury, seizure, and even death. Nutritional management for all fatty acid oxidation disorders includes both avoidance of fasting and aggressive treatment with oral or enteral carbohydrate-rich foods or intravenous dextrose, 10%, during illness and during increased metabolic stress or required fasting, such as for surgery. Whether to supplement with carnitine is controversial.[8]

Peroxisomal disorders occur because of absence or dysfunction of the peroxisomes, cellular organelles responsible for very long-chain fatty acid metabolism. Zellweger syndrome results from the absence of peroxisomes and manifests with severe infantile hypotonia, skeletal dysplasia, sensory deficits, hepatomegaly, and neurological regression. It is usually fatal in infancy. Adrenoleukodystrophy results from the dysfunction of the peroxisomes. It is an X-linked disorder characterized by deficiency in oxidation of very long-chain fatty acids. It typically first manifests in school-aged boys with developmental regression, spasticity, and adrenal failure and progresses to death within a few years of onset of the neurological symptoms. Females affected by adrenoleukodystrophy do not usually have adrenal insufficiency or cerebral disease, but many experience progressive spinal cord disease in adulthood.

Lysosomal storage disorders are both carbohydrate and fat malabsorption disorders. Refer to the "Lysosomal storage disorders" item in Chapter 2, Carbohydrates, for more details.

Nutritional Impact

Evidence suggests that the healthiest fats are polyunsaturated fats, with an understanding that the role of saturated fat intake in human health and cardiovascular disease risk is an area of active investigation and controversy. Ultimately, different saturated fatty acids have variable effects on heart health, which may be further modified by food processing and carbohydrate intake. For example, evidence supports that moderate intake of some minimally processed foods high in saturated fatty acids, such as whole fat dairy, unprocessed meat, and dark chocolate, is not associated with increased risk of cardiovascular disease.[2] A 2020 Cochrane Review of 15 randomized controlled trials showed little or no effect from reducing saturated fat on all-cause mortality, cardiovascular mortality, nonfatal myocardial infarction, cancer mortality, cancer diagnoses, diabetes, HDL cholesterol level, serum triglyceride levels, blood pressure, weight, total cholesterol level, LDL cholesterol level, or body mass index in adults.[9] They did show that replacing dietary saturated fatty acids with polyunsaturated fatty acids and fiber-rich whole grains improves cardiovascular health, although the impact of replacing saturated fats with monounsaturated fats is less clear.[9]

In Sum

- Dietary fats serve as a source of energy and aid in absorption of the fat-soluble vitamins A, D, E, and K. They also serve as structural components of cell membranes and signaling molecules.
- Dietary fats are classified as saturated fat, trans fat, monounsaturated fat, and polyunsaturated fat. Polyunsaturated fats provide the most numerous health benefits. The polyunsaturated omega-6 fatty acid linoleic acid and the omega-3 fatty acid ALA are the only essential fats.
- Fat contains 9 Cal/g. Children and adolescents aged 4 to 18 years should obtain about 25% to 35% of their total daily calories from fat. Children aged 1 to 3 years need 30% to 40% of their total daily calories from fat. There is no established recommended dietary allowance for total fat intake. There is an established AI for total fat of 31 g/d for infants aged 0 to 6 months and 30 g/d for infants aged

6 to 12 months. The infant AI is based on the fat composition in human milk, which optimizes nutrition for growth and development in infancy.

References

1. Briggs MA, Petersen KS, Kris-Etherton PM. Saturated fatty acids and cardiovascular disease: replacements for saturated fat to reduce cardiovascular risk. *Healthcare (Basel)*. 2017; 5(2):29 PMID: 28635680 doi: 10.3390/healthcare5020029
2. Astrup A, Magkos F, Bier DM, et al. Saturated fats and health: a reassessment and proposal for food-based recommendations: JACC state-of-the-art review. *J Am Coll Cardiol*. 2020;76(7):844–857 PMID: 32562735 doi: 10.1016/j.jacc.2020.05.077
3. Schanler RJ, Krebs NF, Mass SB, eds. *Breastfeeding Handbook for Physicians*. 2nd ed. American Academy of Pediatrics, American College of Obstetricians and Gynecologists; 2014
4. Innis SM. Dietary omega 3 fatty acids and the developing brain. *Brain Res*. 2008;1237: 35–43 PMID: 18789910 doi: 10.1016/j.brainres.2008.08.078
5. Newberry SJ, Chung M, Booth M, et al. Omega-3 fatty acids and maternal and child health: an updated systematic review. *Evid Rep Technol Assess (Full Rep)*. 2016;(224):1–826 PMID: 30307735 doi: 10.23970/AHRQEPCERTA224
6. Institute of Medicine. *Dietary Reference Intakes for Energy, Carbohydrate, Fiber, Fat, Fatty Acids, Cholesterol, Protein, and Amino Acids*. National Academies Press; 2005
7. Lee H, Padhi E, Hasegawa Y, et al. Compositional dynamics of the milk fat globule and its role in infant development. *Front Pediatr*. 2018;6:313 PMID: 30460213 doi: 10.3389/fped.2018.00313
8. Merritt JL II, Norris M, Kanungo S. Fatty acid oxidation disorders. *Ann Transl Med*. 2018;6(24):473 PMID: 30740404 doi: 10.21037/atm.2018.10.57
9. Hooper L, Martin N, Jimoh OF, Kirk C, Foster E, Abdelhamid AS. Reduction in saturated fat intake for cardiovascular disease. *Cochrane Database Syst Rev*. 2020;8(8):CD011737 PMID: 32827219

CHAPTER 5

Vitamins

Infants, children, and adolescents need to consume a variety of vitamins in recommended amounts to ensure typical growth and development. Vitamins are present in human (breast) milk and a variety of nutrient-dense foods, such as fruits, vegetables, and whole grains. By definition, vitamins are carbon-containing, noncaloric micronutrients that are essential for typical functioning and that must be consumed in the diet. There are a few exceptions to the definition, including vitamin K and biotin, both of which can be produced by typical intestinal flora; vitamin D, which is technically a prohormone because it can be self-produced with sun exposure; niacin, which can be synthesized from the essential amino acid tryptophan; and vitamin A, which can be synthesized from the provitamin beta carotene, a component of many orange-pigmented plants. **Table A-2** in the Appendix shows recommended dietary intakes of vitamins by age; **Table A-4**, tolerable upper intake levels. Of note, breast milk generally contains adequate amounts of each of the vitamins, except for vitamins K and D, although its overall vitamin composition is affected by maternal diet and nutritional status.[1] Because vitamin D is of particular concern in pediatrics and vitamin K is of special concern in infancy, both vitamins are additionally detailed later in this chapter.

Water-soluble Vitamins

Water-soluble vitamins include thiamin (vitamin B_1), riboflavin (vitamin B_2), niacin (vitamin B_3), pantothenic acid (vitamin B_5), pyridoxine (vitamin B_6), biotin (vitamin B_7 or H), folate (vitamin B_9), cobalamin (vitamin B_{12}), and vitamin C. Most of the B vitamins serve as cofactors of enzymes involved in energy metabolism, while vitamin C plays important roles in collagen, bone, and neurotransmitter synthesis; folate metabolism; and iron absorption.

Water-soluble vitamins are not stored in the body, so they must be regularly consumed in the diet. However, it takes varying amounts of time for each to become deficient. For example, clinical signs of niacin deficiency occur after only a couple of weeks of insufficient intake, those of vitamin C deficiency occur after 1 to 6 months of insufficient intake, and those of vitamin B_{12} deficiency occur only after years of insufficient intake. Refer to **Table 5-1** for more information about each water-soluble vitamin.

Water-soluble vitamins are abundant in fruits and vegetables, but many are susceptible to damage and nutrient losses during storage, preparation, and cooking. **Box 5-1** lists tips that clinicians can share with patients and families for decreasing these nutrient losses.

Table 5-1. Water-soluble Vitamins

Vitamin	Function	Signs of deficiency	Food sources	Clinical considerations	Recommended/adequate intake
Thiamin (B$_1$)	• Carbohydrate metabolism • Muscle contraction • Axonal conduction	• Low appetite • Weight loss • Impaired cardiac and neurological function leading to beriberi (mental confusion, muscular wasting, peripheral neuropathy, and tachycardia), cardiomegaly	• Enriched rice and cereal • Nuts and seeds • Lean and organ meats • Legumes • Whole grains	• Deficiency in children and adolescents is rare. Rarely, deficiency may occur in breastfeeding infants between 2 and 6 mo of age whose mothers have inadequate vitamin B$_1$ intake. • Deficiency may be diagnosed with erythrocyte transketolase activation assay or erythrocyte thiamine pyrophosphate concentration.	RDA • 0–6 mo: 0.2 mg • 7–12 mo: 0.3 mg • 1–3 y: 0.5 mg • 4–8 y: 0.6 mg • 9–13 y: 0.9 mg • Males, 14+ y: 1.2 mg • Females, 14+ y: 1.1 mg
Riboflavin (B$_2$)	• Macronutrient metabolism • Antioxidant	Ariboflavinosis (characterized by skin disorder, hyperemia of mouth and throat, angular stomatitis and cheilosis, hair loss, eye dysfunction, and liver and nervous system dysfunction)	• Meat • Eggs • Dairy • Green leafy vegetables	• Supplementation (400 mg/d) may help prevent migraine headaches, even in the absence of deficiency. • Deficiency is rare. It is more common with a vegan diet, cystic fibrosis, and post-bariatric surgery. • Deficiency is confirmed with measurement of erythrocyte glutathione reductase concentration or 24-h urinary excretion of vitamin B$_2$.	RDA • 0–6 mo: 0.3 mg • 7–12 mo: 0.4 mg • 1–3 y: 0.5 mg • 4–8 y: 0.6 mg • 9–13 y: 0.9 mg • Males, 14+ y: 1.3 mg • Girls, 14–18 y: 1.0 mg • Women, 18+ y: 1.1 mg

Vitamin	Function	Signs/Symptoms	Food Sources	Notes	RDA/AI
Niacin (B₃)	Macronutrient metabolism	Pellagra (characterized by the 4 Ds: dermatitis, dementia, diarrhea, and, eventually, death)	• Lean meats and poultry • Fish • Legumes • Yeast • Fortified cereals	• Deficiency may occur after a few weeks of inadequate intake. • Deficiency may be confirmed with measurement of nicotinamide adenine dinucleotide concentration or 24-h urinary excretion of niacin and N1-methylnicotinamide.	RDA • 0–6 mo: 2 mg • 7–12 mo: 4 mg • 1–3 y: 6 mg • 4–8 y: 8 mg • 9–13 y: 12 mg • Males, 14+ y: 16 mg • Females, 14+ y: 14 mg
Pantothenic acid (B₅)	Synthesis of coenzyme A (fatty acid synthesis)	• Paresthesias • Headache • Fatigue • Irritability and restlessness • Nausea, vomiting, diarrhea	Nearly all plant and animal foods	• Deficiency is exceedingly rare and occurs only in the case of severe malnutrition. • There is no standard laboratory test to diagnose deficiency.	AI • 0–6 mo: 1.7 mg • 7–12 mo: 1.8 mg • 1–3 y: 2 mg • 4–8 y: 3 mg • 9–13 y: 4 mg • 14+ y: 5 mg
Pyridoxine (B₆)	• Coenzyme in protein, carbohydrate, and fat metabolism • Red blood cell production • Conversion of tryptophan to niacin • Neurotransmitter formation • Immune system function	• Microcytic anemia • Neurological abnormalities • Dermatitis and cheilosis • Glossitis • Depression • Confusion • Weakened immune system	• Fish • Organ meats • Starchy vegetables • Chickpeas • Non-citrus fruits	• In children, kidney disease, malabsorption syndromes such as celiac disease and inflammatory bowel disease, and homocystinuria are risk factors for deficiency. • Deficiency is diagnosed by measurement of plasma pyridoxal 5′-phosphate concentration or 24-h urinary excretion of 4-pyridoxic acid.	RDA • 0–6 mo: 0.1 mg • 7–12 mo: 0.3 mg • 1–3 y: 0.5 mg • 4–8 y: 0.6 mg • 9–13 y: 1.0 mg • Males, 14+ y: 1.3 mg • Girls and young women, 14–18 y: 1.2 mg • Women, 19+ y: 1.3 mg

Continued

Table 5-1 (*continued*)

Vitamin	Function	Signs of deficiency	Food sources	Clinical considerations	Recommended/adequate intake
Biotin (B$_7$ or H)	Ultimate "helper vitamin" in macronutrient metabolism of other vitamins	• Thinning hair with progression to loss of all hair on the body • Scaly, red rash around body openings (eyes, nose, mouth, and perineum) • Conjunctivitis • Ketolactic acidosis • Aciduria • Seizures • Skin infection • Brittle nails • Hypotonia, lethargy, and developmental delay in infants	• Most foods contain variable amounts of biotin. • Liver • Salmon • Egg • Sunflower seeds • Almonds • Soybeans	• Deficiency is rare. Severe deficiency has never been reported in individuals eating a typical mixed diet. • Deficiency is diagnosed with laboratory evaluation of vitamin B$_7$.	AI • 0–6 mo: 5 mcg • 7–12 mo: 6 mcg • 1–3 y: 8 mcg • 4–8 y: 12 mcg • 9–13 y: 20 mcg • 14–18 y: 25 mcg • 19+ y: 30 mcg

Vitamin	Function	Deficiency	Sources	Notes	RDA
Folate (B₉)[a]	• DNA production • Amino acid metabolism	• Spina bifida and neural tube defects caused by folate deficiency early in pregnancy • Megaloblastic anemia • Skin lesions • Poor growth	• Dark green leafy and green vegetables, especially spinach, asparagus, and brussels sprouts • Fruit • Nuts • Beans • Seafood • Eggs • Dairy products • Meat • Poultry • Grains	• Named for its abundance in plant foliage • Deficiency is common because of inadequate intake and because folate is easily lost during cooking and food preparation. • The Centers for Disease Control and Prevention recommends that all women of childbearing age take a 400-mcg folic acid supplement daily. • Excessive intake can mask vitamin B₁₂ deficiency. • Deficiency is diagnosed with laboratory evaluation of folate.	RDA • 0–6 mo: 65 mcg • 7–12 mo: 80 mcg • 1–3 y: 150 mcg • 4–8 y: 200 mcg • 9–13 y: 300 mcg • 14+ y: 400 mcg
Cobalamin (B₁₂)	• Red blood cell formation • Neurological function • DNA synthesis	• Megaloblastic anemia • Neurological disorders	• Animal products including fish, meat, poultry, eggs, milk, and milk products • Fortified breakfast cereal • Nutritional yeast	• Supplementation is recommended for those who follow a vegan diet. • Low serum vitamin B₁₂ levels suggest deficiency. Deficiency can be confirmed with measurement of serum homocysteine or urinary or serum methylmalonic acid concentration.	RDA • 0–6 mo: 0.4 mcg • 7–12 mo: 0.5 mcg • 1–3 y: 0.9 mcg • 4–8 y: 1.2 mcg • 9–13 y: 1.8 mcg • 14+ y: 2.4 mcg

Continued

Table 5-1 (*continued*)

Vitamin	Function	Signs of deficiency	Food sources	Clinical considerations	Recommended/ adequate intake
C	● Neurotransmitter synthesis ● Protein metabolism ● Collagen formation ● Antioxidant ● Iron absorption	Scurvy: fatigue, malaise, gum inflammation, petechiae, poor wound healing	● Citrus fruits ● Tomatoes ● Potatoes ● Red and green peppers	● Severe deficiency is uncommon. ● Vitamin C deficiency is a clinical diagnosis.	RDA ● 0–6 mo: 40 mg (AI) ● 7–12 mo: 50 mg (AI) ● 1–3 y: 15 mg ● 4–8 y: 25 mg ● 9–13 y: 45 mg ● Boys, 14–18 y: 75 mg ● Men, 18+ y: 65 mg ● Girls and young women, 14–18 y: 65 mg ● Women, 19+ y: 75 mg

Abbreviations: AI, adequate intake; RDA, recommended dietary allowance.

Note: Needs are increased during pregnancy and lactation, and these recommended amounts are not included in this table.

[a] Also known as *folic acid* when given as supplement.

Derived from reference 2.

CLINICAL PRACTICE TIP

Box 5-1. How to Decrease Nutrient Losses in Fruits and Vegetables

Clinicians can share the following tips with patients and families to help optimize nutritional value of fresh fruits and vegetables and whole grains.

- Purchase: When purchasing fresh produce, choose locally grown produce whenever possible. Nutrient value begins to decline shortly after harvest. Frozen produce is picked at its ripest and immediately frozen, retaining maximal nutrient content.
- Storage: Eat fresh produce as soon after purchase as possible. Cold temperatures help slow vitamin degradation. Use the refrigerator drawer in which humidity is highest to maximize nutrient retention. Use more perishable vegetables (eg, spinach, lettuce, cucumbers) earlier in the week and save heartier vegetables (eg, brussels sprouts, cauliflower) for the end of the week.
- Preparation: Whenever possible, trim or chop produce immediately before eating it to prevent nutrient losses.
- Cooking: Water-soluble vitamins leach out of cooked foods, especially those heated for >2 h, although levels of fiber, minerals, and vitamin A, riboflavin, and niacin are retained. To retain the highest nutrient value possible during cooking, use cooking methods such as pressure cooking, steaming, and microwaving instead of boiling, because boiling leads to losses of water-soluble vitamins from the food into the water. When boiling, a minimal amount of cooking liquid should be used, and the nutrient-rich liquid can be used later for soups and stocks.

Fat-soluble Vitamins

Vitamins A, D, E, and K are fat-soluble vitamins, generally occurring naturally in fat-containing foods and stored in the liver or adipose tissue until needed. This storage capacity not only increases the risk of toxicity from overconsumption but also decreases the risk of deficiency. Refer to **Table 5-2** for more information about each fat-soluble vitamin.

Vitamin D

Vitamin D is detailed more because of its importance in bone health for children, its increased risk for deficiency, and the potential confusion on when and how to assess for vitamin D deficiency in pediatric clinical care.

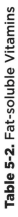

Table 5-2. Fat-soluble Vitamins

Vitamin	Function	Signs of deficiency	Food sources	Clinical considerations	Recommended/adequate intake
A	• Vision, as an essential component of rhodopsin • Cell growth and differentiation • Regulatory role in cellular immune response and humoral immune processes • Support of male and female reproduction and embryonic development	Xerophthalmia progressing to night blindness, followed by full blindness	• Liver • Milk • Eggs • Green leafy and yellow-orange vegetables[a]	• Deficiency is a risk factor for measles and diarrheal disease mortality. • Excess intake of preformed vitamin A in pregnant women, but not provitamin A (beta carotene), increases risk of birth defects. • High intake of provitamin A can turn skin orange, although this effect is nontoxic. • Serum retinol level is used to diagnose vitamin A deficiency.	RDA • 0–6 mo: 400 mcg • 7–12 mo: 500 mcg • 1–3 y: 300 mcg • 4–8 y: 400 mcg • 9–13 y: 600 mcg • Males, 14+ y: 900 mcg • Females, 14+ y: 700 mcg

| D (calciferol) | • Calcium absorption and maintenance of calcium and phosphate concentrations
• Bone growth and remodeling | • Rickets
• Osteomalacia | • Fatty fish (trout, salmon, tuna, and mackerel)
• Fish liver oils
• Beef liver, cheese, egg yolk
• Fortified dairy and plant milk alternatives (120 IU [3 mcg] per 8 fl oz [237 mL])
• Refer to **Table 5-3** for more detailed information. | • The American Academy of Pediatrics recommends that all infants who breastfeed and infants who consume <32 fl oz (1 L) of formula per day take a 400-IU (10-mcg) vitamin D supplement.
• Obesity is associated with lower vitamin D levels.
• Vitamin D's role beyond bone health is currently under investigation.
• Low serum 25-hydroxyvitamin D levels indicate deficiency.
• Refer to the Vitamin D section starting earlier in this chapter for more information. | RDA
• 0-12 mo: 400 IU (10 mcg)
• 1+ y: 600 IU (15 mcg)
Or
• 5-15 min of sun exposure from 10:00 am-3:00 pm, 2-3 times per week[b]
UL
• 0-6 mo: 1,000 IU (25 mcg)
• 7-12 mo: 1,500 IU (38 mcg)
• 1-3 y: 2,500 IU (63 mcg)
• 4-8 y: 3,000 IU (75 mcg)
• 9+ y: 4,000 IU (100 mcg) |

Continued

Table 5-2 (*continued*)

Vitamin	Function	Signs of deficiency	Food sources	Clinical considerations	Recommended/ adequate intake
E	• Antioxidant • Immune processes	• Peripheral neuropathy • Ataxia • Skeletal myopathy • Impaired immune response	• Nuts • Seeds • Vegetable oils, especially sunflower, safflower, and soybean	Deficiency may be confirmed by low serum alpha tocopherol or low serum alpha tocopherol to total plasma lipid ratio.	RDA • 0–6 mo: 4 mg (AI) • 7–12 mo: 5 mg (AI) • 1–3 y: 6 mg • 4–8 y: 7 mg • 9–13 y: 11 mg • 14+ y: 15 mg
K	• Blood clotting • Bone metabolism	Bleeding and hemorrhage	• Green leafy vegetables, especially broccoli, cabbage, turnip greens, and dark lettuce • Vegetable oils, especially soybean and canola • Natto (fermented soybean [Japan]) • Gut bacteria	• Refer to **Box 5-2** for discussion of vitamin K deficiency bleeding in the newborn (previously referred to as *classic hemorrhagic disease of the newborn*). • Vitamin K toxicity is rare. At doses of about 1,000 times the AI, vitamin K can cause severe jaundice in infants and hemolytic anemia. • Deficiency can be confirmed by prolonged prothrombin time or international normalized ratio that corrects after vitamin K injection or by measurement of vitamin K–dependent factors (II, VII, IX, and X).	AI • 0–6 mo: 2 mcg • 7–12 mo: 2.5 mcg • 1–3 y: 30 mcg • 4–8 y: 55 mcg • 9–13 y: 60 mcg • 14–18 y: 75 mcg • Men, 19+ y: 120 mcg • Women, 19+ y: 90 mcg

Abbreviations: AI, adequate intake; RDA, recommended dietary intake; UL, tolerable upper intake level.

a Vitamin A is present in these foods as provitamin beta carotene.

b Sun protection factor 8+ blocks vitamin D–producing UV rays from the sun.

Derived from reference 2.

Vitamin D is obtained either dietarily or endogenously from cholesterol activated by UV rays from sunlight. The vitamin D obtained from sun exposure, foods, and supplements is biologically inert and must undergo hydroxylation 2 times, first in the liver from vitamin D to 25-hydroxyvitamin D (calcidiol). 25-Hydroxyvitamin D is the major circulating form of vitamin D, has a half-life of 2 to 3 weeks, and is generally a good indicator of vitamin D stores. Thus, it is the most accurate laboratory indicator of vitamin D status.

In the kidney, 25-hydroxyvitamin D is converted to the physiologically active 1,25-dihydroxyvitamin D (calcitriol). Calcitriol binding to the vitamin D receptors triggers a metabolic cascade that results in increased calcium and phosphorus absorption and subsequent calcium deposition in bones. If too little vitamin D is available in the body, bone mineralization is impaired, a state potentially leading to rickets and bowing of the weight-bearing large bones in young children and osteopenia and reduced peak bone mass in older children and adolescents. Blood levels of 1,25-dihydroxyvitamin D do not correlate with vitamin D stores; thus, clinicians should not order this laboratory test. Sources of vitamin D are listed in **Table 5-3**.

Although vitamin D may provide health benefits beyond its role in bone health, evidence to date has been inconclusive. Additionally, although vitamin D deficiency is more likely to develop in some children, such as those who have obesity, have darker-pigmented skin, have little or no sun exposure, have absorption disorders, or are breastfeeding (infants), routine screening for vitamin D levels is not recommended, given its high cost and the absence of evidence that screening reduces fracture risks. Rather, when clinicians suspect that a patient is at increased risk for vitamin D deficiency, families should be counseled about appropriate vitamin D supplementation to meet the Dietary Reference Intakes (400 IU [10 mcg] per day for infants and 600 IU [15 mcg] per day for children and adults 1 year and older). The American Academy of Pediatrics recommends screening children when they experience recurrent fractures or when there is suspicion for osteopenia or rickets. Although there is some discrepancy about the threshold for vitamin D deficiency, a 25-hydroxyvitamin D level greater than 20 mg/dL is generally considered sufficient and supplementation is not indicated.[3]

The American Academy of Pediatrics recommends a 400-IU (10-mcg) vitamin D supplement for all infants who consume less than 32 fl oz (1 L) of formula per day and children who consume less than 400 IU of vitamin D per day. Vitamin D comes in 2 forms: vitamin D_3, or cholecalciferol, from sunlight, animal products, and certain supplements, and vitamin D_2, or ergocalciferol, from plant sources and certain supplements. Both forms are similar structurally and functionally. Recommended treatment regimens for vitamin D deficiency are shown in **Table 5-4**.

Vitamin Digestion and Absorption

Like most nutrients, vitamins are primarily absorbed in the small intestine (water-soluble in the jejunum and fat-soluble in the ileum). Following absorption, fat-soluble vitamins are carried by chylomicrons and other blood lipoproteins to the body's cells and to the adipose tissue and the liver for absorption. Colonic bacteria can produce vitamins K, B_{12}, B_1, and B_2. When they do, the vitamins are absorbed from the large intestine into the bloodstream.

Table 5-3. Sources of Vitamin D

Source	Quantity	Amount of vitamin D (IU)	Clinical considerations
Sunlight	5–15 min, 2–3 times per week from 10:00 am–3:00 pm for light skin Dark skin requires 3–5 times' longer exposure.	3,000	Increased risk of skin cancer outweighs benefits. Not as effective for darker-pigmented skin. SPF 8+ prevents transmission of UV-B radiation and blocks vitamin D_3 synthesis.
Fatty fish	Salmon, wild, 3.5 oz Salmon, farmed, 3.5 oz Tuna, canned, 3.5 oz	600–1,000 100–250 240	
Mushrooms	Raw, various, exposed to UV light, ½ c	60–600	When exposed to UV radiation (ie, sunlight, UV lamp), mushrooms generate significant amounts of bioavailable vitamin D.
Egg	1 large	40	
Fortified drinks	Cow milk, 8 fl oz Infant formula, 8 fl oz Fortified juice, 8 fl oz	100	
Fortified foods	Yogurt, 8 fl oz Cheese, 3 oz Breakfast cereal, 1 serving	100 100 40–100	
Supplement	Ergocalciferol (vitamin D_2, nonproprietary), plant-derived, 1 cap Drisdol (vitamin D_2, proprietary), liquid, 1 mL Multivitamin, 1 mL Cholecalciferol (vitamin D_3), mammal-derived, varied	50,000 8,000 400; 500; 1,000 400; 800; 1,000; 2,000; 5,000; 10,000; 50,000	Supplementation should not exceed the UL.

Abbreviation: UL, tolerable upper intake level.

Adapted from reference 3.

Table 5-4. Treatment of Vitamin D Deficiency

Age	Preparation and dose[a]
Infants, 0–12 mo	Ergocalciferol or cholecalciferol (vitamin D_2 or D_3), 50,000 IU weekly for 6 wk Or Vitamin D_2 or D_3, 2,000 IU daily for 6 wk Followed by a maintenance dose of 400–1,000 IU daily
Children and adolescents, 1–18 y	Vitamin D_2 or D_3, 50,000 IU weekly for 6–8 wk Or Vitamin D_2 or D_3, 2,000 IU daily for 6–8 wk Followed by a maintenance dose of 600–1,000 IU daily

[a] Vitamin D_3 may be more potent than vitamin D_2.
Adapted from reference 3.

CLINICAL PRACTICE TIP
Box 5-2. Vitamin K at Birth

When newborns are not treated with vitamin K at birth, vitamin K deficiency bleeding in the newborn (previously referred to as *classic hemorrhagic disease of the newborn*) is more likely to develop because vitamin K does not cross the placenta and is present in negligible amounts in human (breast) milk. Vitamin K deficiency can lead to catastrophic bleeding up to 6 mo after delivery. This is easily preventable with a single 1-mg vitamin K injection given within 6 h of birth for newborns weighing >1,500 g and 0.3–0.5 mg/kg for newborns weighing ≤1,500 g.[4] The injection is extremely safe and effective at preventing early and late vitamin K deficiency bleeding. Oral vitamin K not only requires an inconvenient dosing schedule (2 mg given at birth, 4–6 d after birth, and 4–6 wk of age) but is not effective in preventing late-onset vitamin K deficiency bleeding and is not US Food and Drug Administration approved in the United States.

Malabsorption Syndromes

Several medical conditions can disrupt the absorptive lining of the small intestine and interfere with typical vitamin absorption. These conditions include intestinal bacterial, viral, or parasitic infection; celiac disease; cystic fibrosis; Crohn disease; bariatric surgery complications; and intestinal resection complications. Additionally, vitamin absorption can be impaired if there is any deficiency or malfunction in any number of transport mechanisms required for typical absorption. Chronic diarrhea is a common sign of malabsorption.

Antioxidants and Phytochemicals

Vitamin C, beta carotene, vitamin E, and the mineral selenium are antioxidants. Antioxidants help undo cell damage that results from long-term oxygen exposure. Although antioxidant supplementation is unlikely to benefit health, consumption of a diet high in fruits and vegetables, which naturally contain many antioxidant vitamins, is associated with a lower risk of chronic disease. The decreased risk of chronic disease associated with fruit and vegetable consumption could be from any number of nutrients, including antioxidants naturally present in the food, fiber, monounsaturated fatty acids, or B vitamins.

Refer to **Box 5-3** for more information on multivitamins and guidelines for specific supplementation.

CLINICAL PRACTICE TIP

Box 5-3. Multivitamin Supplementation

Multivitamin use is common in pediatrics, with about one-third of children and adolescents reporting taking a dietary supplement in the past 30 d. Multivitamin-mineral supplements are the most commonly used products.[5] Although supplements may help increase overall nutrient intake, nutritional needs are best met through consumption of a healthy and varied diet. However, in some cases specific supplementation is warranted.

- **Vitamin D:** All infants breastfeeding, infants consuming < 32 fl oz (1 L) of formula daily, and children and adolescents consuming < 400 IU (10 mcg) of vitamin D daily through food intake should take a 400-IU vitamin D supplement.
- **Folic acid:** All female adolescents who could become pregnant should take a 400-mcg folic acid supplement.
- **Iron:** Infants fed human (breast) milk should receive an iron supplement: 2 mg/kg/d for preterm infants and 1 mg/kg/d for full-term infants from 4 mo until the introduction of iron-rich solid foods.[6] Some toddlers with poor intake of iron-rich foods, and menstruating adolescents, may also benefit from supplementation. Iron is detailed in Chapter 6, Minerals.

In Sum

- Vitamins are present naturally in nutrient-rich foods such as fruits, vegetables, whole grains, nuts and seeds, dairy products, meat, and fish. They are needed in small amounts for optimal metabolic function and health. If inadequate amounts of vitamins are consumed in the diet, vitamin deficiencies may occur, which can cause metabolic dysfunction and severe health consequences.
- Vitamins are divided into 2 categories: fat-soluble (A, D, E, and K) and water-soluble (B and C). Water-soluble vitamins pose a higher risk for deficiency because they cannot be stored in the body, whereas fat-soluble vitamins pose a higher risk for toxicity because of their storage capacity in fat tissue.
- Food sources of vitamins are preferable to supplements. Children who eat a balanced and varied diet do not usually need to take a multivitamin or supplements.
- Three vitamins are of special concern in pediatrics: vitamin D, vitamin K, and folate. Infants who breastfeed and all children and adolescents who do not consume at least 400 IU (10 mcg) of vitamin D per day require vitamin D supplementation to prevent rickets and optimize bone health. Newborns require injection with vitamin K at birth to prevent vitamin K deficiency bleeding. Female adolescents who could become pregnant require folate supplementation to prevent the risk of spina bifida in a developing fetus, should these adolescents become pregnant.

References

1. Schanler RJ, Krebs NF, Mass SB, eds. *Breastfeeding Handbook for Physicians.* 2nd ed. American Academy of Pediatrics, American College of Obstetricians and Gynecologists; 2014
2. National Institutes of Health. Dietary supplement fact sheets. Accessed September 15, 2022. https://ods.od.nih.gov/factsheets
3. Golden NH, Abrams SA, Daniels SR, et al; American Academy of Pediatrics Committee on Nutrition. Optimizing bone health in children and adolescents. *Pediatrics.* 2014;134(4):e1229–e1243 PMID: 25266429 doi: 10.1542/peds.2014-2173
4. Hand I, Noble L, Abrams SA. Vitamin K and the newborn infant. *Pediatrics.* 2022;149(3):e2021056036 PMID: 35190810 doi: 10.1542/peds.2021-056036
5. Stierman B, Mishra S, Gahche JJ, Potischman N, Hales CM. Dietary supplement use in children and adolescents aged ≤19 years—United States, 2017–2018. *MMWR Morb Mortal Wkly Rep.* 2020;69(43):1557–1562 PMID: 33119556 doi: 10.15585/mmwr.mm6943a1
6. Baker RD, Greer FR; American Academy of Pediatrics Committee on Nutrition. Diagnosis and prevention of iron deficiency and iron-deficiency anemia in infants and young children (0–3 years of age). *Pediatrics.* 2010;126(5):1040–1050 PMID: 20923825 doi: 10.1542/peds.2010-2576

CHAPTER 6

Minerals

Infants, children, and adolescents require appropriate intake of a variety of minerals to ensure typical growth and bodily functioning. Minerals are present naturally in human milk and many food products, such as nuts and seeds, beans and lentils, dark green leafy vegetables, fish and shellfish, meat, and dairy products. They serve many critical roles in the human body, such as regulating enzyme activity, maintaining acid-base balance, and assisting with muscle contraction and growth. While an overview of each of the minerals is described in this chapter, 3 minerals of special concern in pediatrics (calcium, iron, and sodium) are discussed more in depth. **Table A-3** in the Appendix shows recommended dietary intakes of minerals by age; **Table A-5**, tolerable upper intake levels.

Minerals are categorized as macrominerals (major elements needed in amounts of ≥100 mg/d) and microminerals (trace elements needed in amounts of only <20 mg/d).

Macrominerals

Macrominerals include calcium, phosphorus, magnesium, and the electrolytes sodium, chloride, and potassium (**Table 6-1**).

Calcium

Calcium is the most abundant mineral in the human body, with 99% stored in bone, providing bones with structure and strength. The other 1% is critical for many metabolic functions. Children and adolescents commonly underconsume this mineral, placing their current and future bone health at risk. Peak bone mineral accretion occurs around age 12.5 years for girls and age 14.1 years for boys; 95% of adult bone mass has been attained by 4 years following the peak bone accretion.[2] When there is not enough calcium available through dietary intake, bone stores can become compromised, a state weakening the bones and decreasing peak bone mass. When dietary calcium intake meets needs (**Table 6-1**), enough calcium is available for typical physiological function and increased bone storage, provided there is also adequate supply of vitamin D, which is required for the bone to effectively absorb calcium. Dietary sources of calcium are highlighted in **Table 6-2**.

Although it is preferable that children obtain the recommended dietary allowance (RDA) for calcium through dietary intake, a calcium supplement may be given to those unable to obtain the RDA otherwise. Calcium supplements are available as calcium carbonate and calcium citrate. Calcium carbonate is most bioavailable when consumed with food, whereas calcium citrate may be given with or without food.

Table 6-1. Macrominerals (Major Elements), Including Electrolytes

Mineral	Function	Signs of deficiency	Food sources	Clinical considerations	Recommended intake
Calcium	• Bone and teeth mineralization • Muscle contraction • Nerve transmission • Blood clotting • Blood pressure control • Immunity	Osteopenia or osteoporosis	• Dairy products • Small fish with bones (eg, canned sardines or salmon) • Green leafy vegetables (eg, Chinese cabbage, kale, broccoli) (Spinach contains calcium, but because it is high in oxalates, it is less readily absorbed and is poorly bioavailable.) • Soy • Refer to **Table 6-2** for more detailed information.	• Insufficient intake in adolescence leads to decreased peak bone mass. • 99% of the body's calcium supply is stored in bones and teeth. Sufficient dietary calcium is important to maintain this supply. • Preterm infants are born with low calcium stores (refer to phosphorus "Clinical considerations" later in this table). • Refer to the Calcium section earlier in this chapter for more information.	• 0–6 mo: 200 mg • 7–12 mo: 260 mg • 1–3 y: 700 mg • 4–8 y: 1,000 mg • 9–18 y: 1,300 mg • 19–70 y: 1,000 mg
Chloride	Electrolyte	NA	Salt in foods	Chloride is generally overconsumed; thus, overt deficiencies do not occur.	• 0–6 mo: 0.18 g • 7–12 mo: 0.57 g • 1–3 y: 1.5 g • 4–8 y: 1.9 g • 9–50 y: 2.3 g

| Magnesium | • Cofactor in >300 enzyme systems • Protein synthesis, oxidative phosphorylation and glycolysis • Muscle and nerve function • Blood glucose control • Blood pressure regulation • DNA and RNA synthesis | • Loss of appetite • Nausea, vomiting • Fatigue • Weakness progressing to cramps and seizure • Atypical heart rhythm | • Green leafy vegetables • Legumes • Nuts • Seeds • Whole grains | • Magnesium therapy might help prevent migraines, regardless of the presence or absence of deficiency. • People with type 2 diabetes are at increased risk for magnesium deficiency caused by increased urinary magnesium excretion resulting from increased glucose level in the kidneys. | RDA • 0–6 mo: 30 mg (AI) • 7–12 mo: 75 mg (AI) • 1–3 y: 80 mg • 4–8 y: 130 mg • 9–13 y: 240 mg • Boys and young men, 14–18 y: 410 mg • Men, 19–30 y: 400 mg • Girls and young women, 14–18 y: 360 mg • Women, 19–30 y: 310 mg |

Continued

Table 6-1 (*continued*)

Mineral	Function	Signs of deficiency	Food sources	Clinical considerations	Recommended intake
Phosphorus	• Component of bone, teeth, DNA, and RNA • Component of cell membrane and adenosine triphosphate structure • Regulation of gene transcription • Enzyme activation • pH regulation • Energy storage	• Anorexia • Anemia • Proximal muscle weakness • Bone pain, rickets, and osteomalacia • Increased infection risk • Paresthesias • Ataxia and confusion	• Dairy products • Meats and poultry • Eggs • Nuts • Legumes • Vegetables • Grains	• Phosphorus deficiency is rare and almost never caused by low intake. • Preterm infants are born with low phosphorus stores because two-thirds of bone mineral content is acquired in the third trimester. Low levels of phosphorus and calcium cause osteopenia of prematurity. Thus, preterm formula is usually fortified with higher amounts of calcium and phosphorus. • Refeeding hypophosphatemia can occur 2–5 d after enteral or parenteral feedings in a child or adolescent who is severely malnourished. • Phosphate additives are present in many processed foods to preserve moisture or color or stabilize frozen foods. These additives contribute to overall phosphorus intakes.	RDA • 0–6 mo: 100 mg • 7–12 mo: 275 mg • 1–3 y: 460 mg • 4–8 y: 500 mg • 14–18 y: 1,250 mg • 19+ y: 700 mg

| Potassium | Electrolyte | • Hypertension
• Kidney stones
• Increased bone turnover
• Salt sensitivity
• Severe deficiency resulting from potassium losses, not generally low dietary intake, leads to hypokalemia. | • Many fruits and vegetables
• Soybeans
• Meat
• Poultry
• Fish
• Dairy
• Nuts | Potassium is a "nutrient of public health concern" in that most people do not consume the recommended amount. Nutrients of public health concern are detailed in Chapter 11, Dietary Guidelines and Principles of Healthy Eating. | • 0–6 mo: 400 mg
• 7–12 mo: 860 mg
• 1–3 y: 2,000 mg
• 4–8 y: 2,300 mg
• Boys, 9–13 y: 2,500 mg
• Boys and young men, 14–18 y: 3,000 mg
• Men, 19+ y: 3,400 mg
• Girls and young women, 9–18 y: 2,300 mg
• Women, 19+ y: 2,600 mg |
| Sodium | • Electrolyte functions
— Water balance and distribution
— Osmotic equilibrium
— Acid-base balance
— Intracellular/extracellular differentials | Hyponatremia characterized by nausea, vomiting, headaches, altered mental state/confusion, lethargy, seizures, and coma resulting from excess sodium losses from medications; excess sweating, vomiting, or diarrhea; or excessive water consumption | Salt in foods | • Sodium is generally over-consumed; thus, overt dietary deficiencies do not occur.
• Refer to the Sodium section later in this chapter for more information. | AI
• 0–6 mo: 110 mg
• 7–12 mo: 370 mg
• 1–3 y: 800 mg
• 4–8 y: 1,000 mg
• 9–13 y: 1,200 mg
• 14+ y: 1,500 mg |

Abbreviations: AI, adequate intake; NA, not applicable; RDA, recommended dietary allowance.

Adapted with permission from reference 1.

Table 6-2. Dietary Sources of Calcium

Food category	Source and quantity	Amount of calcium (mg)
Dairy	Milk, 8 fl oz	275–300
	Cheese, 1.5 oz	300–350
	Yogurt, 8 fl oz	350–400
Fatty fish	Salmon, canned with bones, 3 oz	210
	Sardines, canned, 3 oz	325
Green leafy vegetables	Broccoli, 1 c	100
	Spinach, cooked, 1 c	250
	Tomatoes, canned, 1 c	85
Beans	Chickpeas (garbanzo beans), 1 c	210
	White beans, cooked, 1 c	190
	Baked beans, canned, 1 c	120
Fortified foods	Orange juice, 100% with calcium added, 8 fl oz	350
	Tofu, prepared with calcium sulfate, ½ c[a]	860
	Soy milk, calcium-fortified, 8 fl oz[a]	300

[a] Bioavailability of calcium from nondairy sources such as soy milk or plant-based alternatives may be less than that from milk.

Derived from US Department of Agriculture. FoodData Central. Accessed September 15, 2022. https://fdc.nal.usda.gov/index.html.

Sodium

Sodium is the most abundantly consumed mineral in the diet of most children and adolescents, starting in the first few years after birth. Sodium intake in toddlers exceeds the recommended upper level in nearly 80% of children aged 1 to 3 years.[3] Most sodium comes from eating processed and prepared foods, rather than from adding table salt to foods. In the current food environment, there is no shortage of salt-laden foods. A study of the sodium content of commonly consumed toddler foods showed that 72% of toddler dinners were high in sodium.[3]

Because dietary preferences start early, infants and young children exposed to salty foods are likely to prefer and seek out these foods as they grow older. Although sodium serves important functions, it is needed in much smaller amounts than those typically consumed. Too much dietary salt is associated with high blood pressure in children, which can lead to increased risk of cardiovascular disease and stroke in adulthood. To help lower sodium intake in children and adolescents, pediatricians can advise parents to minimize the purchase of processed foods and read the Nutrition Facts label and choose items that are low in sodium.

Microminerals

Microminerals include iodine, iron, selenium, zinc, and fluoride (**Table 6-3**).

Iron

Iron plays several critical roles in human health and typical physiological function. These roles, which follow, are particularly important during the rapid growth that occurs in infancy, childhood, and adolescence.

- Cell growth and differentiation
- An essential component of hemoglobin, the protein that carries inhaled oxygen from the lungs to the tissues
- An essential component of myoglobin, the protein responsible for making oxygen available for muscle contraction

Iron comes in the following 2 forms:

- Heme: Derived from hemoglobin and myoglobin in animal sources (meat, seafood, and poultry). Heme iron is more readily absorbed (bioavailability: 10%–35%).
- Nonheme: Derived from plants and iron-fortified foods. Nonheme iron is less readily absorbed (bioavailability: 1%–10%).

Excellent food sources of iron are listed in **Table 6-4**.

Inhibitors of iron absorption include

- Phytate, found in many plant-based foods
- Polyphenols, notably present in herbal and black teas, legumes, cereals, fruits, and vegetables
- Calcium, found in dairy products, legumes, and green leafy vegetables
- Soy, casein, whey, and egg white proteins
- Oxalic acid, found in spinach, chard, beans, and nuts
- Proton pump inhibitors (eg, omeprazole), which decrease the acidity of the stomach environment, decreasing conversion of ferric iron to ferrous iron, thus decreasing absorption of iron
- Conditions that impair the small intestinal mucosa, thus limiting absorption, including celiac disease, inflammatory bowel disease, and duodenal ulcers

The great enhancer of iron absorption is vitamin C, which can overpower all inhibitors. It forms a chelate with ferric iron in the stomach and remains soluble in the alkaline environment of the duodenum. Consuming foods high in vitamin C (eg, citrus fruits, dark green leafy vegetables, peppers, melons, strawberries) at the same time as foods rich in iron helps increase iron absorption.

Iron deficiency anemia is the most common micronutrient deficiency in the world. It is particularly common in pediatric patients, especially young children who drink large amounts of milk, which is very low in iron, and adolescents, who generally consume low amounts of iron-rich foods. Female adolescents experience further iron losses through menstruation. Signs of iron deficiency include fatigue, poor work performance, and decreased immunity.

Table 6-3. Microminerals (Trace Elements)

Mineral	Function	Signs of deficiency	Food sources	Clinical considerations	Recommended intake
Fluoride	Prevention and reversal of initiation and progression of dental caries	Dental caries	• Fluoridated water • Brewed tea	For children whose water contains little or no fluoride, the American Dental Association recommends fluoride supplementation.	AI • 0-6 mo: 0.01 mg • 7-12 mo: 0.5 mg • 1-3 y: 0.7 mg • 4-8 y: 1 mg • 9-13 y: 2 mg • 14-18 y: 3 mg • Men, 19+ y: 4 mg • Women, 19+ y: 3 mg
Iodine	Thyroid function, specifically triiodothyronine and thyroxine formation	Goiter	• Iodized salt • Seaweed (nori) • Fish • Eggs	Most table salt is iodized. Some sea salts and kosher salt are not.	• 0-6 mo: 110 mcg • 7-12 mo: 130 mcg • 1-8 y: 90 mcg • 9-12 y: 120 mcg • 14+ y: 150 mcg

Iron	• Component of hemoglobin
	• Component of myoglobin
	• Physical growth
	• Neurological development
	• Cellular function
	• Hormone function
		• Weakness
		• Fatigue
		• Difficulty concentrating
		• Decreased immune function
		• Decreased exercise capacity
			• Heme
			  – Meat
			  – Seafood
			  – Poultry
			• Nonheme
			  – Plants (nuts, beans, and vegetables)
			  – Iron-fortified food (bread, cereal, and grains)
				• Human milk contains highly bioavailable iron, but in insufficient amounts for infants aged >4-6 mo.
				• Iron supplementation of 1 mg/kg/d in preterm infants reduces risk of iron deficiency.
				• The American Academy of Pediatrics recommends iron supplementation of 1 mg/kg for breastfed infants from 4 mo until the introduction of iron-containing complementary foods and 2 mg/kg/d for preterm infants aged 1-12 mo who are fed human milk.
				• Refer to the Iron section starting earlier in this chapter for more information.
					RDA
					• 0-6 mo: 0.27 mg (AI)
					• 7-12 mo: 11 mg
					• 1-3 y: 7 mg
					• 4-8 y: 10 mg
					• 9-13 y: 8 mg
					• Boys and young men, 14-18 y: 11 mg
					• Men, 19+ y: 8 mg
					• Girls and young women, 14-18 y: 15 mg
					• Women, 18-50 y: 18 mg

	Functions	Deficiency	Sources	Notes	RDA
Selenium	• Human reproductive function • Thyroid hormone metabolism • DNA synthesis • Antioxidant	• Decreased immunity • Male infertility	• Brazil nuts • Seafood • Meat • Cereal • Dairy products		• 0-6 mo: 15 mcg (AI) • 7-12 mo: 20 mcg (AI) • 1-3 y: 20 mcg • 4-8 y: 30 mcg • 9-13 y: 40 mcg • 14+ y: 55 mcg
Zinc	• >100 enzyme functions • Typical growth and development • Immune function • Protein and DNA synthesis • Wound healing	• Growth restriction • Decreased appetite • Impaired immune function	• Oysters • Red meat • Poultry • Beans • Nuts • Seafood (eg, crab, lobster) • Whole grains • Fortified grains • Dairy	• Phytates (present in grains and legumes) bind zinc and inhibit absorption. • Human milk is a good source of zinc at birth and in early infancy, but the level of zinc in human milk sharply declines over time, requiring infants to meet needs primarily through complementary foods after 6 mo of age.	• 0-6 mo: 2 mg (AI) • 7 mo-3 y: 3 mg • 4-8 y: 5 mg • 9-13 y: 8 mg • Males, 14+ y: 11 mg • Girls and young women, 14-18 y: 9 mg • Women, 19+ y: 8 mg

Abbreviations: AI, adequate intake; RDA, recommended dietary allowance.

Adapted with permission from reference 1.

Table 6-4. Iron-Rich Foods

Food	Amount of iron (mg)
Oysters, cooked, 3 oz	7.8
Hearts of palm, 1 c	4.6
Beef, bottom round, cooked, 3 oz	2.5
Clams, canned, drained, 3 oz	2.3
Chicken, broilers or fryers, flesh and skin, 3 oz	1.1
Tuna, in water, canned, drained, 3 oz	0.8
Egg, 1 grade A large, whole	0.8
Shrimp, 3 oz	0.4
Lentils,[a] cooked, 1 c	6.6
Black beans,[a] canned, 1 c	5.0
Chickpeas (garbanzo beans),[a] cooked, boiled with salt, 1 c	4.7
Tofu,[a] raw, firm, prepared with calcium sulfate, ½ c	3.4
Infant oatmeal,[a] iron-fortified, 1 tbsp	3.0
Rice cereals,[a] iron-fortified, 1 tbsp	2.2
Baked potato,[a] medium, baked, flesh and skin	1.9
Cashews,[a] 1 oz	1.9
Breads,[a] whole grain and enriched, 1 slice	1.8
Spinach and dark leafy vegetables,[a] 1 c	0.8

[a] These are nonheme sources of iron. To improve iron absorption, these foods should be eaten with a vitamin C–rich food.

Derived from US Department of Agriculture FoodData Central. Accessed September 15, 2022. https://fdc.nal.usda.gov/index.html.

Iron deficiency anemia is diagnosed through a series of laboratory abnormalities. The abnormalities include low hemoglobin level caused by lack of available iron, low iron level, low ferritin level, low mean corpuscular volume, low reticulocyte count caused by lack of available hemoglobin, and higher total iron-binding capacity (**Table 6-5**). Some people have laboratory results that do not show iron deficiency but may indicate iron depletion without anemia. Iron depletion without anemia is indicated by within–reference range hemoglobin but low iron and ferritin levels. The American Academy of Pediatrics recommends routinely screening for anemia in children by checking a hemoglobin level at 12 months of age and, if risk factors are present, at other times during childhood and adolescence. Risk factors for iron deficiency include food insecurity,

Table 6-5. The Iron Deficiency Workup

Laboratory test[a]	Function	Result indicating iron deficiency
Hemoglobin level	Iron-containing, oxygen-carrying compound	Low[b]
Hematocrit	Proportion of total blood made up of red blood cells	Low
Mean corpuscular volume	Average volume of a red blood cell	Low
Ferritin level	Measure of iron stores in liver and heart	Low
Iron level	Amount of iron carried in blood by transferrin	Low
Total iron-binding capacity	Measure of available iron-binding sites on transferrin	High
Reticulocyte count	Measure of immature red blood cells	Low

SI conversion factor: To convert g/dL to g/L, multiply by 10.

[a] Refer to Chapter 9, Clinical and Biochemical Evaluation, for reference range values for each laboratory test listed.

[b] Values are considered low at 2 SDs below the mean for age. For hemoglobin level, the cutoff is as follows: 6 mo–2 y, 10.5 g/dL; 2–6 y, 12.5 g/dL; 6–12 y, 11.5 g/dL; and 12–18 y, males, 13 g/dL, and females, 12 g/dL.

breastfeeding, vegetarian or vegan diet, prolonged or heavy menstrual bleeding, or prior diagnosis of iron deficiency anemia.[4]

In addition to increasing dietary intake of iron, most children with iron-deficiency anemia should take an iron supplement of approximately 3 mg/kg/d for 3 to 6 months to replenish iron stores. Potential adverse effects of iron supplements include nausea, vomiting, constipation, diarrhea, dark-colored stools, and abdominal pain. Excessive iron intake can cause severe weakness and fatigue, unexplained joint and abdominal pain, diabetes, changed skin color, liver toxicity, and, in severe cases, death.

Mineral Digestion and Absorption

Micronutrient digestion begins in the mouth, as a person chews, and continues in the stomach, as hydrochloric acid and stomach enzymes further extract nutrients from foods. Most minerals are absorbed in the small intestine, except for sodium and potassium, which are absorbed in the large intestine.

In general, mineral absorption occurs in 3 stages: intraluminal, translocation, and mobilization. In the *intraluminal stage,* positively charged minerals such as calcium, iron, zinc, magnesium, and potassium dissolve in the acidic stomach chyme. Except for iron, which can be absorbed in its ferrous state (ferrous iron; nonheme iron) or bound by heme (heme iron), minerals are absorbed in their ionic state, unbound to organic molecules and complexes. Stomach acidity is important for the conversion of insoluble ferric acid (ferric iron) to absorbable ferrous (ferrous iron) ions. As chyme passes to the less-acidic solution in the duodenum, the minerals form insoluble compounds with hydroxide molecules and protein carriers (chelation compounds). In the *translocation stage,* chelation compounds cross the small intestinal border through facilitated diffusion and/or active transport. Some of the mineral complexes are not absorbed across the small intestinal border and, instead, are sequestered within the absorptive cell for later use. During the *mobilization stage,* minerals and mineral complexes pass into the portal circulation to the liver for processing and then systemic distribution.

Minerals are classified as having low, medium, and high bioavailability, as follows:

- Low bioavailability (1%–10% absorption): iron (nonheme), zinc, chromium, and manganese
- Low-medium bioavailability (10%–30% absorption): iron (heme)
- Medium bioavailability (30%–40% absorption): calcium and magnesium
- High bioavailability (>40% absorption): sodium, potassium, chloride, iodide, and fluoride

Factors affecting bioavailability for any given mineral include

- The presence or absence of other minerals. Carrier proteins required for facilitated diffusion and active transport are nonspecific. Thus, a high intake of a particular mineral may outcompete another mineral for absorption. For example,
  — Zinc absorption is decreased through iron supplementation.
  — Copper absorption is decreased through excess iron and zinc intake.
  — Zinc and manganese absorption are decreased through excess calcium intake.
  — Iron absorption is decreased through excess calcium, zinc, magnesium, and copper intake.

  This factor is especially important to note for children who take mineral supplements.

- The availability of the protein that binds with the mineral to form the chelation complex. For example, iron requires transferrin for absorption, whereas many other minerals require albumin. In most cases, these protein carriers are undersaturated. However, if the mineral is consumed in excess, the mineral can overwhelm the carrier sites and lead to toxicity. Mineral absorption can also be impaired if minerals bind to free fatty acids in the intestinal lumen or if a mineral is present in very high concentrations and forms a nonabsorbable precipitate. Of note, the macrominerals in human milk are more bioavailable than those in infant formula because they are bound to digestible proteins rather than fatty acids and exist in mineral complexes and ionized states that are more readily absorbed.

In Sum
- Minerals are present naturally in many foods, such as nuts and seeds, beans and lentils, dark green leafy vegetables, fish and shellfish, meat, dairy products, and human milk. They serve many critical roles in the human body, such as regulating enzyme activity, maintaining acid-base balance, assisting with muscle contraction, and helping with growth.

- Minerals are divided into 2 categories: macrominerals, or major elements, and microminerals, or trace elements. Calcium, phosphorus, magnesium, and the electrolytes sodium, potassium, and chloride are macrominerals. Microminerals include iodine, selenium, zinc, and fluoride.
- Three minerals are of special concern in pediatrics: calcium, iron, and sodium. Potassium is a "nutrient of public health concern," discussed further in Chapter 11, Dietary Guidelines and Principles of Healthy Eating. Calcium, present primarily in dairy products, human milk, fish with bones, green leafy vegetables, beans, and fortified foods, is important for bone strength. Many children do not obtain the RDA for calcium. Iron is important for neurological development, typical blood functioning, and growth. It is present in 2 forms—the more bioavailable heme iron contained in meat, seafood, and poultry and the less bioavailable nonheme iron contained in nuts, beans, vegetables, and iron-fortified grains. Iron deficiency anemia is the most common micronutrient deficiency in the world. Sodium is present in excess in the food supply, primarily in processed and packaged foods. Excess sodium consumption contributes to hypertension, which is a leading cause of cardiovascular disease and stroke in adulthood.
- Bioavailability of minerals depends on many factors, including the presence or absence of other minerals. For example, iron supplementation decreases zinc absorption; excess iron and zinc intake decreases copper absorption; excess calcium intake reduces zinc and manganese absorption; and excess calcium, zinc, magnesium, and copper intake decreases iron absorption. The impact of mineral-mineral interactions on mineral bioavailability has implications for children who are given mineral supplements that exceed the RDA of intake for a given mineral.

References

1. Institute of Medicine. *Dietary Reference Intakes for Energy, Carbohydrate, Fiber, Fat, Fatty Acids, Cholesterol, Protein, and Amino Acids.* National Academies Press; 2005
2. Weaver CM, Gordon CM, Janz KF, et al. The National Osteoporosis Foundation's position statement on peak bone mass development and lifestyle factors: a systematic review and implementation recommendations. *Osteoporos Int.* 2016;27(4):1281–1386 PMID: 26856587 doi: 10.1007/s00198-015-3440-3
3. Cogswell ME, Gunn JP, Yuan K, Park S, Merritt R. Sodium and sugar in complementary infant and toddler foods sold in the United States. *Pediatrics.* 2015;135(3):416–423 PMID: 25647681 doi: 10.1542/peds.2014-3251
4. Hagan JF Jr, Shaw JS, Duncan PM, eds. *Bright Futures: Guidelines for Health Supervision of Infants, Children, and Adolescents.* 4th ed. American Academy of Pediatrics; 2017 doi: 10.1542/9781610020237

Water and Hydration

Water is the largest component of the human body, comprising 75% of body weight in infants and 50% to 60% of body weight in children, adolescents, and adults.[1] It helps regulate body temperature, protect vital organs, support nutrient absorption, serve as a medium for biochemical reactions, and maintain blood volume. Food and drink intake; sweat, urine, feces, and vomitus excretion; metabolism; breathing; and exercise all influence body water volume.

Water Needs

The National Academy of Medicine has established a total water adequate intake, which includes water from foods, beverages, and drinking water (refer to **Table A-1** in the Appendix). The percentage of total water needed from fluid intake varies by age and sex and is summarized in **Table 7-1**. Although fluid can be obtained from sources other than water (eg, human [breast] milk or formula in infants, milk and other drinks in children), clean, uncontaminated plain water is an important source of hydration. Note that although breast milk or formula is an infant's primary fluid source, water can and should be introduced around 6 months of age.

Most of the time, it is unnecessary for parents or clinicians to keep a tally of how much fluid children and adolescents are drinking, because youth are able to ensure sufficient fluid intake by responding to feelings of thirst with water or other beverages. However,

Table 7-1. Daily Fluid Needs by Age and Sex

Age (sex)	Adequate intake
0–6 mo (boys and girls)	24 fl oz (3 c/0.7 L; from human [breast] milk or formula)
7–12 mo (boys and girls)	20 fl oz (2.5 c/0.6 L; mostly from breast milk or formula)
1–3 y (boys and girls)	30 fl oz (3.5 c/0.9 L)
4–8 y (boys and girls)	40 fl oz (4.5 c/1.2 L)
9–13 y (boys)	60 fl oz (7.5 c/1.8 L)
9–13 y (girls)	54 fl oz (7 c/1.6 L)
14–18 y (boys)	88 fl oz (11 c/2.6 L)
14–18 y (girls)	61 fl oz (8 c/1.8 L)

Derived from reference 1.

attention to fluid intake becomes more important during illness; in hot climates in which a considerable volume of water may be lost through perspiration for evaporative cooling and further lost with increased humidity; and during physical exertion. Infants and toddlers are more susceptible to dehydration than older children and more likely to experience insufficient fluid intake because of their inability to ask for or seek out fluids in response to thirst mechanisms and, therefore, their reliance on caregivers to offer fluids. Recipes that clinicians can share with parents, other caregivers, and patients to help make water more appealing, such as fruit- and herb-infused water, flavored sparkling water, and fruity ice cubes, are available in Part 5, Frequently Asked Questions, Case Studies, and Recipes.

Dehydration

The body maintains water balance effectively despite moderate daily variation in water intake and needs. It retains more water during decreased hydration, resulting in more concentrated urine. During excess water consumption, unneeded water is excreted in very dilute urine. However, a large discrepancy between water consumption and water needs can result in dehydration during underconsumption or hyponatremia during overconsumption. Infants and young children are most susceptible to these variations because of their large surface area relative to their weight. This risk is greatest during gastrointestinal illness leading to fluid and electrolyte losses from vomiting and/or diarrhea. However, poor oral intake and increased insensible losses, especially in newborns and young infants, also lead to dehydration.

The most accurate way to evaluate dehydration is amount of weight loss compared to baseline. Each gram of weight loss equates to 1 mL of water loss. Given that an accurate pre-illness weight is rarely available, clinicians generally estimate the extent of fluid loss on the basis of clinical signs such as those shown in **Table 7-2**. In the outpatient setting, clinicians are most likely to encounter mild (3%–5% volume loss) and moderate (6%–9% volume loss) dehydration. Children with signs of severe dehydration (≥10% volume loss) require emergency department or inpatient evaluation and treatment.

Serum Sodium Levels

Serum sodium levels can vary depending on whether a child has isonatremic, hyponatremic, or hypernatremic dehydration. Isonatremic dehydration (sodium level of 130–150 mEq/L [130–150 mmol/L]) results from equal proportion of water and solute loss, such as in the case of secretory diarrhea. Hyponatremic dehydration (sodium level of <130 mEq/L [130 mmol/L]) results from replacement of diarrheal losses with hypotonic fluids. Hypernatremic dehydration (sodium level of >150 mEq/L [150 mmol/L]) occurs from water loss exceeding solute loss, such as in the case of viral gastroenteritis or inadequate breastfeeding of infants with diarrheal and insensible losses.

Table 7-2. The Classification and Management of Dehydration

	Mild dehydration (3%–5%)	Moderate dehydration (6%–9%)	Severe dehydration (≥10% volume loss)
Clinical signs	Decreased urine output	Decreased urine output Decreased tearing Dry mucous membranes Decreased skin turgor Tachycardia Decreased capillary refill time Deep respirations Sunken fontanelle in infants	Lethargy Tachycardia Hypotension Hypernea Prolonged capillary refill time Cool and mottled extremities
Laboratory findings	Within reference range (laboratory evaluation not needed)	Within range (laboratory evaluation usually not needed)	Decreased serum bicarbonate level Elevated serum urea nitrogen level Low, within range, or high sodium level Elevated creatinine level Low potassium level (stool losses) or high (with worsening metabolic acidosis) Metabolic acidosis Increased urinary specific gravity Low urinary sodium level High urinary osmolality
Treatment	Replenish volume deficit and ongoing losses, and ensure intake of maintenance fluid needs. The volume deficit can be estimated from clinical signs. In general, volume deficit replacement includes 10 mL/kg per watery stool and 2 mL/kg per vomitus. Give ondansetron to help stop vomiting and allow for oral rehydration.		Isotonic intravenous fluids

Continued

Table 7-2 (*continued*)

	Mild dehydration (3%–5%)	Moderate dehydration (6%–9%)	Severe dehydration (≥10% volume loss)
Caregiver instructions	Do • Continue breastfeeding, if applicable. • Use appropriate oral rehydration solutions (eg, Pedialyte, Enfalyte, CeraLyte, World Health Organization solution). • Replace fluids with 1 tsp (5 mL) every few minutes. • Allow foods, and normalize diet as soon as possible. Do not • Restrict lactose intake. • Change or dilute formula, if applicable. • Rehydrate with apple juice, tea, ginger ale, cola, chicken broth, or sports drinks.		Seek medical attention urgently.

Adapted from reference 2.

Fluid Replacement

The aims of fluid replacement are as follows:

- Restore any existing water and electrolyte deficits. Replace 10 mL/kg of body weight for each watery stool and 2 mL/kg of body weight for each vomitus. With a typical illness, this approach generally results in 50 to 100 mL/kg of body weight being replaced slowly over 2 to 4 hours.
- Provide maintenance fluids, according to general fluid needs described previously.
- Replace ongoing losses. Replace losses milliliter for milliliter with fluids of similar electrolyte composition as the fluid losses. For example, replace a 100-mL vomitus with a 100-mL oral rehydration solution.

Most fluids such as apple juice, sports drinks, ginger ale, and chicken broth do not contain the appropriate glucose to sodium ratio for adequate rehydration and should not be used. Solutions such as Pedialyte, Enfalyte, CeraLyte, and World Health Organization rehydration solution are appropriate for rehydration (**Table 7-3**).[2]

Table 7-3. Composition of Oral Rehydration Solutions and Commonly Used Beverages

Solution	Carbohydrate (g/L)	Sodium (mEq/L)	Potassium (mEq/L)	Base (mEq/L)	Osmolarity (mOsm/kg)
Pedialyte (dextrose)	25	45	20	30	250
Enfalyte (corn syrup)	32	50	25	30	200
CeraLyte (rice)	40	70	20	10	235
World Health Organization (glucose)	13.5	75	20	30	245
Inappropriate for rehydration					
Gatorade sports drink	45	20	3	3	280–360
Powerade sports drink	58	10	3	1	403
Apple juice	100–150	3	20	0	700
Tea	0	0	0	0	5
Ginger ale	90	3.5	0.1	3.6	565
Cola	100–150	2	0.1	13	550
Chicken broth	0	250	5	0	450

Adapted from reference 2.

In Sum

- Water serves vital roles including to regulate body temperature, protect vital organs, support nutrient absorption, serve as a medium for biochemical reactions, and maintain blood volume. Food and drink intake; sweat, urine, feces, and vomitus excretion; metabolism; breathing; and exercise all influence body water volume.
- Total water needs can be met through beverage, food, and free water intake. The approximate amount of free water intake needed varies by age and sex. Generally, newborns and infants aged 0 to 6 months need about 24 fl oz (3 c/0.7 L) per day, from breast milk or formula, and infants aged 7 to 12 months need about 20 fl oz (2.5 c/0.6 L) per day, mostly from breast milk or formula plus some free water. Toddlers aged 1 to 3 years need about 30 fl oz (3.5 c/0.9 L) per day, children aged 4 to 8 years need about 40 fl oz (4.5 c/1.2 L) per day, boys aged 9 to 13 years need about 60 fl oz (7.5 c/1.8 L) per day, girls aged 9 to 13 years need about 54 fl oz

(7 c/1.6 L) per day, male adolescents aged 14 to 18 years need about 88 fl oz (11 c/2.6 L) per day, and female adolescents aged 14 to 18 years need about 61 fl oz (8 c/1.8 L) per day. Needs increase with increased physical activity or exercise and during illness, especially illness associated with fever, vomiting, and/or diarrhea.

● In the outpatient setting, clinicians are most likely to encounter mild (3%–5% volume loss) and moderate (6%–9% volume loss) dehydration. Oral rehydration solutions (eg, Pedialyte, Enfalyte, CeraLyte, World Health Organization rehydration solution) are appropriate for prevention of dehydration and for rehydration. Most fluids such as apple juice, sports drinks, ginger ale, and chicken broth do not contain the appropriate glucose to sodium ratio for adequate rehydration and should not be used. The goal of rehydration is to replace fluid losses. With a typical gastrointestinal illness, this approach generally results in 50 to 100 mL/kg of body weight being replaced slowly over 2 to 4 hours.

References

1. Institute of Medicine. *Dietary Reference Intakes for Energy, Carbohydrate, Fiber, Fat, Fatty Acids, Cholesterol, Protein, and Amino Acids.* National Academies Press; 2005
2. Powers KS. Dehydration: isonatremic, hyponatremic, and hypernatremic recognition and management. *Pediatr Rev.* 2015;36(7):274–285 PMID: 26133303 doi: 10.1542/pir.36.7.274

PART 2

Nutritional Assessment

Pediatric clinicians complete a form of a nutritional assessment every time they care for a patient at a health supervision visit or monitor growth and development. Although the assessment is often brief and focused, being well versed in how to conduct a full nutritional assessment can help clinicians more effectively establish a diagnosis of nutrition-related concerns, such as malnutrition and iron deficiency anemia; elucidate a potential nutrition-related cause of other common pediatric conditions, such as constipation and lactose intolerance; inform a nutrition-related treatment plan for an already established diagnosis, such as obesity or disordered eating; or tailor nutritional guidance by a child's age and stage of development and nutritional status.

Clinicians can monitor for healthful nutrition habits and nutrition-related health concerns by using the "ABCD" approach to the nutritional assessment: Anthropometric measures, Biochemical markers, Clinical factors, and Dietary and social histories. Chapter 8, Anthropometric Measures, describes how to measure, evaluate, and monitor important anthropometric measures, such as growth and body mass index percentiles. Chapter 9, Clinical and Biochemical Evaluation, outlines key biochemical markers and clinical factors that play a role in assessing nutritional status. Chapter 10, Dietary History, Social History, and Food Insecurity Screening, describes key components of the dietary and social histories to help assess baseline nutrition behaviors and underlying social, psychological, and cultural factors that influence dietary intake.

CHAPTER 8

Anthropometric Measures

The first part of the nutritional assessment is the collection and interpretation of anthropometric measures, including growth measures such as height and weight, which allow for assessment of weight-for-length, body mass index (BMI), and growth velocity. Sometimes body circumference (waist, hip, and limbs) and skinfold thickness are also used to help assess body composition. Using anthropometric measures to monitor a child's growth provides clinicians with essential information about development and health status. An aberration in typical growth can be an early indicator of a health concern, including a nutrition-related problem such as malnutrition or obesity. Key features and considerations of each of these growth measures are shown in **Table 8-1**.

Growth Charts

Standardized growth charts allow clinicians to track a child's growth over time and compare their growth to that of patients of the same age and sex. The Centers for Disease Control and Prevention (CDC) growth charts were most recently updated in 2000 on the basis of data collected in 5 cross-sectional, nationally representative health examination surveys, spanning from 1963 to 1994. The 2000 CDC BMI charts, which are currently in widespread use in clinical settings, are based on data only through 1980 for children 6 years and older. They exclude the survey results from 1988 to 1994 to prevent normalizing the excess weight gain resulting from the current childhood obesity epidemic that began in the 1980s. This decision explains how it is possible that greater than 30% of children currently have a BMI equal to or greater than the 85th percentile and 18.5% of children currently have a BMI equal to or greater than the 95th percentile.

The World Health Organization (WHO) growth charts are preferable to the CDC growth charts from birth to 24 months of age because these charts are based on growth patterns in infants in 6 countries throughout the world who were predominately breastfed for at least 4 months and still breastfeeding at 12 months. The WHO growth charts represent the optimal growth pattern for infants. The CDC growth charts for newborns, infants, and toddlers aged 0 to 2 years do not represent optimal growth because the weight data were unavailable between birth and 3 months of age, the sample sizes were small for the first 6 months of age, and many infants were primarily formula fed. The CDC charts are references that reflect how infants grew during a specified period, whereas the WHO charts are standards that show how children should grow in an ideal environment. Recognizing the limitations of the CDC birth to 24 months growth charts, the CDC advises clinicians to use the WHO growth charts for children younger than 2 years.[1]

All standardized growth charts follow a normal distribution and include z scores, which indicate 1 SD from the mean. A positive z score of 1 is 1 SD above the mean, whereas

Table 8-1. Standard Growth Measures

Measure	Indication	Clinical considerations	Clinical indicators of concern
Weight	All visits, all ages	• First measure to reflect disruption in health or nutritional status • Average expected weight gain —0–3 mo: 25–30 g/d —3–6 mo: 15–20 g/d —6–12 mo: 10–15 g/d —0–1 y: triple birth weight —1–5 y: approximately 5 lb (2 kg) per year —6–11 y: approximately 7 lb (3 kg) per year	• Crossing of weight-for-age percentiles over time • Atypical weight gain or atypical weight loss
Length	All health supervision visits	• Clinicians can estimate genetic potential (midparental height) with the following equation, if the heights of the biological father and mother are known: Boys: (paternal height + [maternal height + 5 inches or 13 cm]) / 2 Girls: (maternal height + [paternal height − 5 inches or 13 cm]) / 2 Target range: midparental height ± 4 inches or 10 cm • Undernutrition causes poor linear growth. • Overnutrition may result in early maturation and accelerated linear growth, leading to earlier achievement of adult height.	• Crossing of length-for-age percentiles over time • Projected adult height 2 inches (5 cm) below or above midparental height, especially if measured height >97th percentile or <3rd percentile • Growth <1.75 inches (5 cm) per year between the age of 3 and onset of puberty

Weight-for-length	All health supervision visits for newborns, infants, and toddlers aged 0–2 y	• Indicator of underweight, typical weight, or overweight for those up to age 2 y • Identifier of malnutrition	• If weight-for-length is <5th percentile and decreasing over time, malnutrition should be suspected. • If weight-for-length is >95th percentile and increasing over time, overnutrition should be suspected.
BMI	All health supervision visits for children and adolescents aged ≥2 y	• BMI peaks at 6–12 mo of age, declines to nadir at 5–6 y of age, and then increases progressively throughout childhood and adolescence. This period is referred to as the *adiposity rebound.* • An early or pronounced adiposity rebound is associated with increased adiposity in adolescence and adulthood. • An increased BMI percentile tends to persist over time.	• BMI ≤5th percentile = underweight. • BMI ≥85th and <95th percentiles = overweight. • BMI ≥95th percentile = obesity. Class I obesity: 100%–120% of the 95th percentile Class II obesity: ≥120% of the 95th percentile or BMI ≥35, whichever is lower Class III obesity: ≥140% of the 95th percentile or BMI ≥40, whichever is lower
Head circumference	All health supervision visits for newborns, infants, and toddlers aged 0–2 y	Indicator of brain growth. Brain growth can be affected by chronic undernutrition.	• Head circumference <5th percentile indicates microcephaly. • Head circumference >95th percentile indicates macrocephaly.

Continued

Table 8-1 (*continued*)

Measure	Indication	Clinical considerations	Clinical indicators of concern
Growth velocity	As needed for growth concerns	• Typical growth velocity — <1 y: 10 inches (25 cm) per year — 1–2 y: 4.0 inches (10 cm) per year — 2–3 y: 3.2 inches (8 cm) per year — 3–4 y: 2.8 inches (7 cm) per year — 4–10 y: 2.0–2.4 inches (5–6 cm) per year • Prepuberty nadir — Girls: 2.2 inches (5.5 cm) per year — Boys: 1.9 inches (4.9 cm) per year • Pubertal acceleration — Girls: 3.2–4.7 inches (8–12 cm) per year — Boys: 3.9–5.5 inches (10–14 cm) per year	Growth velocity <1.75 inches (5 cm) per year
Body circumference (waist and midarm)	• Obesity • Malnutrition	• Waist circumference is an index of pediatric obesity that best predicts fat mass and metabolic risk. • Midarm circumference is used in the evaluation of malnutrition.	• Waist circumference >90th percentile for age • Midarm circumference <5th percentile for age
Skinfold thickness	Infrequently used in pediatric clinical practice because it requires use of calipers and high technical expertise for accurate measurement; however, may be included as part of an evaluation in an obesity or multidisciplinary clinic	Assessor of muscle and fat mass	Use age-based reference tables.[a]

Abbreviation: BMI, body mass index.

[a] Available at the National Center for Health Statistics website (www.cdc.gov/nchs/data/series/sr_11/sr11_252.pdf).

a negative z score of -1 is 1 SD below the mean. Approximately 68.27% of the population falls within 1 SD (z score of ±1); 95.45%, within 2 SDs (z score of ±2); and 99.73%, within 3 SDs (z score of ±3). Measurements more than 2 SDs above or below the mean (3rd percentile [$z = -2$] and 97th percentile [$z = +2$]) often indicate increased risk for adverse health conditions affecting growth and therefore require further evaluation and possible intervention. Many electronic health record systems automatically calculate z scores on pediatric growth charts.

Specialized growth charts are available for many conditions that affect growth, including preterm birth, severe obesity, Down syndrome, Turner syndrome, achondroplasia, Marfan syndrome, Prader-Willi syndrome, cerebral palsy, and sickle cell anemia (**Box 8-1**).

Typical Growth

Pediatric growth patterns are divided into 4 stages: infancy/toddlerhood (0–2 years), preschool (3–5 years), middle childhood (6–11 years), and adolescence (12–18 years). Characteristics of each phase of growth are highlighted in **Table 8-2**.

Nutritional Causes of Atypical Growth

Nutritional causes of atypical growth result from malnutrition (insufficient caloric intake) or overnutrition (excess caloric intake) as compared with metabolic needs. Nearly any chronic condition can cause atypical growth by contributing to inadequate or excess caloric intake, malabsorption, or increased or decreased metabolic and caloric needs.

Malnutrition

Malnutrition is defined as an "imbalance between nutrient intakes and requirements [that] results in cumulative deficits of energy, protein, or micronutrients."[3] Malnutrition occurs when caloric or nutrient availability is insufficient, whether through

---

CLINICAL PRACTICE TIP

Box 8-1. PediTools

PediTools (https://peditools.org) is a free online resource with numerous useful tools, including a growth chart calculator for infants who experienced preterm birth, a growth chart for children who have Down syndrome, CDC and WHO reference standards for triceps and subscapular skinfold thickness, and a CDC and WHO calculator for midarm circumference percentile and z score.

Abbreviations: CDC, Centers for Disease Control and Prevention; WHO, World Health Organization.

Table 8-2. Pediatric Growth Stages and Typical Growth Patterns

Stage of growth	Key characteristics
Infancy/toddlerhood (0–2 y)	<ul><li>This is a period of very rapid growth.</li><li>Infants double their birth weight by 4–5 mo of age and triple their birth weight by 1 y of age.</li><li>Infants grow 1.5 times their height in the first year.</li><li>Head circumference, a measure of brain growth, increases by 1.3 times in the first year.</li><li>The brain doubles in weight by 12 mo of age.</li><li>Children grow approximately 4.7 inches (12 cm) from 1–2 y of age.</li><li>Children gain approximately 5 lb (2 kg) from 1–2 y of age.</li><li>One-third of infants cross percentiles upward in growth measures in the first 2 y. This growth often occurs for a small infant with tall parents. One-third of infants maintain a consistent growth percentile. One-third of infants cross percentiles downward. This growth often occurs for a large infant with shorter parents.</li><li>Rapid weight gain in the first 2 y increases the risk of childhood obesity. *Rapid weight gain* is defined as a *z* score increase in weight-for-age > 0.67 in 2 time points during the first 2 y after birth.[2]</li></ul>
Preschool (3–5 y)	<ul><li>Children grow approximately 3 inches (8 cm) per year.</li><li>Children gain approximately 5 lb (2 kg) per year.</li><li>The brain triples from birth size by 3 y of age, at which time it is 85% of its adult size.</li></ul>
Middle childhood (6–11 y)	<ul><li>Children grow approximately 2.5 inches (6.4 cm) per year.</li><li>Children gain approximately 4.5 lb (2.0 kg) per year initially, increasing to 8 lb (4 kg) per year as they near ages 10–11 y.</li><li>Girls tend to grow slightly faster and gain slightly more weight than boys at this age.</li></ul>

Table 8-2 (*continued*)

Stage of growth	Key characteristics

Adolescence (12–18 y)	• Girls
	  — Start puberty between ages 8 and 13 y, with menarche occurring at a mean age of 12.5 y
	  — Experience a growth spurt between 11 and 14 y of age
	  — Reach their final adult height approximately 2 y after their first menstrual period
	  — Have an average peak height velocity of approximately 3.25 inches (8.26 cm) per year
	  — Finish growing in height at a bone age of 16 y
	  — Add more body fat than boys during this stage
	• Boys
	  — Start puberty between ages 9 and 14 y
	  — Experience a growth spurt between 13 and 16 y of age, which is of longer duration than the growth spurt experienced by girls
	  — Finish growing in height at a bone age of 18 y
	  — Have an average peak height velocity of 3.5–4.0 inches (8.9–10.2 cm) per year
	  — Add more muscle mass than girls during this stage

low intake, excess intestinal losses, or a combination of the two. When caloric intake is too low, the body naturally compensates by decreasing physical activity and, eventually, slowing growth. If chronic undernutrition occurs, stunting can occur in which a child has short stature or low weight-for-age. Malnutrition can result in decreased school performance, delayed bone age, and increased susceptibility to infection.[4]

Malnutrition manifests first with poor weight gain, but if it persists, linear height can be negatively affected. Brain growth is generally spared; thus, head circumference is the last anthropometric measure to be affected by chronic malnutrition in children aged 0 to 2 years. Malnutrition is classified as mild, moderate, or severe on the basis of anthropometric data shown in **Table 8-3**. Clinicians commonly refer to poor weight gain or very low weight/length or BMI as *failure to thrive;* however, this term is no longer advised (**Box 8-2**).

Overnutrition

The effects of overnutrition are generally classified as atypical weight gain, overweight, and class I, II, and III obesity, as shown in **Table 8-4**. Class II and III obesity are considered to be "severe obesity." Rather than *z* scores, percentage of the 95th percentile on extended BMI growth charts is used to classify obesity severity.

Table 8-3. Classifying the Severity of Pediatric Malnutrition

Primary indicator	Mild malnutrition z score	Moderate malnutrition z score	Severe malnutrition z score
Weight-for-height	−1 to −1.9	≥ −2 to −2.9	At or below −3
Body mass index–for-age	−1 to −1.9	≥ −2 to −2.9	At or below −3
Length-/height-for-age	No data	No data	At or below −3
Midarm circumference	≥ −1 to −1.9	≥ −2 to −2.9	At or below −3
Weight gain velocity (< 2 y of age)	< 75% of norm for expected weight gain	< 50% of norm for expected weight gain	< 25% of norm for expected weight gain
Deceleration in weight-for-length z score	Decline of 1 z score	Decline of 2 z scores	Decline of 3 z scores
Percentage weight loss (usual body weight − current body weight × 100)	5%	7.5%	10%
Inadequate nutrient intake	51%–75% estimated energy/protein needs	26%–50% estimated energy/protein needs	≤ 25% estimated energy/protein needs

Adapted with permission from reference 5.

A BMI greater than the 85th percentile for age and sex (overweight), especially a BMI greater than the 95th percentile for age and sex (obesity), is associated with increased risk of chronic diseases such as type 2 diabetes, hypertension, coronary heart disease, stroke, gallbladder disease, osteoarthritis, and some types of cancer. Of note, although BMI is a commonly used method of approximating body composition in practice, assessment of body composition with skinfold thickness measurements, bioelectrical impedance analysis, or dual-energy x-ray absorptiometry more accurately indicates body fat. However, pediatricians rarely have access to these tools. Childhood overweight, obesity, and related health conditions are detailed in Chapter 20, Obesity and Related Health Conditions.

IN GREATER DEPTH

Box 8-2. *Failure to Thrive*

In the past, poor weight gain and growth was referred to as *failure to thrive,* but this term is no longer advised. The eighth edition of the American Academy of Pediatrics book *Pediatric Nutrition* advises that "failure to thrive as a diagnostic 'label' has been viewed as inappropriate for some time. Parents do not appreciate the term 'failure' and health care professionals know that it is a vague descriptive term that provides no distinct diagnostic direction." The book's previous edition describes failure to thrive as "an imprecise, archaic term that refers to children whose growth is significantly lower than the norms for age and gender ... the underlying cause of failure to thrive is malnutrition."[3] *Malnutrition* is the preferred term, which can be further classified as mild, moderate, or severe on the basis of the criteria in **Table 8-3**.

Table 8-4. Indicators of Pediatric Overnutrition

Primary indicator	Percentile	Percentage of the 95th percentile
Overweight	85th–94th	Not applicable
Class I obesity	≥95th	100%–120% of the 95th percentile
Class II obesity		≥120% of the 95th percentile or body mass index ≥35, whichever is lower
Class III obesity		≥140% of the 95th percentile or body mass index ≥40, whichever is lower
Weight gain velocity	Crossing of 2 major percentiles	Not applicable

Tip: Use "extended body mass index" growth charts in the electronic health record to classify class II and III obesity as the percentage of the 95th percentile.

Derived from reference 6.

In Sum

- Collection and interpretation of anthropometric measures are the first part of the nutritional assessment. Anthropometric measures include height, weight, and head circumference. Plotting accurate anthropometric measures over time provides the clinician with essential information about a newborn's, infant's, child's, or adolescent's growth, development, and health status.

- Healthy newborns, infants, children, and adolescents generally follow a typical growth pattern.
  - Infancy is a period of very rapid growth. Infants generally double their birth weight by 4 to 5 months of age and triple their birth weight by 1 year of age. They grow 1.5 times their birth height in the first year. Brain weight doubles and head circumference increases by 1.3 times in the first year.
  - From 1 to 2 years of age, children grow approximately 4.7 inches (12 cm) and gain approximately 5 lb (2 kg). Rapid weight gain in the first 2 years increases the risk of childhood obesity.
  - From 3 to 5 years of age, children grow approximately 3 inches (8 cm) and gain approximately 5 lb (2 kg) per year. The brain triples from birth size by 3 years of age, at which time it is 85% of its adult size.
  - From 6 to 11 years of age, children grow approximately 2.5 inches (6.4 cm) per year. They gain approximately 4.5 lb (2.0 kg) per year initially, increasing to 8 lb (4 kg) per year as they near ages 10 to 11 years. Girls tend to grow slightly faster and gain slightly more weight than boys at this age.
  - Girls start puberty between ages 8 and 13 years, with the mean age of menarche occurring at 12.5 years. They experience a growth spurt between 11 and 14 years of age, with an average peak height velocity of approximately 3.25 inches (8.26 cm) per year. Typically, girls reach their final adult height approximately 2 years after their first menstrual period and finish growing in height at a bone age of 16 years.
  - Boys start puberty between ages 9 and 14 years. They experience a growth spurt between 13 and 16 years of age, with an average peak height velocity of 3.5 to 4.0 inches (8.9–10.2 cm) per year. Their growth spurt is of longer duration than the growth spurt experienced by girls, and most boys finish growing in height at a bone age of 18 years.
- An aberration in typical growth can be an early indicator of a health concern, including a nutrition-related problem such as malnutrition or overnutrition.

References

1. National Center for Health Statistics. WHO growth charts. Reviewed September 9, 2010. Accessed September 22, 2022. https://www.cdc.gov/growthcharts/who_charts.htm
2. Shin YL. The timing of rapid infant weight gain in relation to childhood obesity. *J Obes Metab Syndr.* 2019;28(4):213–215 PMID: 31909363 doi:10.7570/jomes.2019.28.4.213
3. Kleinman RE, Greer FR, eds. American Academy of Pediatrics Committee on Nutrition. *Pediatric Nutrition.* 8th ed. American Academy of Pediatrics; 2019
4. Institute of Medicine. *Dietary Reference Intakes for Energy, Carbohydrate, Fiber, Fat, Fatty Acids, Cholesterol, Protein, and Amino Acids.* National Academies Press; 2005
5. Becker PJ, Nieman Carney L, Corkins MR, et al. Consensus statement of the Academy of Nutrition and Dietetics/American Society for Parenteral and Enteral Nutrition: indicators recommended for the identification and documentation of pediatric malnutrition (undernutrition). *J Acad Nutr Diet.* 2014;114(12):1988–2000 PMID: 25458748 doi: 10.1016/j.jand.2014.08.026
6. Skinner AC, Ravanbakht SN, Skelton JA, Perrin EM, Armstrong SC. Prevalence of obesity and severe obesity in US children, 1999–2016. *Pediatrics.* 2018;141(3):e20173459 PMID: 29483202 doi: 10.1542/peds.2017-3459

CHAPTER 9

Clinical and Biochemical Evaluation

A patient history, physical examination, and laboratory assessment provide important data points in conducting a nutritional assessment and developing a care plan.

Clinical Evaluation

The clinical evaluation component of the nutritional assessment includes a comprehensive patient history and physical examination.

Clinical History

A medical, family, and social history can offer clues to the potential cause of nutritional concerns. Health status is a helpful component of the patient history, including past illness; current illness or chronic disease; prenatal period and birth; breastfeeding, including components of maternal history that can affect human (breast) milk supply; family health; mental health and social activity; and medication and supplement use. Several health conditions are nutritional risk factors for children (**Table 9-1**). Some medications in particular can affect nutritional status, as shown in **Table 9-2**.

Physical Examination

A nutrition-focused physical examination can provide important clues to potential nutrient deficiencies or excesses. Note that many of the physical examination findings could also occur because of nonnutrition-related conditions. Specific physical examination considerations are shown in **Table 9-3**.

Biochemical Evaluation

Laboratory evaluation is valuable to assess hematologic, protein, hydration, and individual nutrient status. Several commonly assessed nutritional markers and their significance are shown in **Table 9-4**. Of note, although albumin and prealbumin tests had been thought to be indicators of nutritional status, they are markers of inflammation rather than protein-energy malnutrition and should not be used as nutritional markers.[4] As such, they are not included in **Table 9-4**.

Table 9-1. Conditions That Are Nutritional Risk Factors for Children

Condition	Risk category							
	Growth			Diet			Medical	
	Underweight	Overweight	Short stature	Low energy needs	High energy needs	Feeding difficulty	Malnutrition	Medications that affect nutrition
Autism spectrum disorder	X	X				X	X	X
Bronchopulmonary dysplasia	X		X		X	X	X	X
Celiac disease	X		X			X	X	
Cerebral palsy	X	X	X	X	X	X	X	X
Chronic kidney failure	X	X	X			X	X	X
Cystic fibrosis[a]	X		X		X	X	X	X
Down syndrome (trisomy 21 syndrome)	X	X	X	X		X	X	X
Eating disorders	X	X	X		X		X	
Heart disease (congenital)	X		X		X	X	X	X

Condition						
Inflammatory bowel disease	X	X		X	X	X
Liver failure	X	X	X	X		X
Neonatal abstinence syndrome	X	X	X	X	X	X
Prader-Willi syndrome		X	X		X	X
Preterm birth	X	X	X	X		X
Seizure disorder	X					X
Short bowel syndrome	X	X	X	X	X	X

[a] There is an increasing incidence of overweight and obesity that is associated with the new medications being used to treat cystic fibrosis; increased energy needs are present only during acute illness.

Adapted with permission from reference 1.

Table 9-2. Common Drug-Nutrient Interactions

Medication	Nutrients affected	Overall effect	Prevention strategies
Antibiotics	Minerals, fats, proteins	Temporarily decrease absorption Destroy beneficial intestinal bacteria	Advise that patients consider increasing intake of acidophilus and other probiotics from foods or supplements because this *may* counteract loss of intestinal flora.
Anticonvulsants	Vitamins D, K, B_6, and B_{12}; folate; calcium	Decrease nutrient absorption or stores	Encourage a diet high in these nutrients (refer to Chapters 5, Vitamins, and 6, Minerals). Consider vitamin/mineral supplementation.
Antipsychotics	Sodium, potassium	Decrease nutrient absorption Increase weight gain	Monitor weight and laboratory values.
Corticosteroids	Calcium, phosphorus, glucose, vitamin D, protein, sodium, water, zinc, vitamin C, potassium	Stunt growth over the long term Deplete calcium and phosphorus, leading to bone loss Increase glucose level Increase appetite and weight gain Retain fluid	Monitor weight and laboratory values. Supplement with ergocalciferol/ cholecalciferol and calcium.
Diuretics	Potassium, magnesium, calcium, folate	Eliminate or deplete nutrient stores	Encourage foods high in potassium and magnesium (refer to Chapters 5, Vitamins, and 6, Minerals).

Laxatives	Fat-soluble vitamins	May deplete fat-soluble vitamins over the long term	Encourage a high-fiber diet, and increase fluids to help treat constipation. Encourage weight-bearing exercise to improve constipation and support bone strength.
Reflux medications	Vitamin B_{12}, iron, calcium	Eliminate these nutrients over the long term	Encourage a diet high in vitamin B_{12}, iron, and calcium (refer to Chapters 5, Vitamins, and 6, Minerals). Monitor laboratory values.
Stimulants	Calories and overall intake	Decrease appetite and may cause weight loss	Advise patients to eat before each dose. Encourage larger meals at times the patient feels most hungry to offset decreased appetite and intake at other times during the day.

Derived from reference 2.

Table 9-3. Physical Examination Findings That May Be Associated With Nutritional Deficiencies and Excesses

Signs	Possible nutrition-related causes
Integumentary findings	
Skin	
Acanthosis nigricans	Insulin resistance caused by obesity
Decreased subcutaneous tissue	Prolonged protein-calorie deficit
Delayed wound healing	Vitamin C, zinc, or protein deficit
Dermatitis	Zinc or niacin deficiency
Dryness	Vitamin A or essential fatty acid deficit
Edema	Protein-calorie deficiency
Follicular hyperkeratosis	Vitamin A or D deficiency
Orange/yellow pigmentation	Beta carotene excess
Pallor	Iron, vitamin B_{12}, vitamin C, folate, and/or vitamin B_6 deficiency
Pellagrous dermatosis (swollen red pigmentation)	Niacin deficiency, secondary vitamin B_6 deficiency
Petechiae	Vitamin C or K deficiency
Poor skin turgor	Dehydration, sodium deficit
Psoriasis	Biotin deficiency
Purpura	Vitamin C or K deficiency, vitamin E excess
Hair	
Alopecia	Protein, iron, zinc, or biotin deficiency
Corkscrew-shaped hair	Vitamin C deficiency
Depigmentation or color changes	Protein-calorie, copper, manganese, or selenium deficiency
Dull, dry, thin, brittle hair	Protein-calorie or essential fatty acid deficiency
Lanugo (fine, soft hair)	Calorie deficiency

Table 9-3 (*continued*)

Signs	Possible nutrition-related causes
Integumentary findings (*continued*)	
Nails	
Ridges	Central ridges: iron, folate, or protein deficiency Transverse ridges: zinc, protein, or calcium deficiency
Soft, brittle, weak nails	Protein-calorie or magnesium deficiency, vitamin A or selenium excess
Spoon shape	Iron or protein deficiency
Cranial findings	
Delayed suture fusion	Vitamin D deficiency
Flattened skull, prominent frontal bones	Vitamin D deficiency
Hard, tender lumps in occipital region and bulging fontanelle	Vitamin A excess
Headache	Thiamin (vitamin B_1) or vitamin A excess
Sunken fontanelle	Dehydration
Endocrine finding	
Enlarged thyroid gland	Iodine deficiency
Ocular findings	
Angular blepharitis (inflammation of the eyelids)	Riboflavin (vitamin B_2), biotin, vitamin B_6, or zinc deficiency
Angular palpebritis (ie, redness, fissuring at corner of eyes)	Niacin, riboflavin, vitamin B_6, or iron deficiency
Night blindness	Vitamin A deficiency
White or gray spots (Bitot spots) on cornea	Vitamin A deficiency
Xanthelasmas (yellowish cholesterol deposit under skin)	Hyperlipidemia
Oral findings	
Mouth/lips	
Angular stomatitis or cheilitis	Riboflavin, niacin, iron, vitamin B_6, or vitamin B_{12} deficiency; vitamin A excess

Continued

Table 9-3 (*continued*)

Signs	Possible nutrition-related causes
Oral findings (*continued*)	
Tongue	
Decreased taste	Zinc deficiency
Glossitis (swollen, sore, smooth red tongue)	Riboflavin, folate, niacin, vitamin B_6, vitamin B_{12}, or iron deficiency
Magenta color, soreness, burning	Riboflavin deficiency
Paleness	Vitamin B_{12}, folate, or iron deficiency
Raw, swollen beefy-red tongue	Folate or niacin deficiency
Teeth and gums	
Caries	Excess carbohydrates, insufficient fluoride, vitamin D deficiency
Defective enamel	Insufficient vitamin A, vitamin C, calcium, or phosphorus
Mottled enamel, brown spots, pits	Excess fluoride
Reddened gingiva	Vitamin A excess
Spongy, prone to bleeding, receding gums	Vitamin C deficiency
Cardiovascular findings	
Arrhythmia	Insufficient magnesium or potassium, niacin or potassium excess
Decreased blood pressure	Insufficient thiamin, dehydration
Palpitations	Insufficient thiamin
Rapid pulse	Insufficient potassium, dehydration
Gastrointestinal findings	
Constipation	Inadequate fiber or fluids, excess calcium
Diarrhea	Excess juice, high fruit intake, vitamin B_{12} or B_6 deficiency, vitamin C excess
Musculoskeletal findings	
Beading on ribs	Vitamin C or D deficiency
Bleeding into joints, pain	Vitamin C deficiency

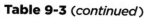

Table 9-3 (continued)

Signs	Possible nutrition-related causes
Musculoskeletal findings (continued)	
Bone demineralization	Calcium, phosphorus, or vitamin D deficiency; vitamin A excess
Calf tenderness, foot drop	Thiamin deficiency
Genu valgum (knock knee), genu varum (bowleg), epiphyseal enlargement	Vitamin D deficiency
Muscle atrophy, dependent edema	Protein-calorie deficiency
Muscle cramps	Calcium, vitamin D, chloride, sodium, potassium, or magnesium deficiency; dehydration
Muscle pain	Biotin or vitamin D deficiency
Peripheral neuropathy	Folate, vitamin B_6, pantothenic acid, vitamin B_{12}, thiamin, or phosphate deficiency; vitamin B_6 toxicity
Tetany	Calcium, vitamin D, or magnesium deficiency; magnesium or vitamin B_6 excess
Neurological findings	
Diminished reflexes	Thiamin deficiency
Listlessness, irritability, lethargy	Protein-calorie, thiamin, niacin, iron, or vitamin B_6 deficiency
Seizures	Thiamin, vitamin B_6, vitamin D, or calcium deficiency; phosphorus excess
Tetany	Magnesium deficiency
Unsteadiness, numbness in hands and feet	Vitamin B_6 excess
Sexual maturity findings	
Delayed sexual maturation	Vitamin A, vitamin D, or protein-calorie deficiency

Derived from reference 3.

Table 9-4. Commonly Assessed Nutritional Markers and Nutrition-Related Health Conditions

Laboratory test	Purpose	Situations causing increase in marker level	Situations causing decrease in marker level	Reference range by age[a,b]
Amylase	Digestive enzyme produced in salivary glands and pancreas and released when either is inflamed	Induced vomiting	Low carbohydrate intake	
Blood urea nitrogen (mg/dL)	Indicator of kidney function	● Dehydration ● Starvation ● Excessive protein intake	● Starvation ● Overhydration	● 0–2 y: 2–19 ● 3–12 y: 5–17 ● 13–18 y: 7–18 ● 19–20 y: 8–21
Calcium[c]		Vitamin D toxicity	● Malnutrition ● Magnesium deficiency ● Vitamin D deficiency	
Complement C3	Indicator of nutritional status		Protein-calorie malnutrition	

Electrolytes (sodium, potassium, and chloride)	Markers of hydration and acid-base balance	● Dehydration
		● Kidney disease
		● Excess dietary intake
			Diuretics, heart failure, liver or kidney disease, laxative use, severe over-hydration	● Sodium (mEq/L)
				  — All ages: 135–145
				● Potassium (mEq/L)
				  — 0–1 mo: 4.5–7.2
				  — 1 to <3 mo: 4.0–6.2
				  — 3 mo–1 y: 3.7–5.6
				  — ≥1–18 y: 3.4–4.7
				● Chloride (mEq/L)
				  — 0–1 mo: 96–106
				  — 1 mo–18 y: 90–110

	Indicator of nutritional status	Pernicious anemia	• Malnutrition • Celiac disease	All ages: >6–7
Folate, serum (ng/mL)				
Iron markers (hemoglobin, mean corpuscular volume, ferritin, iron, serum total iron-binding capacity, transferrin saturation and concentration, and reticulocyte count [absolute and percentage])	Indicators of nutritional status, with hemoglobin being the most sensitive indicator of iron status	• Vitamin B_{12} deficiency • Excessive iron intake • Hypoxia	• Inadequate dietary iron intake • Kidney disease • Blood loss	• Hemoglobin (g/dL) — Newborn: 13.5–19.5 — 1–29 d: 14.5–22 — 1–2 mo: 10–18 — 3–5 mo: 9.5–13.5 — 6–23 mo: 10.5–13.5 — 2–5 y: 11.5–13.5 — 6–11 y: 11.5–15.5 — Boys, 12–17 y: 13–16 — Girls, 12–17 y: 12–16

Continued

Table 9-4 (*continued*)

Laboratory test	Purpose	Situations causing increase in marker level	Situations causing decrease in marker level	Reference range by age[a,b]
Iron markers (*continued*)				● Mean corpuscular volume (mcm^3) — All ages: 80-100 ● Serum ferritin (ng/mL) — Boys, 0-6 mo: 6-400 — Girls, 0-6 mo: 6-430 — Boys, 7 mo-2 y: 12-57 — Girls, 7 mo-2 y: 12-60 — Boys, 3-14 y: 14-80 — Girls, 3-14 y: 12-73 — Boys, 15-19 y: 20-155 — Girls, 15-19 y: 12-90 ● Serum iron (mcg/dL) — 0-6 wk: 100-250 — 7 wk-11 mo: 40-100 — 1-10 y: 50-120 — Males, ≥11 y: 50-170 — Females, ≥11 y: 30-160 ● Serum total iron-binding capacity (mcg/dL) — 0-2 mo: 59-175 — 3 mo-17 y: 250-400 — ≥18 y: 240-450 ● Serum transferrin saturation (%) — All ages: 20-50

Parameter	Indicator of	Increased with	Decreased with	Reference range
				• Serum transferrin concentration (mg/dL) – All ages: 180–370 • Absolute reticulocyte count (×10³/mcL) – 3 mo–adulthood: 25–75 • Percentage of red blood cells (%) – 3 mo–adulthood: approximately 1.5
Magnesium (mg/dL)	Indicator of kidney and gastrointestinal function	• Dehydration • Laxative use	• Inadequate dietary magnesium intake • Diuretic use • Laxative use • Celiac disease	0–20 y: 1.5–2.5
Phosphorus (mg/dL)	Indicator of nutritional status	• Excessive supplementation • Kidney disease	• Refeeding syndrome • Diuretic use • Laxative use • Untreated diabetes • Malabsorption	• 0–11 mo: 4.8–8.2 • 1–3 y: 3.8–6.5 • 4–6 y: 4.1–5.4 • 7–11 y: 3.7–5.6 • 12–13 y: 3.3–5.4 • 14–15 y: 2.9–5.4 • 16–20 y: 2.7–4.7

Continued

Table 9-4 (*continued*)

Laboratory test	Purpose	Situations causing increase in marker level	Situations causing decrease in marker level	Reference range by age[a,b]
Stool pH	Measure of fermented carbohydrate in stool, indicator of sugar malabsorption		Carbohydrate malabsorption (pH <5.5)	All ages: pH >5.5
Vitamin B_{12} (pg/mL)	Indicator of vitamin B_{12} intake	Excessive intake	<ul><li>Pernicious anemia</li><li>Vegan eating plan</li><li>Post-bariatric surgery</li></ul>	All ages: 200–900
Vitamin D (25-hydroxyvitamin D) (ng/mL)	Indicator of vitamin D status	Excessive intake	<ul><li>Inadequate vitamin D intake</li></ul>	All ages: >20
Zinc (mcg/dL)	Indicator of nutritional status, with zinc deficiency causing altered taste, poor weight gain, and/or signs of depression	Excessive supplementation	<ul><li>Malnutrition</li><li>Poorly planned vegetarian diet</li><li>Excessive exercise</li><li>Post-bariatric surgery</li></ul>	<ul><li>0–16 y: 66–144</li><li>Males, ≥17 y: 75–291</li><li>Females, ≥17 y: 65–256</li></ul>

SI conversion factors: To convert g/dL to g/L, multiply by 10.0; mcg/dL to mcmol/L, by 0.179 (iron and total iron-binding capacity) or 0.153 (zinc); mcm³ to fL, by 1.0; mEq/L to mmol/L, by 1.0; mg/dL to mcmol/L, by 0.123; mg/dL to mmol/L, by 0.357 (blood urea nitrogen), 0.4114 (magnesium), or 0.323 (phosphorus); ng/mL to mcg/L, by 1.0; ng/mL to nmol/L, by 2.266 (folate) or 2.496 (vitamin D); percentage to proportion, by 0.01; pg/mL to pmol/L, by 0.7378; and ×10³/mcL to ×10⁹/L, by 1.0.

[a] If no range is indicated, laboratory reference ranges should be used.

[b] Reference ranges may vary slightly by laboratory.

[c] Blood calcium level does not reflect dietary calcium intake.

Derived from American Academy of Pediatrics Committee on Nutrition. Assessment of nutritional status. In: Kleinman RE, Greer FR, eds. *Pediatric Nutrition.* 8th ed. American Academy of Pediatrics; 2019:723–773 and reference 3.

In Sum

- The patient history and physical examination offer clues to the potential cause of nutritional concerns and indications for further laboratory evaluation to assess nutritional status. Certain health conditions, including many genetic syndromes and chronic diseases and some medication effects, increase nutritional risk.
- A biochemical or laboratory evaluation of nutritional markers provides additional information to help assess hematologic, protein, hydration, and individual nutrient status and targets for nutritional therapy.

References

1. Konek SH, Becker PJ. *Samour & King's Pediatric Nutrition in Clinical Care*. 5th ed. Jones & Bartlett; 2020

2. Behavioral Health Nutrition Dietetic Practice Group, Pediatric Nutrition Practice Group. *Pocket Guide to Children With Special Health Care and Nutritional Needs*. Wittenbrook W, Corkins KG, eds. 2nd ed. Academy of Nutrition and Dietetics; 2021

3. Leonberg B. *Pocket Guide to Pediatric Nutrition Assessment*. 3rd ed. Academy of Nutrition and Dietetics; 2020

4. Evans DC, Corkins MR, Malone A, et al; ASPEN Malnutrition Committee. The use of visceral proteins as nutrition markers: an ASPEN position paper. *Nutr Clin Pract*. 2021;36(1):22–28 PMID: 33125793 doi: 10.1002/ncp.10588

CHAPTER 10

Dietary History, Social History, and Food Insecurity Screening

Obtaining a dietary and social history and screening for food insecurity are important parts of the nutritional assessment. A complete history includes an estimate of the quantity, quality, and timing of dietary intake and an understanding and consideration of a family's norms around food and food intake and the social determinants of health that affect dietary intake. Incorporating food insecurity screening into clinical practice provides an opportunity to identify children at high risk for nutritional problems and to connect families to community and public health resources to support optimal nutrition.

Obtaining a Dietary History

At the minimum, a dietary history should aim to capture

- All the foods, beverages, medications, and supplements that a child consumes on a typical day
- The portions consumed
- The quality of the foods and beverages consumed
- Time of consumption, including time of day and the duration
- Location of consumption, including where in the home, if eaten at home, or where outside the home, if eaten elsewhere

Table 10-1 shows common methods of obtaining a dietary history.

Most pediatric clinicians will not have the time or desire to obtain and analyze a detailed 3-day food record, although it may be feasible to collect a basic diet history, such as a 24-hour recall, in a short clinical visit. The American Academy of Pediatrics (AAP) *Bright Futures Nutrition* and *Bright Futures Nutrition Pocket Guide* include age-specific dietary history questionnaires that clinicians can use (https://brightfutures.aap.org). Additionally, patients can find many online tools and apps they can use to assess their own dietary intake, or pediatricians may consider referring a patient to a registered dietitian nutritionist for a more detailed dietary assessment and treatment plan (**Box 10-1**).

Obtaining a Social History

A child's dietary intake is influenced by social determinants of health. The social determinants of health are the conditions in the environments in which people are born, live, work, play, learn, and age that affect health, quality of life outcomes, and risks. The social determinants of health are often categorized into 5 key determinants, as shown in **Figure 10-1**.

Table 10-1. Common Methods of Obtaining a Dietary History

Name	Description	Advantages	Disadvantages
Diet interview	This is a subjective measure using open- and closed-ended questions. Trained clinician or registered dietitian nutritionist collects a detailed nutritional history of the type and amount of all food and beverages consumed in a specified period.	• Assesses typical dietary intake in detail • Comprehensive review of factors affecting dietary intake • May be steered by the interviewer to help the family or patient recall and quantify intake	• Requires trained interviewer • Subject to possible bias associated with interviewing and self-reporting • Time consuming
24-h recall	This is a subjective measure using open-ended questions. From child or caregiver, trained interviewer solicits recall of the type, amount, and timing of food and beverage intake in the previous 24 h or typical intake in any 24-h period.	• Relatively quick and easy to obtain • Provides a snapshot of typical dietary intake • Minimal respondent burden; does not require record keeping by the patient or family	• Requires trained interviewer. • Subject to possible bias associated with interviewing and self-reporting. • Prior 24-h intake may not reflect usual intake. • Relies on recollection. • Tends to underestimate intake.

Method	Description	Advantages	Disadvantages
3-d food record or food diary	This is a subjective measure using open-ended questions. Child or caregiver is asked to record actual intake consecutively for 3 d. Child or caregiver may be provided with a form to record intake or may be asked to keep a food diary or use an app or photo log to record intake. Record should include 1 d on weekend to account for differing consumption patterns.	• Does not require an interviewer • Data gathered in real time and prospectively • Includes actual (reported) amounts of food consumed • Provides a more comprehensive picture of usual intake than a 24-h recall • Reduced possibility of recall bias • Suitable for computer analysis	• Relatively significant respondent burden; requires record keeping by child/caregiver. • Subject to possible bias associated with self-reporting. • Completion of nutritional assessment may be delayed to allow patient adequate time to complete food record. • Family may change diet pattern because they know it is being monitored; thus, food record may not reflect typical diet.
Food frequency questionnaire	This is a subjective measure using a predefined format. Child or caregiver completes a questionnaire designed to gather data on frequency of eating and amount of foods eaten.	• Decreases the time required for interview • Can provide a more detailed picture of nutrient adequacy than a 24-h recall	• Difficult to assess unique details of diet • Overreporting of intake common • May not have certain cultural foods listed in templated questionnaire

Derived from reference 1 and Shim JS, Oh K, Kim HC. Dietary assessment methods in epidemiologic studies. *Epidemiol Health.* 2014;36:e2014009.

CLINICAL PRACTICE TIP

Box 10-1. Finding a Pediatric Registered Dietitian Nutritionist

Pediatric registered dietitian nutritionists (RDs or RDNs for short) are specially trained in the nutritional assessment and counseling of children, adolescents, and their families to help achieve nutrition goals. In most states, they are licensed allied health professionals. The Academy of Nutrition and Dietetics offers an online search tool to find a registered dietitian nutritionist by either zip code or city and state (www.eatright.org).

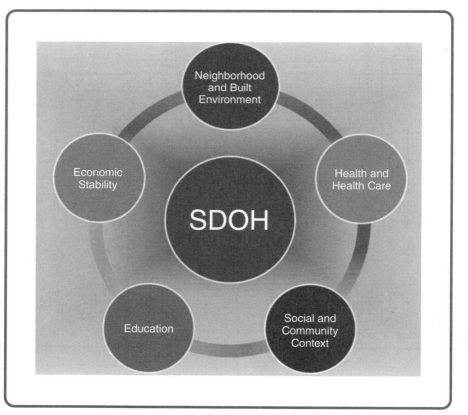

Figure 10-1. The social determinants of health (SDOH).

Reproduced from reference 2.

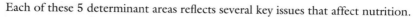

Each of these 5 determinant areas reflects several key issues that affect nutrition.

- Economic stability: employment, food insecurity, housing instability, and poverty
- Education: early childhood education and development, high school graduation, higher education enrollment, language, and literacy
- Social and community context: civic participation; discrimination; incarceration; and social cohesion
- Health and health care: health care access, primary care access, and health literacy
- Neighborhood and built environment: access to foods that support healthy eating patterns; crime and violence; environmental conditions; and housing quality[2]

The history can touch on each of these nutrition-related social determinants of health by including questions that elucidate social factors such as the availability of resources and supports at home and in neighborhoods and communities; the quality of the educational system and school food environment; the nature and quality of social experiences; relationships; exposures to media; culture and beliefs about nutrition and food; understanding of underlying health concerns and knowledge of nutrition; the safety and walkability of neighborhoods; the cleanliness of water, food, and air; and access to healthful, affordable, high-quality foods. Screening for food insecurity is particularly important when discussing pediatric nutrition and the role that clinicians can play in helping improve nutrition.

Assessing Food Security

Food security is a measure of economic stability. Food insecurity is a household-level economic and social condition of limited or uncertain access to adequate food. It includes very low food security and low food security[3] (**Figure 10-2**).

More than 1 in 7 children experience food insecurity, with up to 1 in 4 children affected during the COVID-19 pandemic.[4] Families affected by poverty, inadequate wages, housing insecurity, food deserts, and structural racism are more likely to experience food insecurity. These families may be working poor, single-parent, rural, or Black or Hispanic/Latino, American Indian, or Alaska Native, although any family can be affected.[4] Public health interventions such as the Supplemental Nutrition Assistance Program (SNAP) and the Special Supplemental Nutrition Program for Women, Infants, and Children (WIC) are focused on helping ensure that all families can access healthful foods. However, not all families with food insecurity participate in these programs. At least 16% of families with food insecurity do not receive federal supports.

Food insecurity is associated with many health harms for children and their families, including poorer overall health, more hospitalizations, higher iron deficiency rates, lower bone density, obesity, poor cognitive performance, developmental and behavioral concerns, emotional distress, worsened adolescent mental health, and increased risk of chronic diseases such as diabetes, hyperlipidemia, and cardiovascular disease as an adult.[5]

At the family level, food insecurity may manifest with food anxiety, diet monotony, and decreased nutritional quality.[4] As money for food runs low, families may purchase more inexpensive shelf-stable, highly processed, calorically dense foods rather than more

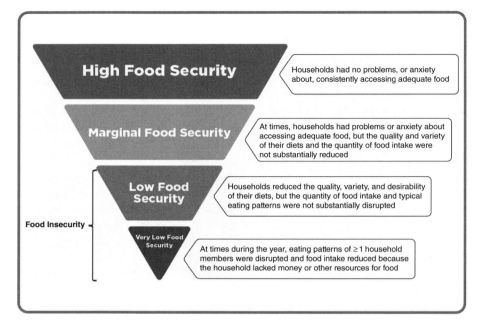

Figure 10-2. Classification of food security.

Adapted with permission from Hunger + Health/Feeding America. What is food insecurity? Accessed September 22, 2022. https://hungerandhealth.feedingamerica.org/understand-food-insecurity.

costly nutrient-dense foods. Adults may decrease their own food intake by eating less food and skipping meals to prioritize feeding their children. This contributes not only to worsened nutrition but toxic and chronic stress. Although pediatricians might emphasize consuming healthful whole foods, families with food insecurity may be struggling to obtain enough food.

In its joint toolkit with the Food Research & Action Center, the AAP recommends that clinicians follow 3 steps to address food insecurity[4]:

1. Screen and identify.
2. Connect.
3. Advocate.

Screen and Identify

Pediatricians are encouraged to screen for food insecurity at clinical visits and as part of the nutritional assessment by using the Hunger Vital Sign (**Box 10-2**). The AAP recommends deploying the Hunger Vital Sign at health supervision visits, visits for nutrition-related conditions, emergency department visits, hospital admissions, and newborn care before discharge.[4]

CLINICAL PRACTICE TIP

Box 10-2. Food Insecurity Screening: The Hunger Vital Sign

Food insecurity screening with the Hunger Vital Sign consists of 2 statements. An "often true" or a "sometimes true" response to either statement identifies food insecurity with a sensitivity of 97% and a specificity of 83%.[5] Generally, routinely administering the screening by electronic or written means, rather than verbal, helps decrease a feeling of shame, embarrassment, or stigma.

1. Within the past 12 months, we worried whether our food would run out before we got money to buy more (often true, sometimes true, never true, or don't know/refused).

2. Within the past 12 months, the food we bought just didn't last and we didn't have money to get more (often true, sometimes true, never true, or don't know/refused).

Hunger Vital Sign reproduced from Hager ER, Quigg AM, Black MM, et al. Development and validity of a 2-item screen to identify families at risk for food insecurity. *Pediatrics.* 2010;126(1):e26–e32.

Connect

Pediatricians are advised to connect families experiencing food insecurity to federal nutrition programs or other state and local community resources in a supportive and nonjudgmental way. In their toolkit for pediatricians to address food insecurity, the Food Research & Action Center and the AAP recommend doing so by discussing responses and next steps when the child is distracted, by noting that assistance is available and most people need it at some point, and by noting that help benefits all family members but especially the children.[4] In many cases, providing families with the recommendation to call 211 or search Google's Find Food Support is the easiest way to way to connect families with resources (**Box 10-3**).

Advocate

Pediatricians can advocate for patients to have increased access to healthful foods by aligning with stakeholders to support policies that address food insecurity at its root causes and support access to healthful, affordable foods in all communities.

Assessing Participation in Food Assistance Programs

As part of the nutritional assessment, clinicians should identify whether patients are eligible for participation in food assistance programs and, if so, whether they currently participate. The federal and state governments sponsor several nutrition assistance

---

CLINICAL PRACTICE TIP

Box 10-3. 211 and Google's Find Food Support

Most counties in the United States offer 211 service, which can link eligible patients to federal nutrition programs and community and public health resources, such as food pantries and food banks. Clinicians can help patients and families connect with resources by encouraging them to call 211 or visit 211.org. In some cases, 211 can directly assist families in enrolling in food assistance programs such as the Supplemental Nutrition Assistance Program and the Special Supplemental Nutrition Program for Women, Infants, and Children (refer to the following sections on these programs). The Federal Communications Commission notes that 211 is available to approximately 309 million people, which is 94.6% of the total US population.[6] Additionally, in 2021, Google launched the website Find Food Support locator tool (https://findfoodsupport.withgoogle.com), which families can use to find the nearest food bank, food pantry, or school lunch pickup site by entering their address.

---

programs that help reduce food insecurity and negative health outcomes among recipients. Except for SNAP, the programs provide food assistance aligned with the *Dietary Guidelines for Americans* (refer to Chapter 11, Dietary Guidelines and Principles of Healthy Eating). Additionally, other community resources such as food pantries and soup kitchens help provide safety net food resources. A patient handout from the Food Research & Action Center and AAP food insecurity toolkit that highlights typically available resources is shown in **Box 10-4**.

Special Supplemental Nutrition Program for Women, Infants, and Children

The Special Supplemental Nutrition Program for Women, Infants, and Children (WIC) is a federally funded, state-administered program that provides food vouchers and health education for pregnant and postpartum women, infants, and children up to their fifth birthday on the basis of eligibility and low income. WIC-authorized foods include infant cereal, baby foods, iron-fortified cereal, fruits and vegetables, vitamin C–rich fruit or vegetable juice, eggs, milk, cheese, yogurt, soy-based beverages, tofu, peanut butter, dried and canned beans/peas, canned fish, and whole wheat bread and other whole grain options. Participants also receive health screening, nutritional and breastfeeding counseling, immunization screening and referral, and substance use resources. In 2009, the WIC food package benefits were changed so program participants were able to purchase more fruits and vegetables, less juice, more whole grains instead of refined grains, and low-fat or skim milk. These changes have been associated with decreased childhood

CLINICAL PRACTICE TIP

Box 10-4. Food Assistance Programs

The following resource was produced as part of the Food Research & Action Center and American Academy of Pediatrics toolkit for pediatricians to address food insecurity[4] and can be downloaded (https://frac.org/research/resource-library/federal-nutrition-programs-emergency-food-referral-chart) and edited to provide as a handout to patients:

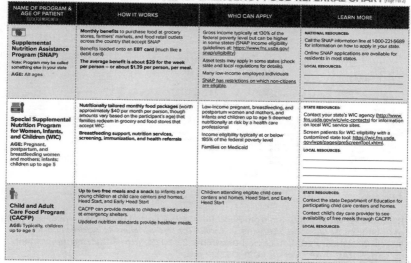

FEDERAL NUTRITION PROGRAMS AND EMERGENCY FOOD REFERRAL CHART (Page 1 of 2)

NAME OF PROGRAM & AGE OF PATIENT (CLICK FOR MORE INFO)	HOW IT WORKS	WHO CAN APPLY	LEARN MORE
Supplemental Nutrition Assistance Program (SNAP) Note: Program may be called something else in your state AGE: All ages	**Monthly benefits** to purchase food at grocery stores, farmers' markets, and food retail outlets across the country that accept SNAP. Benefits loaded onto an **EBT card** (much like a debit card). **The average benefit is about $29 for the week per person – or about $1.39 per person, per meal.**	Gross income typically at 130% of the federal poverty level but can be higher in some states (SNAP income eligibility guidelines at: https://www.fns.usda.gov/snap/eligibility) Asset tests may apply in some states (check state and local regulations for details). Many low-income employed individuals SNAP has restrictions on which non-citizens are eligible.	**NATIONAL RESOURCES:** Call the SNAP information line at 1-800-221-5689 for information on how to apply in your state. Online SNAP applications are available for residents in most states. **LOCAL RESOURCES:** _____ _____ _____
Special Supplemental Nutrition Program for Women, Infants, and Children (WIC) AGE: Pregnant, postpartum, and breastfeeding women and mothers; infants; children up to age 5	**Nutritionally tailored monthly food packages** (worth approximately $40 per month per person, though amounts vary based on the participant's age) that families redeem in grocery and food stores that accept WIC. **Breastfeeding support, nutrition services, screening, immunization, and health referrals**	Low-income pregnant, breastfeeding, and postpartum women and mothers, and infants and children up to age 5 deemed nutritionally at risk by a health care professional Income eligibility typically at or below 185% of the federal poverty level Families on Medicaid	**STATE RESOURCES:** Contact your state's WIC agency (http://www.fns.usda.gov/wic/wic-contacts) for information on local WIC service sites. Screen patients for WIC eligibility with a customized state tool: https://wic.fns.usda.gov/wps/pages/preScreenTool.xhtml. **LOCAL RESOURCES:** _____ _____ _____
Child and Adult Care Food Program (CACFP) AGE: Typically, children up to age 5	**Up to two free meals and a snack** to infants and young children at child care centers and homes, Head Start, and Early Head Start CACFP can provide meals to children 18 and under at emergency shelters. Updated nutrition standards provide healthier meals.	Children attending eligible child care centers and homes, Head Start, and Early Head Start	**STATE RESOURCES:** Contact the state Department of Education for participating child care centers and homes. Contact child's day care provider to see availability of free meals through CACFP. **LOCAL RESOURCES:** _____ _____ _____

FRAC
Food Research & Action Center Copyright © 2022 Food Research & Action Center

USDA NATIONAL HUNGER HOTLINE
1-866-3-HUNGRY/866-348-6479 or **1-877-8-HAMBRE**/877-842-6273
Monday through Friday

American Academy of Pediatrics
DEDICATED TO THE HEALTH OF ALL CHILDREN®

Continued

CLINICAL PRACTICE TIP

Box 10-4 (continued)

FEDERAL NUTRITION PROGRAMS AND EMERGENCY FOOD REFERRAL CHART (Page 2 of 2)

NAME OF PROGRAM & AGE OF PATIENT (CLICK FOR MORE INFO)	HOW IT WORKS	WHO CAN APPLY	LEARN MORE
National School Lunch Program AND **School Breakfast Program** AGE: Children at participating schools	Free, reduced-priced, or paid school meals in participating schools. Meals meet federal nutrition standards, which require schools to serve more whole grains, fruits, and vegetables.	Children of families at low or moderate income levels can qualify for free or reduced-price meals. Free to all students at schools adopting community eligibility, which allows schools with high numbers of low-income children to offer free breakfast and lunch to all students without collecting school meal applications	Contact child's school to see availability of free breakfast and lunch and application process, if any. Contact the state Department of Education for a list of participating schools. LOCAL RESOURCES:
Fresh Fruit and Vegetable Program AGE: Elementary school-age students	The Fresh Fruit and Vegetable Program **provides federal funding** to elementary schools to serve fruits and vegetables as snacks to help young students improve their diets and establish healthy eating habits. Limited federal funding is available in all states.	Elementary schools with high numbers of low-income students	LOCAL RESOURCES:
Afterschool Nutrition Programs (Available through CACFP or the National School Lunch Program) AGE: Children 18 and under	Free, healthy snacks and/or meals meeting federal nutrition standards in enrichment programs running afterschool, on weekends, or during school holidays	Children can access free meals at participating enrichment programs offered at community sites, including schools, park and recreation centers, libraries, faith-based organizations, or community centers.	Contact child's school to check participation in afterschool meals or knowledge of local participating organizations. Contact the state Department of Education for participating sites. LOCAL RESOURCES:
Summer Nutrition Programs AGE: Children 18 and under	Up to two free meals at approved school and community sites during summer vacation. Meals must meet approved federal nutrition standards.	Children can access meals at participating community sites, which can include schools, park and recreation centers, libraries, faith-based organizations, or community centers. There is no need to show identification.	LOCAL RESOURCES:
The Emergency Food Assistance Program (TEFAP) AND **The Emergency Food Network** AGE: All ages	Through TEFAP, participating food banks distribute U.S. commodities to local partners, including pantries, food shelves, soup kitchens, social service agencies, and faith-based groups. Additionally, many emergency food sites purchase food or receive food donations. Many food banks are committing to distributing more fresh produce in addition to shelf-stable foods.	Access depends on site requirements; some sites require referrals.	LOCAL RESOURCES:

FRAC Food Research & Action Center Copyright © 2022 Food Research & Action Center

USDA NATIONAL HUNGER HOTLINE
1-866-3-HUNGRY/866-348-6479 or 1-877-8-HAMBRE/877-842-6273
Monday through Friday

American Academy of Pediatrics
DEDICATED TO THE HEALTH OF ALL CHILDREN®

Reproduced with permission from Food Research & Action Center, American Academy of Pediatrics. *Screen and Intervene: A Toolkit for Pediatricians to Address Food Insecurity*. January 2021. Accessed December 21, 2022. https://frac.org/wp-content/uploads/FRAC_AAP_Toolkit_2021_032122.pdf.

obesity[7] and improved neurocognitive outcomes.[8] Refer to Part 5, Frequently Asked Questions, Case Studies, and Recipes, for recipes and sample meal plans based on the WIC food package.

Supplemental Nutrition Assistance Program

The Supplemental Nutrition Assistance Program (SNAP) is a federally funded, state-administered entitlement program that provides nutrition assistance and nutrition education to 45 million families with very low income, including 23 million children. It is the only government feeding program that does not have nutrition standards to address diet quality. The maximum SNAP allotment for a family of 4 in 2023 is $939/mo (US dollar). This is approximately $31/d or $8 per person per day. The funding is based on the US Department of Agriculture Thrifty Food Plan. Family benefit amounts are calculated by subtracting 30% of a household's net monthly income from the maximum allotment, because SNAP households are expected to spend approximately 30% of their own resources on food. This is a very limited food budget for even the most cost-conscious SNAP recipients, who are expected to implement the following strategies to stretch this food budget to meet caloric and nutritional needs:

- Eat at home for nearly all meals and snacks.
- Plan ahead when grocery shopping, by being aware of foods on hand in the refrigerator and pantry, having a shopping list, and accounting for bulk, coupon, and in-store savings. Choose low-cost nutrient-dense foods such as canned tuna and salmon, eggs, and dry beans and grains.
- Choose fruits and vegetables that are most likely to be eaten or have a long shelf life to minimize food waste, selecting canned and frozen produce most of the time, because they are usually less expensive than fresh produce.

Box 10-5 shows 1 days' worth of breakfast, lunch, dinner, and snacks that can feed a family of 4 for approximately $31, the Thrifty Food Plan and SNAP allotment. Refer to Part 5, Frequently Asked Questions, Case Studies, and Recipes, for recipes to accompany this meal plan. The recipes help save money and optimize nutritional value by substituting vegetables and meats on the basis of what is in season or on sale. Pantry items such as salt, pepper, and olive oil are listed at the end of the ingredient lists and are not factored into the price.

National School Breakfast, National School Lunch, and Summer Food Service Programs

The National School Breakfast, National School Lunch, and Summer Food Service Programs are federally funded entitlement programs that provide low-cost or free nutritionally balanced breakfasts and lunches in public and private schools, in residential care institutions, and, during the summer, in designated community locations. Children in households with income below 130% of the federal poverty level or those receiving SNAP qualify for free meals. Although meals must meet federal meal requirements, including meeting one-third of the recommended dietary allowance of necessary nutrients (**Table 10-2**) and following the MyPlate guidance (refer to Chapter 12, Healthy Eating Plans), decisions about what foods to provide and how they are prepared are made locally.

Box 10-5. Recipes: Feeding a Family of 4 on $31/d

- Breakfast: Spinach, Egg, and Cheese Breakfast Pita Pockets (about $4.00)
- Lunch: Grilled Chicken Whole Wheat Pita Wraps With Creamy Ranch Bean Dip (about $13.00)
- Dinner: Turkey and Vegetable Whole Wheat Chow Mein–style Noodles (about $12.00)
- Snack: Carrots and Cucumbers With Creamy Ranch Bean Dip (about $2.00)

Table 10-2. Nutrition Standards in the National School Lunch and School Breakfast Programs

	Breakfast meal pattern			Lunch meal pattern		
	Grades K-5	Grades 6-8	Grades 9-12	Grades K-5	Grades 6-8	Grades 9-12
	Amount of food per week (minimum per day)					
Fruit (cups)	5 (1)	5 (1)	5 (1)	2½ (½)	2½ (½)	5 (1)
Vegetables (cups)	0	0	0	3¾ (¾)	3¾ (¾)	5 (1)
Dark green	0	0	0	½	½	½
Red/orange	0	0	0	¾	¾	1¼
Beans/peas (legumes)	0	0	0	½	½	½
Starchy	0	0	0	½	½	½
Other	0	0	0	½	½	¾
Additional vegetables to reach total	0	0	0	1	1	1½
Grains (oz eq)	7-10 (1)	8-10 (1)	9-10 (1)	8-9 (1)	8-10 (1)	10-12 (2)
Meats/meats alternatives (oz eq)	0	0	0	8-10 (1)	9-10 (1)	10-12 (2)
Fluid milk (cups)	5 (1)	5 (1)	5 (1)	5 (1)	5 (1)	5 (1)
	Other specifications: daily amount based on the average for a 5-day week					
Min-max calories (kcal)	350-500	400-500	450-600	550-650	600-700	750-850
Saturated fat (% of total calories)	<10	<10	<10	<10	<10	<10
Sodium (mg)	≤430	≤470	≤500	≤640	≤710	≤740
Trans fat	Nutrition label of manufacturer specifications must indicate 0 g of *trans* fat per serving.					

Abbreviations: K, kindergarten; max, maximum; min, minimum.

Reproduced from US Department of Agriculture. 7 CFR Parts 210 and 220. Nutrition standards in the National School Lunch and School Breakfast Programs; final rule. *Fed Regist*. 2012;77(17):4088. https://www.govinfo.gov/content/pkg/FR-2012-01-26/pdf/2012-1010.pdf. Accessed September 22, 2022.

Child and Adult Care Food Program

The Child and Adult Care Food Program is a federally funded program that reimburses nutritious meals and snacks to eligible children being cared for in child care centers and child care homes, children participating in after-school programs, children residing in emergency shelters, and adults 60 years and older or living with a disability and enrolled in day care facilities. To receive reimbursement, facilities must meet minimal requirements established by the US Department of Agriculture. For children, this minimum includes at least 1 serving each of milk, fruit or vegetable, and grain or bread at breakfast; 1 serving each of milk, grain, or meat or meat alternative and 2 servings of fruits or vegetables or a combination of fruits and vegetables at lunch and dinner; and at least 1 serving from each of 2 of the 4 meal components (milk, fruit or vegetable, grain or bread, or meat/meat alternative).

Food Pantries and Soup Kitchens

Most communities have food pantries and soup kitchens to help provide food resources beyond federal and state programs. Many food pantries are taking steps to improve the nutritional quality of food items, offer increased nutrition education, display healthier items at the pantry, and seek out healthier food donations. Healthy Eating Research, a national program of the Robert Wood Johnson Foundation, convened an expert panel who published nutrition guidelines to help guide the charitable food system (**Table 10-3**).

Understanding Family and Cultural Nutritional Beliefs and Practices

An important part of the nutritional assessment includes asking open questions and showing genuine interest in learning more about a patient's or family's nutritional and cultural beliefs and practices. This helps clinicians tailor guidance in a way that respects and preserves cultural practices and family structure and routines while helping achieve nutrition or health goals.

The dietary and social aspects of the nutritional assessment can help clinicians understand the family-level factors that influence a patient's or family's daily food choices. These include a child's taste preferences and the caregivers' response to those preferences; parental expectations of mealtime and snack time behavior; nutrition knowledge; caregiver ability to obtain and prepare healthful foods; parent feeding practices; the mealtime environment, including the presence or absence of family meals; a child's screen time, sleep, and physical activity habits, including participation in athletics; and cultural beliefs and traditions. Culture includes traits such as race and ethnicity, country or region of ancestry and current or prior residence, age, gender, spiritual beliefs and practices, language, sexual orientation, level of education, and physical ability. Chapters 12, Healthy Eating Plans, and 13, Culinary Medicine and Strategies for Healthy Eating, include more in-depth discussions of family and cultural considerations in providing nutritional guidance and coaching.

Table 10-3. Robert Wood Johnson Foundation Healthy Eating Research Nutrition Guidelines for Ranking Charitable Food

Food category	Example products	Choose often			Choose sometimes			Choose rarely		
		Saturated fat	Sodium	Added sugar	Saturated fat	Sodium	Added sugar	Saturated fat	Sodium	Added sugar
Fruits and vegetables	Fresh, canned, frozen, and dried fruits and vegetables, frozen broccoli with cheese sauce, apple sauce, tomato sauce, 100% juice, 100% fruit popsicle	≤2 g	≤230 mg	0 g	All 100% juice and plain dried fruit / ≥2.5 g	231–479 mg	1–11 g	≥2.5 g	≥480 mg	≥12 g
Grains	Bread, rice, pasta, grains with seasoning mixes	First ingredient must be whole grain AND meet following thresholds: ≤2 g	≤230 mg	≤6 g	≥2.5 g	231–479 mg	7–11 g	≥2.5 g	≥480 mg	≥12 g
Protein	Animal (beef, pork, poultry, sausage, deli meats, hot dogs, eggs) and plant proteins (nuts, seeds, veggie burgers, soy, beans, peanut butter)	≤2 g	≤230 mg	≤6 g	2.5–4.5 g	231–479 mg	7–11 g	≥5 g	≥480 mg	≥12 g
Dairy	Milk, cheese, yogurt	≤3 g	≤230 mg	0 g	3.5–6 g	231–479 mg	1–11 g	≥6.5 g	≥480 mg	≥12 g
Non-dairy alternatives	All plant-based milks, yogurts and cheeses	≤2 g	≤230 mg	≤6 g	≥2.5 g	231–479 mg	7–11 g	≥2.5 g	≥480 mg	≥12 g

Category	Food examples									
Beverages	Water, soda, coffee, tea, sports drinks, non-100% juice products	0 g	0 mg	0 g	0 g	1-140 mg	1-11 g	≥1 g	≥141 mg	≥12 g
Mixed dishes	Frozen meals, soups, stews, macaroni and cheese	≤3 g	≤480 mg	≤6 g	3.5-6 g	481-599 mg	7-11 g	≥6.5 g	≥600 mg	≥12 g
Processed and packaged snacks	Chips (including potato, corn, and other vegetable chips), crackers, granola and other bars, popcorn	None	If a grain is the first ingredient, it must be a whole grain AND meet following thresholds:		0-2 g	0-140 mg	0-6 g	≥2.5 g	≥141 mg	≥7 g
Desserts	Ice cream, frozen yogurt, chocolate, cookies, cakes, pastries, snack cakes, baked goods, cake mixes	None			None			All desserts		
Condiments and cooking staples	Spices, oil, butter, plant-based spreads, flour, salad dressing, jarred sauces (except tomato sauce), seasoning, salt, sugar	Not ranked								
Miscellaneous products	Nutritional supplements, baby food	Not ranked								

Reproduced with permission from reference 9.

In Sum

- The dietary and social histories provide critical information to help assess baseline nutrition habits, including intake, routines, and cultural practices and beliefs.
- There are several methods that clinicians can use to collect dietary intake information, such as the diet interview, 24-hour recall, and 3-day food record. Although each method includes limitations, all can provide a useful approximation of typical nutrition practices and intake.
- Food security is an important factor in the nutritional assessment and an important predictor of overall child health. Clinicians should screen patients for food insecurity and help connect patients who experience food insecurity with resources such as WIC, SNAP, and local food pantries, as appropriate.

References

1. Leonberg B. *Pocket Guide to Pediatric Nutrition Assessment*. 3rd ed. Academy of Nutrition and Dietetics; 2020

2. Office of Disease Prevention and Health Promotion. Social determinants of health. Accessed May 24, 2021. https://www.healthypeople.gov/2020/topics-objectives/topic/social-determinants-of-health

3. Economic Research Service. Definitions of food security. US Department of Agriculture. Updated September 7, 2022. Accessed September 22, 2022. https://www.ers.usda.gov/topics/food-nutrition-assistance/food-security-in-the-us/definitions-of-food-security.aspx

4. Ashbrook A, Essel K, Montez K, Bennet-Tejes D. *Screen and Intervene: A Toolkit for Pediatricians to Address Food Insecurity*. American Academy of Pediatrics, Food Research & Action Center; 2021

5. Gitterman BA, Chilton LA, Cotton WH, et al; American Academy of Pediatrics Council on Community Pediatrics and Committee on Nutrition. Promoting food security for all children. *Pediatrics*. 2015;136(5):e1431–e1438 PMID: 26498462 doi: 10.1542/peds.2015-3301

6. Federal Communications Commission. Dial 211 for essential community services. Reviewed December 31, 2019. Accessed September 22, 2022. https://www.fcc.gov/sites/default/files/dial_211_for_essential_community_services.pdf

7. Daepp MIG, Gortmaker SL, Wang YC, Long MW, Kenney EL. WIC food package changes: trends in childhood obesity prevalence. *Pediatrics*. 2019;143(5):e20182841 PMID: 30936251 doi: 10.1542/peds.2018-2841

8. Guan A, Hamad R, Batra A, Bush NR, Tylavsky FA, LeWinn KZ. The revised WIC food package and child development: a quasi-experimental study. *Pediatrics*. 2021; 147(2):e20201853 PMID: 33495370 doi: 10.1542/peds.2020-1853

9. Schwartz M, Levi R, Lott M, et al. *Healthy Eating Research Nutrition Guidelines for the Charitable Food System*. Healthy Eating Research; 2020

Nutritional Counseling

Patients and their caregivers rely on pediatricians to provide credible, up-to-date nutrition guidance. Part 3, Nutritional Counseling, focuses on providing clinicians with the knowledge and tools to help patients and families adopt healthy eating patterns. This includes training in health behavior change theories and communication strategies that can be applied to help patients successfully plan and make dietary and health changes.

Chapter 11, Dietary Guidelines and Principles of Healthy Eating, provides a detailed overview of the *Dietary Guidelines for Americans* and evidence-informed principles of healthy eating, and Chapter 12, Healthy Eating Plans, highlights several well-studied healthy eating plans, such as the Dietary Approaches to Stop Hypertension (DASH) eating plan, the healthy vegetarian eating plan, and the healthy Mediterranean-style eating plan. Chapter 13, Culinary Medicine and Strategies for Healthy Eating, helps translate information about healthy eating and healthy eating plans into action with culinary medicine and implemented key strategies for healthy eating. Chapter 14, Theories of Behavior Change and Motivational Interviewing, introduces clinicians to the stages of change model of behavior change and motivational interviewing communication approach as tools to help support patients and their families in making nutritional changes. Chapter 15, SMART Goals and Action Plans, details how to help patients set SMART (Specific, Measurable, Attainable, Relevant, and Time bound) goals and develop action plans to turn intentions to change nutrition practices into action.

CHAPTER 11

Dietary Guidelines and Principles of Healthy Eating

Patients and their families receive nutrition information from myriad sources, including family, friends, neighbors, online searches and social media, news reports, school and work sites, and health care and allied health professionals. Pediatricians are a trusted resource for families and uniquely positioned to provide patients and their families up-to-date, evidence-informed, and actionable nutrition information and counseling. The *Dietary Guidelines for Americans,* Healthy People 2030 nutrition indicators, and guidance from American Academy of Pediatrics policy statements and clinical practice guidelines serve as important sources of this information. Additionally, an emphasis on responsive feeding serves as the foundation for instilling healthy eating habits and a positive relationship with food throughout infancy, childhood, and adolescence.

Dietary Guidelines for Americans

Published by the US Department of Agriculture and the US Department of Health and Human Services every 5 years since 1980, the *Dietary Guidelines for Americans* aim to incorporate the best scientific evidence about what to eat to meet nutrient needs, optimize health, and prevent disease. For the first time, the 2020 to 2025 dietary guidelines include guidance for infants and toddlers in addition to people 2 years and older.

The dietary guidelines are based on a scientific report from the Dietary Guidelines Advisory Committee, which provides a comprehensive overview of the studies reviewed to inform the dietary guidelines and rationale for the recommendations. The full scientific advisory report is available online (www.dietaryguidelines.gov/2020-advisory-committee-report). Although the scientific report informs the dietary guidelines, the content of the published guidelines is subject to the discretion of the US Department of Agriculture and US Department of Health and Human Services, following a comment and feedback period from stakeholders, which includes feedback from industry and corporate stakeholders. After this review process, the guidelines sometimes differ slightly from the advisory committee recommendations. For example, on the basis of the scientific evidence of health harms caused by added sugars consumption, the 2020 advisory committee recommended that people consume no more than 6% of calories from added sugars. The published guidelines recommend no more than 10% of calories from added sugars.

The dietary guidelines are used widely through government-supported nutrition programs and initiatives, including the National School Lunch Program; the Special Supplemental Nutrition Program for Women, Infants, and Children; and state and local health promotion and disease prevention initiatives. The dietary guidelines are available for review and download (https://dietaryguidelines.gov).

Key Recommendations

The dietary guidelines provide science-based recommendations to help families adopt healthy eating patterns that are culturally adaptable and affordable. Clinicians can help families adopt the key recommendations from the 2020 to 2025 dietary guidelines[1] by advising them as follows:

- Follow a healthy eating pattern across the life span. This includes initiating a healthful dietary pattern early in life for infants and young children and following healthful dietary patterns for nutritional needs at each life stage. Clinicians should provide anticipatory guidance at all health supervision visits supporting increased exposure to fruits, vegetables, and other nutrient-dense foods and limiting access to highly processed and sugary foods. They should encourage exclusively feeding human (breast) milk for about the first 6 months after birth, providing iron-fortified infant formula during the first year after birth when breast milk is unavailable, and introducing nutrient-dense complementary foods at about 6 months of age (refer to Part 4, Nutrition Prescription, for developmentally tailored recommendations for providing anticipatory guidance).
- Focus on variety, nutrient density, and amount. Select a wide variety of nutrient-dense foods, and eat them in appropriate portions to meet nutritional needs. Clinicians should support breastfeeding and breast milk consumption in infancy, with gradual introduction of nutrient-rich complementary foods starting around 6 months of age.
- Limit calories from added sugars and saturated fats and reduce sodium intake. Clinicians should encourage families to replace foods and beverages high in added sugars, saturated fats, and sodium with healthier options. In the first 2 years, if not longer, avoid sugary drinks and foods.
- Shift to healthier food and beverage choices that have a higher nutrient density and lower caloric content. Clinicians should help families explore how to incorporate more fruits, vegetables, and whole grains into a family meal plan and fewer processed, sweetened, and salted foods.
- Clinicians should recognize cultural, ethnic, and socioeconomic factors that influence food preferences and access to healthful foods and beverages, as well as the importance of tools and resources for families to plan and monitor their diets. Access to healthful foods and healthy eating patterns should be promoted for all ages where people live, learn, work, play, and gather.

The healthy eating plans recommended in the dietary guidelines are detailed in Chapter 12, Healthy Eating Plans.

Healthy Eating Index

The Healthy Eating Index is a commonly used measure of diet quality that aims to assess adherence to the dietary guidelines. It scores food intake patterns from a range of 0 (lowest dietary quality) to 100 (highest dietary quality). It is made up of 13 components, as shown in **Table 11-1**. The average score is 59 out of 100, with adolescents

Table 11-1. HEI-2015 Components and Scoring Standards

Component	Maximum points	Standard for maximum score[a]	Standard for a minimum score of 0[a]
Adequacy			
Total fruits[b]	5	≥0.8 cup equivalent per 1,000 kcal	No fruit
Whole fruits[c]	5	≥0.4 cup equivalent per 1,000 kcal	No whole fruit
Total vegetables[d]	5	≥1.1 cup equivalent per 1,000 kcal	No vegetables
Greens and beans[d]	5	≥0.2 cup equivalent per 1,000 kcal	No dark-green vegetables or legumes
Whole grains	10	≥1.5 cup equivalent per 1,000 kcal	No whole grains
Dairy[e]	10	≥1.3 cup equivalent per 1,000 kcal	No dairy
Total protein foods[d]	5	≥2.5 cup equivalent per 1,000 kcal	No protein foods
Seafood and plant proteins[d,f]	5	≥0.8 cup equivalent per 1,000 kcal	No seafood or plant proteins
Fatty acids[g]	10	(PUFAs + MUFAs)/ SFAs ≥2.5	(PUFAs + MUFAs)/ SFAs ≤1.2
Moderation			
Refined grains	10	≤1.8 oz equivalent per 1,000 kcal	≥4.3 oz equivalent per 1,000 kcal
Sodium	10	≤1.1 g per 1,000 kcal	≥2.0 g per 1,000 kcal
Added sugars	10	≤6.5% of energy	≥26% of energy
Saturated fats	10	≤8% of energy	≥16% of energy

Abbreviations: HEI, Healthy Eating Index; MUFA, monounsaturated fatty acid; PUFA, polyunsaturated fatty acid; SFA, saturated fatty acid.

[a] Intakes between the minimum and maximum standards are scored proportionately.

[b] Includes 100% fruit juice.

[c] Includes all forms except juice.

[d] Includes legumes (beans and peas).

[e] Includes all milk products, such as fluid milk, yogurt, and cheese, and fortified soy beverages.

[f] Includes seafood, nuts, seeds, soy products (other than beverages), and legumes (beans and peas).

[g] Ratio of PUFAs and MUFAs to SFAs.

Reproduced from Center for Nutrition Policy and Promotion. How the HEI is scored. Food and Nutrition Service. 2022. Accessed October 5, 2022. https://www.fns.usda.gov/how-hei-scored.

scoring the lowest at 51 (**Figure 11-1**). Higher scores are associated with decreased risk of diet-related chronic diseases such as heart disease, type 2 diabetes, and cancer. As shown in **Figure 11-2**, the typical dietary intake in the United States is not, and has not ever been, aligned with the dietary guidelines.

Nutrients of Public Health Concern

The low adherence to the dietary guidelines by the US population as a whole, including among children and adolescents, is for many people a risk factor for inadequate consumption of key nutrients. The dietary guidelines refer to these nutrients as "nutrients of public health concern." They include nutrients such as vitamin D, calcium, fiber, potassium, and, in some age-groups, iron. Underconsumption of key nutrients occurs because of lower-than-recommend intake of fruits and vegetables, dairy products, and whole grains. Additionally, people of all ages tend to overconsume saturated fats (solid fats), added sugars, and sodium (often referred to as "SoFAS"). This excess intake results from high intakes of foods such as red meat, high-fat dairy products, foods that include large amounts of butter and oil, and highly processed foods. For example, excess sugar intake results from high intakes of sugary foods such as sugary drinks, sweet snacks, and breakfast cereals and bars. Excess sodium intake results from high intakes of highly processed frozen and canned foods and salty foods such as chips, crackers, lunch meats, and pizza. **Table 11-2** lists underconsumed and overconsumed nutrients by age-group.

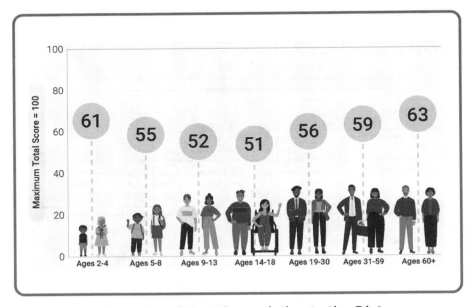

Figure 11-1. Adherence of the US population to the *Dietary Guidelines for Americans* across life stages.

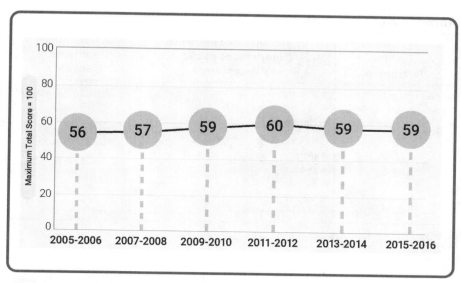

Figure 11-2. Adherence of the US population to the *Dietary Guidelines for Americans* over time.

Reproduced from reference 1.

Table 11-2. Underconsumed and Overconsumed Nutrients of Public Health Concern

Age-group	Underconsumed nutrients ("nutrients of public health concern")	Overconsumed nutrients ("SoFAS")
All ages	• Vitamin D • Calcium • Dietary fiber • Potassium	• Saturated fat • Added sugars • Sodium
Newborns and infants (0–12 mo)	Ages ≥6 mo, inadequate consumption from complementary foods: • Iron (in breastfed infants) • Zinc (in breastfed infants) • Protein (in breastfed infants) • Choline (in all older infants)	
Toddlers (12–24 mo)	Same as for all ages	
Children (2–8 y)	Same as for all ages	

Continued

Table 11-2 (*continued*)

Age-group	Underconsumed nutrients ("nutrients of public health concern")	Overconsumed nutrients ("SoFAS")
Children and adolescents (9-14 y)	• Phosphorus • Magnesium • Choline Only in adolescent girls: • Iron • Protein • Folate • Vitamin B_6 • Vitamin B_{12}	

Derived from reference 1.

Responsive Feeding

In addition to providing education and counseling to support families in what to eat, clinicians play an important role in providing families guidance on how to eat. One of the most impactful ways to do this is by encouraging responsive feeding.

The dietary guidelines define *responsive feeding* as "a feeding style that emphasizes recognizing and responding to the hunger or fullness cues of an infant or young child."[1] It is one of the most important feeding skills that a parent can develop and warrants discussion starting from the first newborn visit. A randomized clinical trial showed that anticipatory guidance in responsive feeding can help prevent parents from using food to soothe and provide more structure to feeding routines.[2] Overall, responsive feeding throughout infancy and childhood helps promote healthful nutrition, healthy growth and body mass index, and healthful family relationships around feeding and mealtimes. Following are several ways for pediatricians to promote responsive feeding. Further guidance tailored to an infant's, child's, or adolescent's age and stage of development is provided in chapters 16, Nutrition in Infancy, and 17, Nutrition in Childhood and Adolescence.

- Help parents recognize and respond to their infant's or child's cues of hunger and fullness. For example, signs of hunger in an infant include increased alertness, rooting and lip smacking, and opening of the mouth. Crying and irritability are later signs.
  - Signs of satiety in an infant include falling asleep and pulling or turning away from the breast, bottle, or spoon.
  - Toddlers are better able to tell parents when they are hungry but may also show signs of hunger by becoming more grumpy or irritable.
- Provide anticipatory guidance around expected developmental feeding stages. Support infants, children, and adolescents to use their body's cues for hunger and

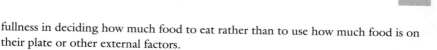

fullness in deciding how much food to eat rather than to use how much food is on their plate or other external factors.

- Encourage parents to develop a feeding routine, especially once complementary foods are introduced.
- Advise parents to resist the urge to offer food "rewards" and comforts or food punishments for young children. Food rewards are usually sugary foods that act on the pleasure centers of the brain. Repeated exposures to these foods paired with a positive memory or experience establish a strong connection in the brain. As a result, later in life when children feel sadness or anxiety, they may seek out these same types of high-sugar foods to recreate the more positive feelings or emotions from childhood, resulting in emotional eating, a habit that can continue into adulthood. Using food as comfort teaches a child to use food to soothe, which can contribute to emotional eating.
- Encourage children to meet fluid needs with water and milk (or breast milk or formula for infants) and avoid other drinks, most of the time. A strong risk factor for the development of childhood weight concerns is the routine consumption of sugary drinks. Additionally, sugary drinks do not contribute to feelings of satiety, increasing risk of overfeeding.
- Remind parents and other caregivers of the power of parental modeling, and encourage them to model a positive relationship with food, such as letting their children observe them eating in a balanced way, listening to their body for feelings of hunger and fullness, incorporating a variety of foods into their diet, and avoiding negative self-talk or dieting.
- Encourage parents and other caregivers to prioritize family meals, whenever possible. Greater frequency of family meals is associated with increased nutrient-dense food intake, a more balanced diet, more food enjoyment, and less fussy and emotional eating in infants and toddlers.[3] Parents might aim for 15- to 20-minute mealtimes with younger children to prevent grazing and frustrations and difficulty staying seated.
- Encourage parents to create a positive experience around food and mealtimes. Focus less on the food and more on the social interactions with children and other family members.

Clinicians can learn more about responsive feeding and access patient education materials through the Building a Foundation for Healthy Active Living portal at the American Academy of Pediatrics Institute for Healthy Childhood Weight website (https://ihcw.aap.org).

Healthy People 2030

The federal government sets data-driven objectives to improve health and well-being in the next decade. Healthy People 2030 consists of 355 objectives; 24 are nutrition objectives. The nutrition objectives that are relevant to infants, children, and adolescents are included in **Table 11-3**. The nutrition objectives to reduce consumption of added sugars and reduce household food insecurity are *leading health indicators,* a classification that gives them the highest priority for action. As such, pediatric clinicians

Table 11-3. Healthy People 2030 Nutrition Objectives

Objective	Summary	Baseline and goal amounts
Reduce consumption of added sugars by people aged ≥2 y[a]	Added sugars in foods and drinks can make it hard for people to get the nutrients they need without getting too many calories. People who eat too much added sugar may be at higher risk for tooth decay and obesity, but many people in the United States consume too much added sugar. Pricing strategies, such as a sugary drink tax, and education interventions in schools may help people limit foods and drinks with added sugars. Encouraging people to use the Nutrition Facts label can also help them track their consumption of added sugars.	Baseline: 13.5% mean calories from added sugars in 2013-2016 Goal: 11.5%
Reduce household food insecurity and, therefore, hunger[a]	Food insecurity is linked to negative health outcomes in children and adults. Giving more people benefits through nutrition assistance programs, increasing benefit amounts, and addressing unemployment may help reduce food insecurity and hunger.	Baseline: 11% in 2018 Goal: 6%
Eliminate very low food security among children	Children in the United States with very low food security often do not have enough to eat. This lack of food is linked to negative health outcomes. Giving more people benefits through nutrition assistance programs, increasing benefit amounts, and reducing unemployment may help reduce very low food security among children.	Baseline: 0.59% in 2018 Goal: 0%
Increase consumption of fruit by people aged ≥2 y	Fruit is recommended as a key part of a healthy diet, and eating fruit is linked to a lower risk for many diseases, but most people in the United States do not eat enough fruit. Evidence suggests that nutritional counseling, school- and workplace-based programs that use >1 strategy, and school nutrition policies can help people eat more fruit.	Baseline: 0.51 c eq per 1,000 kcal in 2013-2016 Goal: 0.56 c eq per 1,000 kcal

Increase consumption of vegetables by people aged ≥2 y	Vegetables are recommended as a key part of a healthy diet, and eating vegetables is linked to a lower risk for many diseases, but most people in the United States do not eat enough vegetables. Evidence suggests that nutritional counseling, school- and workplace-based programs that use >1 strategy, and school nutrition policies can help people eat more vegetables.	Baseline: 0.76 c eq per 1,000 kcal in 2013–2016 Goal: 0.84 c eq per 1,000 kcal
Increase consumption of dark green vegetables, red and orange vegetables, and beans and peas by people aged ≥2 y	Vegetables are recommended as a key part of a healthy diet, and eating vegetables is linked to a lower risk for many diseases. To obtain the most health benefits from vegetables, people should eat a variety of dark green and red and orange vegetables, as well as beans and peas, but most people in the United States do not eat enough vegetables. Evidence suggests that nutritional counseling, school- and workplace-based programs that use >1 strategy, and school nutrition policies can help people eat more vegetables.	Baseline: 0.31 c eq per 1,000 kcal in 2013–2016 Goal: 0.33 c eq per 1,000 kcal
Increase consumption of whole grains by people aged ≥2 y	Whole grains are rich in dietary fiber and other nutrients and are recommended as a key part of a healthy diet. Eating whole grains may help lower the risk for coronary heart disease, but many people in the United States eat too many refined grains and not enough whole grains. Behavior change interventions can help people eat more whole grains to get the recommended amount of dietary fiber.	Baseline: 0.46 oz eq per 1,000 kcal in 2013–2016 Goal: 0.62 oz eq per 1,000 kcal

Continued

Table 11-3 *(continued)*

Objective	Summary	Baseline and goal amounts
Reduce consumption of saturated fat by people aged ≥2 y	People who replace the saturated fat in their diet with unsaturated fat are likely to have a lower cholesterol level, which may reduce the risk of heart problems, but many people in the United States eat too much saturated fat. Nutritional counseling and behavioral interventions can help people eat less saturated fat. Encouraging people to use the Nutrition Facts label can also help them track their consumption of saturated fat.	Baseline: 11.4% mean calories from saturated fat in 2013–2016 Goal: 8.4%
Reduce consumption of sodium by people aged ≥2 y	Eating too much salt (sodium) may increase the risk of high blood pressure and cardiovascular disease, and most people in the United States eat too much salt. Strategies that involve both population-level interventions (eg, reducing the amount of salt in packaged foods) and individual-level interventions (eg, behavioral counseling) seem to be the most effective ways to help people eat less salt. Encouraging people to use the Nutrition Facts label can also help them track their consumption of salt.	Baseline: 3,406 mg was the mean total intake by people aged ≥2 y in 2013–2016. Goal: 2,725 mg
Increase consumption of calcium by people aged ≥2 y	People need calcium for healthy bones, and getting enough calcium may reduce the risk of osteoporosis. Although average calcium consumption has increased in the United States in recent years, many people still do not get enough calcium. Nutritional counseling and behavioral interventions can help people get more calcium. Encouraging people to use the Nutrition Facts label can also help them track their consumption of calcium.	Baseline: 1,077 mg of calcium from foods, dietary supplements, antacids, and drinking water was the mean total intake by people ≥2 y in 2013–2016. Goal: 1,184 mg

Increase consumption of potassium by people aged ≥2 y	People who get enough potassium are less likely to have high blood pressure, but most people in the United States do not get enough potassium. Some dietary interventions that promote eating large amounts of fruits and vegetables, such as the Dietary Approaches to Stop Hypertension diet, may help people get enough potassium. In addition, encouraging people to use the Nutrition Facts label can help them track their consumption of potassium.	Baseline: 2,512 mg of potassium from foods and dietary supplements was the mean total intake by people ≥2 y in 2013–2016. Goal: 2,763 mg
Increase consumption of vitamin D by people aged ≥2 y	Vitamin D helps the body absorb calcium, which is important for healthy bones. People who get enough vitamin D and calcium may also have a lower risk for osteoporosis, but many people in the United States do not get enough vitamin D. Eating foods with added vitamin D and taking supplements can help people get enough vitamin D. Encouraging people to use the Nutrition Facts label can also help them track their consumption of vitamin D.	Baseline: 632 IU (15.8 mcg) of vitamin D from foods and dietary supplements was the mean total intake by people ≥2 y in 2013–2016. Goal: 760 IU (19 mcg)
Reduce iron deficiency in children aged 1–2 y	Young children who do not get enough iron are at higher risk for developmental problems. Giving young children supplements or iron-rich foods can help reduce iron deficiency.	Baseline: 6.3% of children aged 1–2 y had iron deficiency in 2015–2016. Goal: 2.1%
Increase the proportion of adolescents participating in the School Breakfast Program	The School Breakfast Program lowers the risk of food insecurity and helps children eat healthier. Increasing participation in the program can help students do better in school and address behavioral and mental health concerns related to food insecurity. Strategies to provide breakfast after the school day starts and to offer free breakfast to all students can increase participation in the program.	Baseline: 35.4% of students attending schools enrolled in the School Breakfast Program participated in 2017–2018. Goal: 40.2%

Continued

Table 11-3 (*continued*)

Objective	Summary	Baseline and goal amounts
Reduce iron deficiency in females aged 12–49 y	Blood needs iron to carry oxygen through the body, but some people do not have enough iron. Women are more likely than men to have an iron deficiency because they lose blood during menstruation. Pregnancy and childbirth can also cause iron deficiency. Supplements and foods with added iron are effective methods to help women get enough iron. Encouraging people to use the Nutrition Facts label can also help them track their consumption of iron.	Baseline: 11% of females aged 12–49 y had iron deficiency in 2015–2016. Goal: 7.2%
Increase the proportion of infants breastfeeding exclusively through age 6 mo	Breastfeeding is linked to a reduced risk for many illnesses in children and mothers. Exclusive breastfeeding for the first 6 mo after birth is linked to health benefits for infants. Although breastfeeding initiation rates are high in the United States, most women do not breastfeed exclusively for the first 6 mo. Strategies such as peer support, education, longer maternity leaves, and breastfeeding support in the hospital, workplace, and community may help more women breastfeed exclusively.	Baseline: 24.9% of infants born in 2015 were breastfed exclusively through 6 mo of age. Goal: 42.4%
Increase the proportion of infants breastfeeding at age 1 y	Breastfeeding is linked to reduced risk for many illnesses in children and mothers. National guidelines recommend exclusive breastfeeding for the first 6 mo after birth and continued breastfeeding for at least the first year. Although breastfeeding initiation rates are high in the United States, most women do not breastfeed for the entire first year. Strategies such as peer support, education, longer maternity leaves, and breastfeeding support in the hospital, workplace, and community may help more women breastfeed longer.	Baseline: 35.9% of infants born in 2015 were breastfed to any extent at 1 y. Goal: 54.1%

[a] Leading health indicator.

Derived from reference 2.

should also prioritize these indicators, taking steps to help support families in reducing sugar intake, screening for food insecurity, and connecting families with resources to reduce food insecurity (refer to Chapter 10, Dietary History, Social History, and Food Insecurity Screening).

Advocating for Healthier Nutrition

A child's nutrition intake is influenced by a complex interplay of individual, family, community, and societal factors, such as those initially described in Bronfenbrenner's ecological theory of child development in 1977 (**Figure 11-3**).[4]

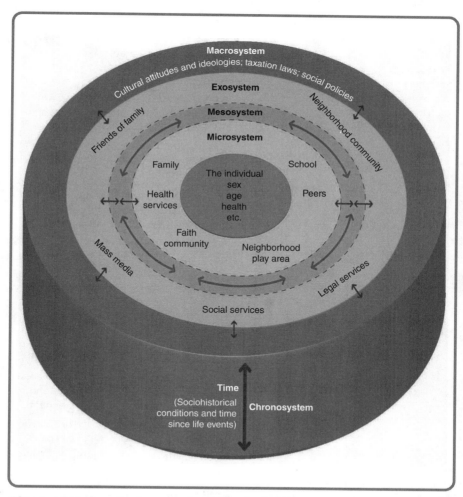

Figure 11-3. Bronfenbrenner's ecological theory of child development.

Reproduced with permission from Lopez M, Ruiz MO, Rovnaghi CR, et al. The social ecology of childhood and early life adversity. *Pediatr Res.* 2021;89(2):353-367.

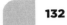

This theory of development has evolved over time but still provides a useful framework to consider key strategies and advocacy opportunities to promote healthful nutrition in each domain. Several suggested strategies using Bronfenbrenner's theory as a framework and based on American Academy of Pediatrics policy statements are highlighted in **Table 11-4**.

Table 11-4. Strategies to Advocate for Healthier Nutrition for Children and Adolescents

System	Agent	Strategies
Microsystem (direct contact with child) Mesosystem (interplay of microsystems with each other)	Family	Encourage families to prioritize family meals.[5]
		Encourage families to practice responsive feeding (Refer to the Responsive Feeding section earlier in this chapter.)
		Encourage purchase and preparation of healthful lunches and snacks.[6]
		Encourage caregivers to talk openly and critically about media, and how advertisements shape wants, from the time that children are young.[7]
	School	Support implementation of US Department of Agriculture guidelines for school meals and competitive foods sold in schools.[6]
		Avoid food "rewards."[6]
		Engage with wellness councils and school health advisory committees.[6]
	Health services	Provide developmentally tailored evidence-informed nutrition information.[8]
		Be knowledgeable about breastfeeding and lactation resources in the community, and help mothers and infants when problems occur.[8,9]
		Encourage enrollment in Special Supplemental Nutrition Program for Women, Infants, and Children services and other eligible benefits.[9]
		Promote a positive body image, and discourage dieting, skipping of meals, or use of diet pills.[5]
		Focus on healthy habits rather than weight.[5]
Exosystem (social structures that influence a child)	Neighborhood and community	Advocate for food pantries to offer healthy options and specifically tailored food packages to address needs of pregnant and breastfeeding women and young children.[9]

Table 11-4 (*continued*)

System	Agent	Strategies
Exosystem (social structures that influence a child) (*continued*)	Mass media	Support reduction in sugary drink marketing.[8] Encourage limits on advertising to children and adolescents.[7,8]
	Social services and health care	Screen for food insecurity.[9] Encourage hospitals and health care facilities to serve as models for healthful food and beverage options.[8] Collaborate with public health entities to identify communities in need of focused interventions, and advocate for healthy environments with access to healthful foods and public health investments to improve individual and population health.[10] Advocate for population-based approaches to health within one's own health care institutions and systems.[10]
	School board	Support healthful food options as the default choice in the school environment, such as school meals and snacks.[6]
	Government agencies	Support funding to federal nutrition programs and linking of nutrition and health assistance programs, such as the Special Supplemental Nutrition Program for Women, Infants, and Children or Supplemental Nutrition Assistance Program and Medicaid.[9] Advocate for federal nutrition assistance programs to ensure access to healthful foods and beverages and limit juice.[8,9,11] Support policies that raise the price of sugary drinks, such as an excise tax.[8] Support required nutrition information on the Nutrition Facts label, restaurant menus, and advertisements.[8]
Macrosystem (culture and cultural factors that influence a child)	Attitudes and ideologies of the culture	Offer early, intensive, and longitudinal educational support with culturally responsive teaching and promotion of health literacy.[12]
Chronosystem (all the changes that occur over a lifetime that influence development)	Environmental and cultural changes that occur over the life course	Assess patients for stressors and social determinants of health associated with racism.[13]

In Sum

- The dietary guidelines provide up-to-date information on nutrition strategies to promote optimal health and nutrition for infants, children, and adolescents. The key recommendations include
  - — Follow a healthy eating pattern across the life span.
  - — Focus on variety, nutrient density, and amount.
  - — Limit calories from added sugars and saturated fats and reduce sodium intake.
  - — Shift to healthier food and beverage choices that have a higher nutrient density and lower caloric content.
  - — Recognize cultural, ethnic, and socioeconomic factors that influence food preferences and access to healthful foods and beverages, as well as the importance of tools and resources for families to plan and monitor their diets.
- There is a notable discrepancy between the dietary guidelines and how children and adolescents actually eat. Any steps toward helping infants, children, and adolescents more closely follow the dietary guidelines will benefit health.
- Nutrients of public health concern for all age-groups include vitamin D, calcium, dietary fiber, and potassium. Breastfed infants are more likely to underconsume iron, zinc, and protein from complementary foods after age 6 months. All older infants are more likely to underconsume choline. Older children ($\geq$ 9 years) and adolescents are more likely to underconsume phosphorus, magnesium, and choline. Female adolescents are more likely to also underconsume iron, protein, folate, vitamin B_6, and vitamin B_{12}.
- The Healthy People 2030 goals include several areas of focus to improve child nutrition. Two nutrition indicators are of highest priority: decreasing added sugars consumption and reducing food insecurity.
- Responsive feeding sets the foundation to support infants, children, and adolescents to make healthier nutrition choices and to have a healthy relationship with food. Pediatricians play an important role in teaching parents about responsive feeding and providing them encouragement and support to practice responsive feeding.

References

1. US Department of Health and Human Services, US Department of Agriculture. *Dietary Guidelines for Americans, 2020–2025.* 9th ed. 2020. Accessed October 5, 2022. https://www.dietaryguidelines.gov/sites/default/files/2020-12/Dietary_Guidelines_for_Americans_2020-2025.pdf

2. Office of Disease Prevention and Health Promotion. Healthy People 2030: nutrition and healthy eating. US Dept of Health and Human Services. Accessed October 5, 2022. https://health.gov/healthypeople/objectives-and-data/browse-objectives/nutrition-and-healthy-eating

3. Global Food Research Program. *Ultra-processed Foods: A Global Threat to Public Health.* University of North Carolina at Chapel Hill; 2021. Accessed October 5, 2022. https://www.globalfoodresearchprogram.org/wp-content/uploads/2021/04/UPF_ultra-processed_food_fact_sheet.pdf

4. Bronfenbrenner U. Toward an experimental ecology of human development. *Am Psychol.* 1977;32(7):513–531 doi: 10.1037/0003-066X.32.7.513

5. Golden NH, Schneider M, Wood C, et al; American Academy of Pediatrics Committee on Nutrition, Committee on Adolescence, and Section on Obesity. Preventing obesity and eating disorders in adolescents. *Pediatrics.* 2016;138(3):e20161649 PMID: 27550979 doi: 10.1542/peds.2016-1649

6. Murray R, Bhatia J, Okamoto J, et al; American Academy of Pediatrics Council on School Health and Committee on Nutrition. Snacks, sweetened beverages, added sugars, and schools. *Pediatrics.* 2015;135(3):575–583 PMID: 25713277 doi: 10.1542/peds.2014-3902

7. Radesky J, Chassiakos YLR, Ameenuddin N, Navsaria D; American Academy of Pediatrics Council on Communication and Media. Digital advertising to children. *Pediatrics.* 2020;146(1):e20201681 PMID: 32571990 doi: 10.1542/peds.2020-1681

8. Muth ND, Dietz WH, Magge SN, et al; American Academy of Pediatrics Section on Obesity and Committee on Nutrition, American Heart Association. Public policies to reduce sugary drink consumption in children and adolescents. *Pediatrics.* 2019;143(4):e20190282 PMID: 30910915 doi: 10.1542/peds.2019-0282

9. Gitterman BA, Chilton LA, Cotton WH, et al; American Academy of Pediatrics Council on Community Pediatrics and Committee on Nutrition. Promoting food security for all children. *Pediatrics.* 2015;136(5):e1431–e1438 PMID: 26498462 doi: 10.1542/peds.2015-3301

10. Kuo AA, Thomas PA, Chilton LA, et al; American Academy of Pediatrics Council on Community Pediatrics and Section on Epidemiology, Public Health, and Evidence. Pediatricians and public health: optimizing the health and well-being of the nation's children. *Pediatrics.* 2018;141(2):e20173848 PMID: 29358481 doi: 10.1542/peds.2017-3848

11. Heyman MB, Abrams SA, Heitlinger LA, et al; American Academy of Pediatrics Section on Gastroenterology, Hepatology, and Nutrition and Committee on Nutrition. Fruit juice in infants, children, and adolescents: current recommendations. *Pediatrics.* 2017;139(6):e20170967 PMID: 28562300 doi: 10.1542/peds.2017-0967

12. Linton JM, Green A, Chilton LA, et al; American Academy of Pediatrics Council on Community Pediatrics. Providing care for children in immigrant families. *Pediatrics.* 2019;144(3):e20192077 PMID: 31427460 doi: 10.1542/peds.2019-2077

13. Trent M, Dooley DG, Dougé J, et al; American Academy of Pediatrics Section on Adolescent Health, Council on Community Pediatrics, and Committee on Adolescence. The impact of racism on child and adolescent health. *Pediatrics.* 2019;144(2):e20191765 PMID: 31358665 doi: 10.1542/peds.2019-1765

CHAPTER 12

Healthy Eating Plans

The best eating plan for any individual child, adolescent, or family will be influenced by many factors, such as culture, taste preferences, food access, food security, social norms, and culinary interest and skill. Recommending a one-size-fits-all approach to eating and mealtimes is unlikely to lead to significant dietary changes or improved health. However, healthy eating plans share common features, such as aligning with the *Dietary Guidelines for Americans*.[1]

Characteristics of a Healthy Eating Plan

The healthiest eating plans include ample amounts of key nutrients and share several common features. They tend to be moderate or high in

- Vegetables
- Fruits
- Legumes
- Whole grains
- Low-fat or nonfat dairy[a]
- Seafood
- Nuts
- Unsaturated vegetable oils

And low in

- Red and processed meats
- Sugar-sweetened foods and drinks
- Salt
- Solid (saturated) fats
- Refined grains
- Ultra-processed foods (**Box 12-1**)

Several of the most well-studied healthy eating plans are described in the following sections, including the Healthy US-Style Dietary Pattern, the Dietary Approaches to Stop Hypertension (DASH) eating plan, the Healthy Vegetarian eating plan, and the Healthy Mediterranean-style eating plan. Each of these are recommended as model healthy eating plans for children 2 years and older in the dietary guidelines.

The Healthy US-Style Dietary Pattern

The Healthy US-Style Dietary Pattern serves as the foundation for the dietary guideline recommendations and the associated MyPlate meal plans intended to help people 2 years and older make healthier meal choices. The Healthy US-Style Dietary Pattern

---

[a] The eating plans advised by the dietary guidelines recommend low-fat or nonfat dairy products. However, there is not evidence that higher-fat dairy is related to obesity or adverse cardiovascular disease outcomes.

IN GREATER DEPTH

Box 12-1. Ultra-processed Foods

Ultra-processed foods are "edible products formulated from food-derived substances, along with additives that heighten their appeal and durability."[2] They include products such as sugary drinks, packaged snacks and cookies, instant soups and noodles, ready-to-eat or ready-to-heat meals, and candy—foods that children and adolescents tend to consume in large amounts. In fact, one study showed that children, adolescents, and young adults aged 2–19 y consume > 60% of total calories from ultra-processed foods.[3] High intake of ultra-processed foods is associated with overconsumption, excess weight gain and obesity, dyslipidemia, type 2 diabetes, premature death, cancer, and depression.[2] Researchers at the Center for Epidemiological Studies in Health and Nutrition at the University of Sao Paulo, Brazil, developed a classification system known as the NOVA Food Classification system (**Figure 12-1**) to differentiate ultra-processed foods from other foods whose processing is generally less detrimental or not detrimental to health. This classification system has been adopted widely in characterizing processed foods.

GROUP 1	GROUP 2	GROUP 3	GROUP 4
Unprocessed/ minimally processed	**Processed culinary ingredients**	**Processed foods**	**Ultra-processed foods**
Foods unaltered or altered by processes such as removing inedible parts, drying, grinding, cooking, pasteurization, freezing, or non-alcoholic fermentation. No substances are added. Processing aims to increase food stability and enable easier or more diverse preparation.	Substances obtained directly from Group 1 foods or from nature, created by industrial processes such as pressing, centrifuging, refining, extracting or mining. Processing aims to create products to be used in preparation, seasoning and cooking of Group 1 foods.	Products made by adding edible substances from Group 2 to Group 1 foods using preservation methods such as non-alcoholic fermentation, canning, or bottling. Processing aims to increase stability and durability of Group 1 foods and to make them more enjoyable.	Formulations of low-cost substances derived from Group 1 foods with little to no whole foods; always contain edible substances not used in home kitchens (e.g., protein isolates) and/or cosmetic additives (e.g., flavors, colors, emulsifiers). Processing involves multiple steps and industries and aims to create products liable to replace all other NOVA groups.
Examples: Fresh or frozen fruits/vegetables, pulses, packaged grains, flours, nuts, plain pasta, pasteurized milk, chilled/frozen meat	*Examples: Butter, vegetable oils, other fats, sugar, molasses, honey, salt*	*Examples: Canned vegetables in brine, freshly made breads or cheeses, cured meats*	*Examples: Packaged snacks, cookies/biscuits, instant soups/ noodles, ready-to-eat/heat meals, candy, soft drinks*

Figure 12-1. The NOVA Food Classification system of food processing.

is high in fruits, vegetables, dairy, fish, poultry, nuts, and whole grains and low in red meat, sweets, and sugary drinks. Thus, it contains high amounts of potassium, magnesium, calcium, protein, and fiber and low amounts of sugar, saturated fat, and sodium. The dietary guidelines note that it is essentially equivalent to the DASH eating plan (described later in this chapter).[1]

MyPlate

MyPlate simplifies the Healthy US-Style Dietary Pattern into an easily understood and implemented graphic: a dinner plate divided into 4 sections—fruits, vegetables, protein, and grains, accompanied by a glass of milk. The goal of this icon is to better visualize a balanced diet that is about 50% fruits and vegetables, with remaining portions made up of lean protein, grains, and dairy (**Figure 12-2**). **Box 12-2** provides more detailed information about MyPlate messaging and shares how clinicians can help their patients obtain their own, individualized, MyPlate plan. The MyPlate Kitchen (www.myplate.gov/myplate-kitchen) includes a variety of resources and recipes, such as recipes celebrating cuisines from around the world.

Refer to Part 5, Frequently Asked Questions, Case Studies, and Recipes, for several mix-and-match MyPlate-consistent meals that can be shared with families to help them translate MyPlate recommendations into changes in consumption patterns.

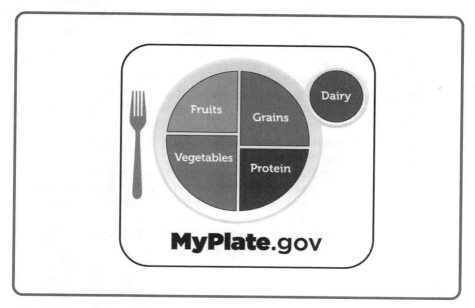

Figure 12-2. MyPlate.

Reproduced from US Department of Agriculture. MyPlate. Accessed October 5, 2022. https://www.myplate.gov.

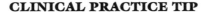

CLINICAL PRACTICE TIP

Box 12-2. MyPlate Plan

Encourage parents and other caregivers who want to help their children follow a healthy eating plan to obtain their individualized MyPlate plan (www.choosemyplate.gov/MyPlateplan).

The key MyPlate messages to share with patients and their families are as follows:

- Find your healthy eating style and maintain it for a lifetime. Aim to eat a variety of foods from the 5 MyPlate food groups to meet caloric and nutrient needs. Remember, healthy eating does not need to be perfect.
- Make half your plate fruits and vegetables. Focus on whole fruits more than juice. Choose fresh, frozen, canned, dried, or pureed versions with little or no added sugars. Vary your vegetables; that is, eat them raw or cooked, fresh, frozen, canned, or dried. Eat all the colors, including red, orange, and dark green, which are high in nutrients.
- Make half your grains whole grains. Choose whole grain breads, cereals, and pasta. Identify whole grains by reading ingredient lists and looking for whole wheat flour, whole grain corn, whole grain brown rice, buckwheat, bulgur, whole rye, and whole oats. Look for products with at least 3 g of fiber per serving. Foods labeled "multigrain," "100% wheat," "seven grain," and "bran" are not usually whole wheat.
- Remember to drink milk or consume a dairy equivalent. The dairy group includes milk, yogurt, and cheese. Fortified soy milk is considered a dairy equivalent. Other plant-based "milks," such as almond milk and rice milk, are not dairy equivalents. Dairy provides important nutrients (eg, calcium, vitamin D, potassium, protein) that help build strong bones.
- Eat a variety of protein foods. Meat, poultry, seafood, beans, eggs, soy, nuts, and seeds all count. When choosing beef, choose lean cuts such as round or sirloin and ground beef that is at least 92% lean. Bake, roast, broil, or grill rather than fry or sauté.
- Make small changes to what you eat and drink that will work for now and in the future. Celebrate each success.

US Department of Agriculture Food Plans

The Healthy US-Style Dietary Pattern is used for the US Department of Agriculture food plans that include sample meals to approximate costs of a healthy eating pattern at the following 4 levels:

- Thrifty Food Plan (minimal cost): The Thrifty Food Plan is the lowest cost of the 4 US Department of Agriculture food plans. This food plan is designed to meet the dietary guidelines for families at the lowest 25th percentile of spending for groceries and food. By law, the cost of this plan serves as the basis for the maximum benefit in the Supplemental Nutrition Assistance Program (SNAP) (refer to Chapter 10, Dietary History, Social History, and Food Insecurity Screening). In 2023, the benefit provides approximately $939/mo (US dollar; about $31/d) for a family of 4. The Agricultural Improvement Act of 2018 required that beginning in 2022, the Thrifty Food Plan must be reevaluated every 5 years on the basis of current food prices, food composition data, consumption patterns, and dietary guidance. Previously, the Thrifty Food Plan was updated at discretion of the Secretary of the US Department of Agriculture. Before a 21% benefit increase in 2021, the Thrifty Food Plan was criticized extensively as impractical and inadequate. For example, the Food Research & Action Center noted that it "include[d] impractical lists of foods; lack[ed] the variety called for in the *Dietary Guidelines for Americans;* unrealistically assume[d] adequate facilities and time for food preparation, food availability, food affordability, and adequate, affordable transportation; underestimate[d] food waste; [wa]s exacerbated in its inadequacy by SNAP benefit calculations; cost[ed] more than the SNAP allotment in many parts of the country; and ignore[d] special dietary needs."[4]
- Low Cost: This food plan is designed to meet the dietary guidelines for families at the 25th to 50th percentile of spending for groceries and food. For this plan, a family of 4 spends approximately $970/mo. Bankruptcy courts use this value to determine the portion of a person's income to allocate to food expenses.[5]
- Moderate Cost: This food plan is designed to meet the dietary guidelines for families at the 50th to 75th percentile of spending for groceries and food. For this plan, a family of 4 spends approximately $1,210/mo.[5]
- Liberal: This food plan is designed to meet the dietary guidelines for families above the 75th percentile of spending for groceries and food. For this plan, a family of 4 spends approximately $1,460/mo on food. The Department of Defense uses this value to determine a Basic Allowance for Subsistence for service members.[5]

These food plans are intended to show that eating healthfully and according to the recommendations can be done on most any budget. However, careful planning and preparing of most or all meals and snacks at home are necessary in many cases, which, as described in the discussion of the Thrifty Food Plan, may be impractical. Chapter 10, Dietary History, Social History, and Food Insecurity Screening, explores strategies to help minimize food costs.

The DASH Eating Plan

Consuming a diet high in vegetables, fruits, whole grains, seafood, nuts, and legumes and limiting sweets, sugar-sweetened beverages, and red meats promote optimal heart health and blood pressure control. Several eating patterns fit this profile; however, the DASH eating plan has been the most studied with the most profound effects on blood pressure.

The DASH eating plan

- Emphasizes vegetables, fruits, and whole grains
- Includes fat-free and low-fat dairy products, fish, poultry, beans, nuts, and vegetable oils
- Limits foods high in saturated fat
- Limits sugary drinks and sweets
- Limits sodium to 2,300 mg (or 1,500 mg, if even further blood pressure reduction is needed)

Table 12-1 shows a standard DASH eating plan at various calorie levels.

Researchers of an umbrella review of systematic reviews and meta-analyses of the DASH eating plan and cardiometabolic risk concluded that the DASH dietary pattern was associated with reduced-incident cardiovascular disease, coronary heart disease, stroke, and diabetes in adults. It decreased systolic blood pressure by 5.2 mm Hg, diastolic blood pressure by 2.6 mm Hg, total cholesterol level by 7.7 mg/dL (0.2 mmol/L), low-density–lipoprotein cholesterol level by 0.10 mmol/L (3.9 mg/dL), hemoglobin A_{1c} level by 0.53% (0.53), and body weight by 3.1 lb (1.42 kg). It did not affect high-density–lipoprotein cholesterol or fasting blood glucose level.[6] A study of children and adolescents showed that adherence to the DASH diet was associated with decreased incidence of hypertension, high level of fasting plasma glucose, and abdominal obesity.[7]

The "Day of DASH" recipes in Part 5, Frequently Asked Questions, Case Studies, and Recipes, can be shared with patients to help make it easier to put the DASH eating plan into practice.

Vegetarian Eating Plan

Many children, adolescents, and their families follow a vegetarian eating plan. A well-planned vegetarian eating plan can optimize nutrition and benefit health while promoting environmental health through use of fewer natural resources and less environmental damage (**Box 12-3**).[8] Vegetarian diets tend to be low in saturated fat and animal protein and high in fiber, folate, vitamins C and E, carotenoids, and some phytochemicals. Children and adolescents who follow a vegetarian eating plan tend to consume greater amounts of fruits and vegetables and less sweets, salty snacks, and saturated fat than their nonvegetarian peers. They also tend to have lower risk for overweight and obesity.[8] Although following a vegetarian eating plan does not seem to be a risk factor for disordered eating, pediatricians should be aware that children and adolescents with eating disorders may choose to follow a vegetarian eating plan as a means of food restriction.[8]

Table 12-1. DASH Eating Plan

Food group	1,200 Cal	1,400 Cal	1,600 Cal	1,800 Cal	2,000 Cal	2,600 Cal	Examples of a single serving	Significance
	Servings per day							
Grains[a]	4-5	5-6	6	6	6-8	10-11	1 slice bread; 1 oz dry cereal[b]; ½ c cooked rice, pasta, or cereal[b]	Major sources of energy and fiber
Vegetables	3-4	3-4	3-4	4-5	4-5	5-6	1 c raw leafy vegetable; ½ c cut-up raw or cooked vegetable; ½ c vegetable juice	Rich sources of potassium, magnesium, and fiber
Fruits	3-4	4	4	4-5	4-5	5-6	1 medium fruit; ¼ c dried fruit; ½ c fresh, frozen, or canned fruit; ½ c fruit juice	Important sources of potassium, magnesium, and fiber
Fat-free or low-fat dairy products[b]	2-3	2-3	2-3	2-3	2-3	3	1 c milk or yogurt; 1½ oz cheese	Major sources of calcium, vitamin D, and protein
Lean meats, poultry, and fish	≤3	≤3-4	≤3-4	≤6	≤6	≤6	1 oz cooked meats, poultry, or fish; 1 egg	Rich sources of protein and magnesium

Continued

Table 12-1 (*continued*)

Food group	1,200 Cal	1,400 Cal	1,600 Cal	1,800 Cal	2,000 Cal	2,600 Cal	Examples of a single serving	Significance
	Servings per day							
Nuts, seeds, and legumes	3 per week	3 per week	3–4 per week	4 per week	4–5 per week	1	⅓ c or 1½ oz nuts 2 tbsp peanut butter 2 tbsp or ½ oz seeds ½ c cooked legumes (dried beans, peas)	Rich sources of energy, magnesium, protein, and fiber
Fats and oils^c	1	1	2	2–3	2–3	3	1 tsp soft margarine 1 tsp vegetable oil 1 tbsp mayonnaise 2 tbsp salad dressing	The DASH study had 27% of calories as fat, including fat in or added to foods.
Sweets and added sugars	≤3 per week	≤3 per week	≤3 per week	≤5 per week	≤5 per week	≤2	1 tbsp sugar 1 tbsp jelly or jam ½ c sorbet, gelatin dessert 1 c lemonade	Sweets should be low in fat.
Maximum sodium limit^d	2,300 mg/d	2,300 mg/d	2,300 mg/d	2,300 mg/d	2,300 mg/d	2,300 mg/d		

Abbreviation: DASH, Dietary Approaches to Stop Hypertension.

[a] Whole grains are recommended for most grain servings as a good source of fiber and nutrients.

[b] For lactose intolerance, try lactase enzyme pills with dairy products or lactose-free or lactose-reduced milk.

[c] Fat content changes the serving amount for fats and oils. For example, 1 tbsp regular salad dressing = one serving; 1 tbsp low-fat dressing = one-half serving; 1 tbsp fat-free dressing = zero servings.

[d] The DASH eating plan has a sodium limit of either 2,300 or 1,500 mg/d.

Adapted from National Heart, Lung, and Blood Institute. Following the DASH eating plan. Accessed October 5, 2022. https://www.nhlbi.nih.gov/education/dash/following-dash.

Box 12-3. An Example of Environmental Benefit When a Person Chooses Vegetarian Protein Sources

Production of 1 kg of protein from kidney beans compared to production of 1 kg of protein from beef requires

- 18 times less land
- 10 times less water
- 9 times less fuel
- 12 times less fertilizer
- 10 times less pesticide

Derived from Ranacharoenpong K, Soret S, Harwatt H, Wien M, Sabaté J. The environmental cost of protein food choices. *Public Health Nutr.* 2015;18(11):2067–2073. Erratum in: *Public Health Nutr.* 2015;18(11):2096.

Types of Vegetarian Eating Plans

Children and adolescents may adopt any of several variations of a vegetarian eating plan, which may or may not include fish, eggs, or dairy products (**Table 12-2**).

A *flexitarian* is not a vegetarian but consumes meat, poultry, and fish infrequently. A *pescatarian* eats fish but avoids meat and poultry. A *lacto-ovo vegetarian* does not eat

Table 12-2. Protein Sources in Different Types of Vegetarian Eating Plans[a]

Eating plan	Food category						
	Meat	**Poultry**	**Fish**	**Eggs**	**Dairy**	**Legumes**	**Vegetables**
Flexitarian	Sparingly	Sparingly	✓	✓	✓	✓	✓
Pescatarian	X	X	✓	✓	✓	✓	✓
Lacto-ovo vegetarian	X	X	X	✓	✓	✓	✓
Lacto-vegetarian	X	X	X	X	✓	✓	✓
Ovo-vegetarian	X	X	X	✓	X	✓	✓
Vegan	X	X	X	X	X	✓	✓

X indicates that the food is not consumed in the eating plan; ✓, that the food is consumed in the eating plan.

[a] All the eating plans include fruits, vegetables, and grains.

meat, poultry, or fish but does eat eggs and dairy products. A *lacto-vegetarian* does not eat eggs, meat, poultry, or fish but does eat dairy. An *ovo-vegetarian* does not eat dairy, meat, poultry, or fish but does eat eggs. A *vegan* does not eat any animal products, including dairy and eggs.

Nutrient Considerations

Well-planned vegetarian eating plans of all types can meet nutritional needs. However, poorly planned vegetarian diets may be a risk factor for inadequate intake of certain nutrients. These nutrients are as follows[8]:

- Calories: Despite risk of insufficient caloric intake, most children and adolescents who follow a vegetarian eating plan consume sufficient calories.
- Protein: Children and adolescents who follow a vegetarian plan tend to attain adequate intake of protein variety and quantity. Regular intake of legumes (eg, beans, peas, lentils, peanuts, soy) ensures adequate intake of protein. Children and adolescents who follow a vegan eating plan may require higher protein intake than nonvegan children because of decreased protein quality. Toddlers may need 30% to 35% more protein, preschoolers may need 20% to 30% more, and older children and adolescents may need 20% more. Plant-based "meats" (eg, Impossible Burger, Beyond Meat) are popular sources of vegetarian protein that taste like meat. These products have made adopting a vegetarian eating plan more accessible for many children, adolescents, and their families. As such, many patients and families may have questions about the nutritional value of these products and whether these alternative protein sources are recommended. A brief primer for these discussions is included in **Box 12-4**.

IN GREATER DEPTH

Box 12-4. The Popularity and Nutritional Value of Vegetarian Meats

Vegetarian "meats" are increasingly popular with children and adolescents, including those who follow a vegetarian or vegan diet and those who aim to decrease the amount of animal-based protein they consume. Most people think the products taste very similar to their animal-based counterparts. They contain a similar amount of protein to meat products, no cholesterol because they are wholly plant based, and high levels of many micronutrients. However, they can be high in saturated fat and sodium and are ultra-processed. Two of the most popular brands include Impossible Burger and Beyond Meat, both of which include a blend of different plant proteins.

IN GREATER DEPTH

Box 12-4 (*continued*)

Impossible Burger patties are made primarily of water, soy protein concentrate, coconut oil, and sunflower oil. They also contain potato protein, methylcellulose, yeast extract, cultured dextrose, modified food starch, soy leghemoglobin, salt, soy protein isolate, mixed tocopherols (vitamin E), zinc gluconate, thiamine hydrochloride (vitamin B_1), sodium ascorbate (vitamin C), niacin, pyridoxine hydrocholoride (vitamin B_6), riboflavin (vitamin B_2), and vitamin B_{12}. The soy leghemoglobin is what makes an Impossible Burger taste "meaty." The soy leghemoglobin is heme derived from soy plants genetically engineered with a yeast. A 4-oz Impossible Burger patty contains 240 Cal, 8 g of saturated fat (40% RDA), 370 mg of sodium (16% RDA), and 19 g of protein (31% RDA). It also includes calcium (15% RDA), iron (25% RDA), potassium (15% RDA), thiamin (2,350% RDA), riboflavin (15% RDA), niacin (50% RDA), vitamin B_6 (20%), folate (30% RDA), and vitamin B_{12} (130% RDA).

Beyond Meat burgers are made of water, pea protein isolate, expeller-pressed canola oil, refined coconut oil, rice protein, natural flavors, cocoa butter, mung bean protein, methylcellulose, potato starch, apple extract, salt, potassium chloride, vinegar, lemon juice concentrate, sunflower lecithin, pomegranate fruit powder, and beet juice extract (for color). A 4-oz Beyond Meat patty contains 260 Cal, 5 g of saturated fat (25% RDA), 350 mg of sodium (15% RDA), 20 g of protein (40% RDA), and 2 g of fiber (7% RDA). It also includes calcium (8% RDA), iron (20% RDA), and potassium (6% RDA).

To compare, a 4-oz beef (80% lean/20% fat) patty contains 284 Cal, 8.5 g of saturated fat (43% RDA), 75 mg of sodium (3% RDA), 19 g of protein (31% RDA), and 80 mg of cholesterol (27% RDA). It also includes calcium (2% RDA), iron (12% RDA), and potassium (6% RDA). The RDA included on the Nutrition Facts label, noted here, is the average daily level of intake sufficient to meet the nutrient requirements of nearly all (97%–98%) healthy people, based on a 2,000-Cal diet.

Abbreviation: RDA, recommended dietary allowance.

- Iron: Iron bioavailability from vegetarian sources (nonheme iron) is lower than that from nonvegetarian sources. Inadequate iron intake is generally common in children and more so common in children who follow a vegetarian eating plan. Risk for iron deficiency should be routinely monitored in children and adolescents who follow a vegetarian eating plan. Children who have iron deficiency should increase iron intake through an iron-rich diet and/or supplementation. Phytates, oxalates, and phenolic compounds are present in many plant foods and inhibit iron absorption, whereas vitamin C enhances iron absorption. On the whole, vegetarians need about 1.8 times higher iron intake than that of nonvegetarians.

- Zinc: Zinc levels may be lower in children and adolescents following a vegetarian diet, although deficiency is rare. Excellent vegetarian sources of zinc include soy, legumes, grains, cheese, seeds, and nuts. Additionally, soaking and sprouting beans, grains, nuts, and seeds and leavening bread can reduce binding of zinc with phytic acid and increase zinc bioavailability. Citric acid can also increase zinc absorption.

- Vitamin B_{12}: Vitamin B_{12} is present naturally primarily in animal products. It is present in very small amounts in some fermented foods, nori, spirulina, chlorella algae, and unfortified nutritional yeast. Although most vegetarian eating plans contain sufficient vitamin B_{12}, children who follow a vegan eating plan should take a vitamin B_{12} supplement or consume fortified foods, such as fortified nutritional yeast. Approximately 1% of ingested supplemental vitamin B_{12} is absorbed, so an appropriate supplement dose is about 100 times the recommended dietary allowance.

- Calcium: Bioavailability of calcium in plant foods can be impaired by oxalates, phytates, and fiber, which are found in many plant foods. For instance, although spinach, beet greens, and Swiss chard contain high levels of calcium, they also contain high levels of oxalates, making them a poor calcium source. Low-level oxalate greens such as kale, turnips, Chinese cabbage, and bok choy are good sources of calcium, as are fortified plant milks and soy, white beans, almonds, tahini, figs, and oranges.

- Vitamin D: Few foods naturally contain vitamin D. Children and adolescents who follow an ovo-vegetarian or vegan eating pattern or who do not obtain recommended levels of dairy or equivalent food products fortified with vitamin D may need to take a 400-IU (10-mcg) vitamin D supplement to meet needs.

- Omega-3 fatty acids: Although intake of alpha-linolenic acid is sufficient in most vegetarian and vegan eating plans, intake of eicosapentaenoic acid and docosahexaenoic acid is generally low in vegetarian (and absent in vegan) eating plans. A small proportion of alpha-linolenic acid is converted to eicosapentaenoic acid and docosahexaenoic acid; thus, higher than recommended alpha-linolenic acid intake may help increase the amount converted.

The Healthy Vegetarian Eating Plan

The dietary guidelines recommend a vegetarian eating plan as an excellent approach to good nutrition for children, adolescents, and adults alike. A sample plan is included in **Table 12-3**.

Table 12-3. Healthy Vegetarian Dietary Pattern for Ages 2 and Older, With Daily or Weekly Amounts From Food Groups, Subgroups, and Components

CALORIE LEVEL OF PATTERN	1,000	1,200	1,400	1,600	1,800	2,000	2,200	2,400	2,600	2,800	3,000	3,200
FOOD GROUP OR SUBGROUP	Daily amount of food from each group (Vegetable and protein foods subgroup amounts are per week.)											
Vegetables (cup eq/day)	1	1½	1½	2	2½	2½	3	3	3½	3½	4	4
Vegetable subgroups in weekly amounts												
Dark-green vegetables (cup eq/wk)	½	1	1	1½	1½	1½	2	2	2½	2½	2½	2½
Red and orange vegetables (cup eq/wk)	2½	3	3	4	5½	5½	6	6	7	7	7½	7½
Beans, peas, lentils (cup eq/wk)	½	½	½	1	1½	1½	2	2	2½	2½	3	3
Starchy vegetables (cup eq/wk)	2	3½	3½	4	5	5	6	6	7	7	8	8
Other vegetables (cup eq/wk)	1½	2½	2½	3½	4	4	5	5	5½	5½	7	7
Fruits (cup eq/day)	1	1	1½	1½	1½	2	2	2	2	2½	2½	2½
Grains (ounce eq/day)	3	4	5	5½	6½	6½	7½	8½	9½	10½	10½	10½
Whole grains (ounce eq/day)	1½	2	2½	3	3½	3½	4	4½	5	5½	5½	5½
Refined grains (ounce eq/day)	1½	2	2½	2½	3	3	3½	4	4½	5	5	5
Dairy (cup eq/day)	2	2½	2½	3	3	3	3	3	3	3	3	3
Protein foods (ounce eq/day)	1	1½	2	2½	3	3½	3½	4	4½	5	5½	6

Continued

Table 12-3 (continued)

CALORIE LEVEL OF PATTERN	1,000	1,200	1,400	1,600	1,800	2,000	2,200	2,400	2,600	2,800	3,000	3,200
Protein foods subgroups in weekly amounts												
Eggs (ounce eq/wk)	2	3	3	3	3	3	3	3	3	4	4	4
Beans, peas, lentils (cup eq/wk)	1	2	4	4	6	6	6	8	9	10	11	12
Soy products (ounce eq/wk)	2	3	4	6	6	8	8	9	10	11	12	13
Nuts, seeds (ounce eq/wk)	2	2	3	5	6	7	7	8	9	10	12	13
Oils (grams/day)	**15**	**17**	**17**	**22**	**24**	**27**	**29**	**31**	**34**	**36**	**44**	**51**
Limit on calories for other uses (kcal/day)	**170**	**140**	**160**	**150**	**150**	**250**	**290**	**350**	**350**	**350**	**390**	**500**
Limit on calories for other uses (%/day)	17%	12%	11%	9%	8%	13%	13%	15%	13%	13%	13%	16%

In general, 1 cup of raw or cooked vegetables or vegetable juice, or 2 cups of raw leafy greens, can be considered 1 cup from the vegetable group.

In general, 1 cup of fruit or 100% fruit juice, or ½ cup of dried fruit, can be considered 1 cup from the fruit group.

In general, 1 slice of bread; 1 cup of ready-to-eat cereal; or ½ cup of cooked rice, cooked pasta, or cooked cereal can be considered a 1 ounce-equivalent from the grains group.

In general, 1 ounce of meat, poultry, or fish; ¼ cup of cooked beans, peas, or lentils; 1 egg; 1 tablespoon of peanut butter; or ½ ounce of nuts or seeds can be considered a 1 ounce-equivalent from the protein group.

Table reproduced from US Department of Health and Human Services, US Department of Agriculture. *Dietary Guidelines for Americans, 2020–2025.* 9th ed. 2020:148. Accessed October 5, 2022. https://dietaryguidelines.gov.

Footnotes source: US Department of Agriculture. https://ask.usda.gov. Accessed October 24, 2022.

The Healthy Mediterranean-style Eating Plan

The dietary guidelines endorse the healthy Mediterranean-style eating plan as an excellent approach to good nutrition for people 2 years and older. There is no single agreed-on "Mediterranean diet"; rather, there are several variations of the Mediterranean-style eating plan that share common qualities, including high intake of vegetables, legumes, fruits, nuts, and whole grains. Olive oil is the primary source of fat, with moderate intake of dairy (mostly cheese and yogurt), moderate intake of fish, low amounts of red meat, and, for adults, moderate consumption of wine with meals. A healthy Mediterranean-style dietary pattern at several calorie levels is shown in **Table 12-4**.

Several measures are being studied to help define adherence to a Mediterranean-style eating plan. One measure that is often used in children is the KIDMED index shown in **Table 12-5**. The KIDMED questionnaire is the most widely used scoring system by researchers, nutritionists, and educators to assess adherence to the Mediterranean-style eating plan in children and adolescents.[10]

Following a Mediterranean-style eating plan offers numerous benefits for adults, such as increased life expectancy and reduced chronic disease risk (eg, cardiovascular disease, cancer, diabetes, obesity, neurodegenerative disease).[11] Although there is limited research investigating the health impacts of the Mediterranean-style eating plan on children and adolescents, and overall adherence among children and adolescents is low, even in Mediterranean countries, some evidence suggests that it is associated with increased physical activity and diet adequacy[10] and reduced asthma risk.[12]

The benefits attributed to the Mediterranean-style eating plan are likely owed to more than a sum of individual dietary components. Rather, they are likely owed to the combination of a healthy, nutrient-packed eating plan that includes locally sourced foods and traditional cooking methods of individual regions (eg, Greece, Italy, Spain, Morocco) and a lifestyle that includes regular physical activity. Refer to Part 5, Frequently Asked Questions, Case Studies, and Recipes, for several sample Mediterranean-style recipes.

Cultural Considerations

Many food and nutrition habits are deeply ingrained components of a patient's or family's culture. Although food provides sustenance, it serves many other roles, such as a show of love or affection, a time for family gathering and shared activity, and celebration.

Clinicians should aim to provide culturally sensitive nutritional guidance, leaning strongly on a family's expertise and knowledge and guiding them in establishing goals that not only are consistent with their beliefs and cultural practices but also can help attain a nutrition objective to improve health. Several strategies for clinicians are highlighted in **Table 12-6**.

Table 12-4. Healthy Mediterranean-style Dietary Pattern for Ages 2 and Older, With Daily or Weekly Amounts From Food Groups, Subgroups, and Components

CALORIE LEVEL OF PATTERN	1,000	1,200	1,400	1,600	1,800	2,000	2,200	2,400	2,600	2,800	3,000	3,200
FOOD GROUP OR SUBGROUP	Daily amount of food from each group (Vegetable and protein foods subgroup amounts are per week.)											
Vegetables (cup eq/day)	1	1½	1½	2	2½	2½	3	3	3½	3½	4	4
	Vegetable subgroups in weekly amounts											
Dark-green vegetables (cup eq/wk)	½	1	1	1½	1½	1½	2	2	2½	2½	2½	2½
Red and orange vegetables (cup eq/wk)	2½	3	3	4	5½	5½	6	6	7	7	7½	7½
Beans, peas, lentils (cup eq/wk)	½	½	½	1	1½	1½	2	2	2½	2½	3	3
Starchy vegetables (cup eq/wk)	2	3½	3½	4	5	5	6	6	7	7	8	8
Other vegetables (cup eq/wk)	1½	2½	2½	3½	4	4	5	5	5½	5½	7	7
Fruits (cup eq/day)	1	1	1½	2	2	2½	2½	2½	2½	3	3	3
Grains (ounce eq/day)	3	4	5	5	6	6	7	8	9	10	10	10
Whole grains (ounce eq/day)	1½	2	2½	3	3	3	3½	4	4½	5	5	5
Refined grains (ounce eq/day)	1½	2	2½	2	3	3	3½	4	4½	5	5	5
Dairy (cup eq/day)	2	2½	2½	2	2	2	2	2½	2½	2½	2½	2½
Protein foods (ounce eq/day)	2	3	4	5½	6	6½	7	7½	7½	8	8	8

Protein foods subgroups in weekly amounts											
Meats, poultry, eggs (ounce eq/wk)	10	14	19	23	23	26	28	31	31	33	33	33
Seafood (ounce eq/wk)	3	4	6	11	15	15	16	16	17	17	17	17
Nuts, seeds, soy products (ounce eq/wk)	2	2	3	4	4	5	5	5	5	6	6	6
Oils (grams/day)	**15**	**17**	**17**	**22**	**24**	**27**	**29**	**31**	**34**	**36**	**44**	**51**
Limit on calories for other uses (kcal/day)	**130**	**80**	**90**	**120**	**140**	**240**	**250**	**280**	**300**	**330**	**400**	**540**
Limit on calories for other uses (%/day)	13%	7%	6%	8%	8%	12%	11%	12%	12%	12%	13%	17%

Reproduced from US Department of Health and Human Services, US Department of Agriculture. *Dietary Guidelines for Americans, 2020–2025*. 9th ed. 2020:149. Accessed October 5, 2022. https://dietaryguidelines.gov.

Table 12-5. KIDMED Index to Assess Child and Adolescent Adherence to the Mediterranean-style Eating Plan

Question	Score for YES answer
1. Eats fruit or drinks fruit juice every day	+1
2. Has a second fruit every day	+1
3. Has fresh or cooked vegetables regularly once a day	+1
4. Has fresh or cooked vegetables more than once a day	+1
5. Consumes fish regularly (at least 2–3 times per week)	+1
6. Eats at a fast-food restaurant >1 time per week	−1
7. Likes legumes (beans, nuts, peas, lentils, or peanuts) and eats them >1 time per week	+1
8. Consumes pasta or rice almost every day (≥5 times per week)	+1
9. Has cereals or grains (eg, bread) for breakfast	+1
10. Consumes nuts regularly (at least 2–3 times per week)	+1
11. Uses olive oil at home	+1
12. Skips breakfast	−1
13. Has a dairy product for breakfast (eg, yogurt, milk)	+1
14. Has commercially baked goods or pastries for breakfast	−1
15. Eats 2 servings of yogurt and/or cheese (1–1.5 oz [40 g]) daily	+1
16. Eats sweets and/or candy several times every day	−1

Scoring:

Add the sum of the values of items 1–16.

A score of >8 indicates an optimal Mediterranean-style diet.

A score of 4–7 indicates that improvement is needed to adjust intake to Mediterranean-style patterns.

A score of ≤3 indicates very low diet quality.

Adapted with permission from reference 9.

Table 12-6. Strategies for Providing Culturally Sensitive Nutritional Guidance

Cultural Consideration	Suggested Approach
Clinician, patient, and caregiver knowledge, attitudes, beliefs, and traditions, as well as the characteristics of the clinician-patient relationship, including communication style, trust, and prejudice, influence the success of that relationship.	Practice empathy. Test assumptions. Be aware of bias and prejudices. Aim to bridge differences in beliefs, communication approach, and decision-making approach. Learn more about a patient and family's culture and food traditions. Resources such as Oldways (https://oldwayspt.org) provide information about many traditional diets from around the world.
Cultural influence on views on healthful nutrition, physical activity, weight, and disease prevention influence the change process.	Ask open-ended questions to assess understanding and beliefs around nutrition and health. Elicit the patient's own motivations to change.
Current and future motivation to change is influenced by social supports, previous experiences, and access to resources that support the change.	Assess the patient's social supports and resources, including family support for change, access to healthful food and physical activity, and health literacy. Ascertain the patient's previous experience or efforts to change nutrition behaviors. Identify additional resources that may help support the patient and family in successfully making the change.
Helping the patient and family change requires negotiation between the patient, caregivers, and clinician.	Practice key communication skills, including open-ended questions, affirmations, reflective listening, and summarizing, to best understand the patient's situation, bring about a patient's change talk, and help the patient bring forth their own motivation for change. This is the practice of motivational interviewing, which is detailed in Chapter 14, Theories of Behavior Change and Motivational Interviewing.

Derived from reference 13.

In Sum
- Healthy eating plans are generally high in whole grains, fruits, and vegetables and low in added sugars, saturated fat, and sodium. The Healthy US-Style, DASH, vegetarian, and Mediterranean-style eating plans are examples of these types of eating patterns. That said, there is no one "healthiest" eating pattern. Rather, families are encouraged to adopt an eating pattern that best fits their preferences, cultural traditions, budget, and lifestyle, while aiming to eat as many whole foods, and minimizing intake of highly processed foods, to the extent possible.
- The MyPlate icon simplifies the Healthy US-Style Dietary Pattern into an easily understood and implemented graphic: a dinner plate divided into 4 sections—fruits, vegetables, protein, and grains accompanied by a glass of milk. The goal of this icon is to better visualize a balanced diet that is about 50% fruits and vegetables, with remaining portions made up of lean protein, grains, and dairy.

References

1. US Department of Health and Human Services, US Department of Agriculture. *Dietary Guidelines for Americans, 2020–2025.* 9th ed. 2020. Accessed October 5, 2022. https://www.dietaryguidelines.gov/sites/default/files/2020-12/Dietary_Guidelines_for_Americans_2020-2025.pdf

2. Global Food Research Program. *Ultra-processed Foods: A Global Threat to Public Health.* University of North Carolina at Chapel Hill. 2021. Accessed October 5, 2022. https://www.globalfoodresearchprogram.org/wp-content/uploads/2021/04/UPF_ultra-processed_food_fact_sheet.pdf

3. Wang L, Martínez Steele E, Du M, et al. Trends in consumption of ultraprocessed foods among US youths aged 2–19 years, 1999–2018. *JAMA.* 2021;326(6):519–530 PMID: 34374722 doi: 10.1001/jama.2021.10238

4. Hartline-Grafton HW, Weill J. *Replacing the Thrifty Food Plan in Order to Provide Adequate Allotments for SNAP Beneficiaries.* Food Research & Action Center; 2012

5. US Department of Agriculture. Official USDA food plans: cost of food at home at three levels, U.S. average, February 2022. Accessed October 5, 2022. https://fns-prod.azureedge.us/sites/default/files/media/file/CostofFoodFeb2022LowModLib.pdf

6. Chiavaroli L, Viguiliouk E, Nishi SK, et al. DASH dietary pattern and cardiometabolic outcomes: an umbrella review of systematic reviews and meta-analyses. *Nutrients.* 2019;11(2):338 PMID: 30764511 doi: 10.3390/nu11020338

7. Asghari G, Yuzbashian E, Mirmiran P, Hooshmand F, Najafi R, Azizi F. Dietary Approaches to Stop Hypertension (DASH) dietary pattern is associated with reduced incidence of metabolic syndrome in children and adolescents. *J Pediatr.* 2016;174:178–184.e1 PMID: 27156186 doi: 10.1016/j.jpeds.2016.03.077

8. Melina V, Craig W, Levin S. Position of the Academy of Nutrition and Dietetics: vegetarian diets. *J Acad Nutr Diet.* 2016;116(12):1970–1980 PMID: 27886704 doi: 10.1016/j.jand.2016.09.025

9. Serra-Majem L, Ribas L, García A, Pérez-Rodrigo C, Aranceta J. Nutrient adequacy and Mediterranean diet in Spanish school children and adolescents. *Eur J Clin Nutr.* 2003;57(suppl 1):S35–S39 PMID: 12947450 doi: 10.1038/sj.ejcn.1601812

10. Iaccarino Idelson P, Scalfi L, Valerio G. Adherence to the Mediterranean Diet in children and adolescents: a systematic review. *Nutr Metab Cardiovasc Dis.* 2017;27(4):283–299 PMID: 28254269 doi: 10.1016/j.numecd.2017.01.002

11. Dinu M, Pagliai G, Casini A, Sofi F. Mediterranean diet and multiple health outcomes: an umbrella review of meta-analyses of observational studies and randomised trials. *Eur J Clin Nutr.* 2018;72(1):30–43 PMID: 28488692 doi: 10.1038/ejcn.2017.58
12. Garcia-Marcos L, Castro-Rodriguez JA, Weinmayr G, Panagiotakos DB, Priftis KN, Nagel G. Influence of Mediterranean diet on asthma in children: a systematic review and meta-analysis. *Pediatr Allergy Immunol.* 2013;24(4):330–338 PMID: 23578354 doi: 10.1111/pai.12071
13. Stuart-Shor EM, Berra KA, Kamau MW, Kumanyika SK. Behavioral strategies for cardio-vascular risk reduction in diverse and underserved racial/ethnic groups. *Circulation.* 2012;125(1):171–184 PMID: 22215892 doi: 10.1161/CIRCULATIONAHA.110.968495

CHAPTER 13

Culinary Medicine and Strategies for Healthy Eating

Culinary medicine combines the art of cooking with the science of medicine. As a discipline, the goal of culinary medicine is to provide hands-on education about the influence of food on health and disease through cooking classes that teach the why and how of healthy eating patterns and low-cost, convenient, health-promoting, delicious home-cooked meals. Although the skills of culinary medicine may not be teachable through a book, this overview aims to provide practical applications to help patients build skills and self-efficacy in preparing healthful, enjoyable, culturally tailored, and cost-effective meals. Additionally, this chapter provides an overview of mindful and intuitive eating to support savoring and enjoyment of food.

Culinary medicine aims to help patients and families prepare, savor, and enjoy food; learn to like new tastes and textures; and incorporate cultural practices and mindfulness into eating routines. Parents and pediatricians are often concerned that children and adolescents refuse to eat in a way consistent with the *Dietary Guidelines for Americans* and the healthy eating patterns described in chapters 11, Dietary Guidelines and Principles of Healthy Eating, and 12, Healthy Eating Plans. Clinicians who apply principles of culinary medicine can help children and adolescents learn to like and prefer healthful foods in the quantities that are likely to promote optimal health and nutrition.

Taste as a Predictor of Intake

Taste is a strong predictor of intake, especially for children.[1] Humans experience 5 tastes: sweet, sour, bitter, salty, and umami (savory). Evolutionarily, humans evolved with a preference for sweet and salty foods and a dislike for bitter and sour foods. Hunter-gatherers needed to be able to distinguish safe and healthful foods from potential toxins. Foods that were sweet, such as berries, were generally safe for consumption, whereas plants that were bitter were more likely to be toxic. On the whole, simple carbohydrates taste sweet, the amino acids glutamate and aspartate taste savory, acids taste sour, and many toxic compounds and some vegetables taste bitter.[2] About 20% of people carry a gene that makes them "supertasters." They have many more taste buds that make them very sensitive to bitter tastes, which they often find to be repugnant. About 30% of people are "nontasters." Nontasters have fewer taste buds on the fungiform papillae than average, causing them to hardly notice bitter tastes.[3] These differences may help explain why some children express pickier eating habits than others. Strategies to prevent and address picky eating are discussed in chapters 17, Nutrition in Childhood and Adolescence, and 19, Mental Health, Behavioral, and Developmental Conditions.

Humans taste mostly with taste buds located on the papillae of the tongue, although there are some taste buds on the soft palate and pharynx. The tongue also contains other bumps on the surface of the anterior two-thirds of the tongue (known as *filiform papillae*) that help detect texture.[2]

At the same time that the brain is processing a food's taste, it is receiving another message from the olfactory center in the posterior nasal cavity. The smell of a food combined with its taste and texture is how humans experience flavor.[4] There are 350 to 400 types of odor receptors and a total of about 40 million smell receptors in the posterior nasal cavity. The sense of smell is powerful. It can differentiate hundreds of distinct odors and is 10,000 times more sensitive than the sense of taste.

An Acquired Taste

Both taste and texture preferences can change with repeated exposures. For example, infants exposed to a wide variety of healthful foods, including bitter and sour tastes— first in utero through amniotic fluid, next through maternal breast milk, and then in the first several months of exposure to solid foods—come to like a wide variety of foods. A toddler has a natural tendency to reject new foods (neophobia) but can learn to like a new food after many repeated exposures. In fact, it can take 8 to 10 or more tries of a food to like it and even more for some children who have more rigid prefer-ences.[5,6] With time and repeated exposures, foods that were once rejected can become not only tolerable but even preferred. To help children acquire a taste for healthful foods, even those that the child has previously rejected, clinicians should encourage parents and other caregivers to repeatedly expose children to these foods and limit access to highly processed and sugary foods. Strategies to help infants, children, and adolescents increase liking of new foods are detailed in chapters 16, Nutrition in Infancy, and 17, Nutrition in Childhood and Adolescence.

Just as a child can come to acquire a taste for bitter and sour foods with repeated expo-sures, there is some evidence that they may decrease a craving or taste for sweet foods and drinks by decreasing sugar in their diet.[7] When a child reduces or eliminates sugar or salt intake, their brain initially craves the sugar and salt more.[8] However, if this craving is ignored, it may eventually lessen, and very sweet or very salty foods no longer taste as good. Parents and other caregivers who are working with a child to reduce sugar and salt intake may help reduce cravings by removing sugary and salty foods from the home and pantry so the child does not have to rely on willpower to avoid these foods.

Taste Enhancers

As caregivers work to help their children increase willingness to try new foods, clini-cians may consider offering suggestions to help improve a child's perception of a food's taste. For example, meals and foods that are brightly colored are generally more ap-pealing than dark- or bland-colored foods, except for green-colored foods, which many children reject because of the association of green with bitter vegetables. Clinicians might encourage parents to plate foods in a way that includes foods of several different colors or foods in shapes or sizes that may seem fun to a child.

Temperature also influences the perception of food taste. The same amount of sugar tastes sweeter at higher temperatures, whereas the opposite is true for salt: the same amount of salt tastes saltier at lower temperatures. The combination of cold and hot temperatures or hot and spicy foods in the same dish enhances flavor. Foods served at their ideal temperature taste better. Clinicians might note to caregivers to aim to serve foods at their ideal temperature whenever possible to help facilitate a child's increased liking of the foods.

Adding a *small amount* of table salt to foods during food preparation enhances sweet taste and reduces bitter taste and generally amplifies a food's tastes. Adding a small amount of black pepper during food preparation adds flavor to a food and enhances the salty taste. Small amounts of spices and herbs can notably enhance the taste of a food or meal. Spices are components of aromatic plants, such as bark, roots, buds, flowers, fruits, and seeds that are grown in the tropics, and add a sweet, spicy, or hot flavor to foods. Herbs are leaves and stems of plants that grow in temperate climates. Seeds such as caraway and sesame, which come from tropical and temperate regions, and dehydrated vegetables (eg, celery, garlic salt) also add flavor to foods.

Nonnutritive Sweeteners

Children and adolescents prefer sweet foods, but, as has been discussed, too much sugar intake is detrimental to health. In an effort to reduce sugar intake while selecting foods and beverages that children like to eat and drink, many caregivers may choose products sweetened with nonnutritive sweeteners, defined as *noncaloric sweeteners* used to increase the palatability of foods. They include the US Food and Drug Administration (FDA)–approved artificial sweeteners saccharin, aspartame, acesulfame potassium, sucralose, and neotame and the plant-based sweeteners stevia and luo han guo, which are generally recognized as safe (GRAS for short) by the FDA. Nonnutritive sweeteners are highly prevalent in the food supply, including foods and beverages targeted to young children. Nonnutritive sweeteners are intensely sweet—180 to 20,000 times sweeter than sugar. There is some concern that early exposure to this degree of sweetness may negatively affect a child's taste preferences, but there are limited data to know whether this is true. Some evidence suggests that when nonnutritive sweeteners are substituted for calorically sweetened foods and beverages, they can support slowed weight gain or weight loss in the short term, but long-term data are lacking.[9] In all, too few studies have been done in children to fully understand the potential effects of artificial noncaloric sweeteners.

Mindful and Intuitive Eating

As important as what children and adolescents eat is how they eat. Increased mindfulness and savoring of food may help patients enjoy food and eating while eating the right portion sizes of foods to support optimal growth and nutrition. Mindfulness includes several key principles to be practiced together.[10]

- Non-judging: being open minded to the new and unfamiliar
- Patience: slowing down and increasing awareness of the moment and the experience

- Beginner's mindset: approaching each experience as if new
- Trust: noticing, appreciating, and accepting one's experience
- Non-striving: savoring the moment
- Acceptance: noticing and accepting one's experience, whether positive or not

Oftentimes, parents express frustrations about how their children eat. For example, some worry that children refuse to try certain foods, overeat other foods, eat too fast, or mindlessly snack or graze on foods throughout the day. Teaching parents, children, and adolescents about the principles of mindful eating can help families establish family rules or norms consistent with these principles. This set of rules or norms can help children grow up to have a positive relationship with food and use their body's cues for hunger and fullness to guide intake. In addition, parents can be particularly influential models in helping their children practice mindful principles.

Mindfulness applied to eating experiences is often referred to as *intuitive eating,* although there are some nuanced differences debated in the literature. Although most of the research and focus of intuitive eating has been on adults, in large part in response to a diet-centric culture, the principles also apply to school-aged children and adolescents. Studies to date suggest that mindful and intuitive eating are associated with improved psychological health,[11] although they may not lead to changes in energy intake or diet quality.[12] The essence of intuitive eating is explained by the oft-cited 10 principles of intuitive eating first described in 1995 by registered dietitians Evelyn Tribole and Elyse Resch.

1. Focus on and encourage healthy habits to promote health and de-emphasize both weight and a focus on weight loss.
2. Advise families to help children recognize their body's cues of hunger and fullness and use those cues to guide intake. Encourage parents to allow their child to determine portion size based on hunger and satiety rather than dictate portions.
3. Encourage a healthy home environment to support healthy choices as default. Encourage families to incorporate all foods into a healthy eating plan, and discourage families from eliminating whole food groups or restricting food, especially if done to lose weight.
4. Encourage families to avoid labeling foods as "good" or "bad," or labeling days as "good" or "bad," on the basis of food intake.
5. Help patients practice savoring their food. Savoring involves using all senses to experience a food. It encourages slowing down and noticing the texture, taste, smell, feel, and sound of the food while eating it (**Box 13-1**). It can be particularly effective in helping children and adolescents practice slowing down while eating, decreasing portion sizes if they tend to overeat, or consuming smaller portions of desserts and sweets.
6. Help patients learn to use tools such as the hunger meter to identify feelings of both hunger and satiety (**Box 13-2**). Patients should practice stopping when content, rather than when uncomfortably full. Strategies such as use of the hunger meter are commonly referred to as *appetite awareness* in the literature and have been shown to effectively support long-term maintenance of a healthier weight when included with family-based behavioral obesity treatment.[13]

Box 13-1. Savoring and the Raisin Meditation

The "raisin meditation" offers an approach to help school-aged children, adolescents, and their families increase mindfulness around eating and practice savoring by paying attention to each of the senses when eating a food. This meditation can also be done with a sweet or preferred food.

Raisin meditation

1. Place a single raisin on a table.
2. Imagine that you have just been dropped on Earth, with no past experiences, including neither having seen nor tasted a raisin. Take a few deep breaths.
3. Look at the raisin carefully. Notice its curves, its wrinkles, its shiny parts, and its dull parts.
4. Pick up the raisin. Feel its weight.
5. Roll the raisin between your fingers. Listen to its sound. Feel its stickiness.
6. Smell the raisin.
7. Notice how you feel about the raisin.
8. Place the raisin into your mouth and hold it there. Do not bite down. What do you taste?
9. Bite down on the raisin one time. What do you notice?
10. Slowly chew. What do you experience with each bite?
11. Chew the raisin until it is liquid in your mouth before you swallow.
12. Swallow the raisin.
13. Close your eyes for a few breaths and consider what you just experienced.

A caregiver may ask the child what they thought of the experience and how it might change the way they approach food. The caregiver could ask the child whether they would be willing to try this experiment with a dessert food the next time they eat dessert. The act of practicing savoring this way may help children be more mindful of what they are eating, enjoy the food more, and be likely to be satisfied with a smaller portion of food or dessert in the future.

Adapted with permission from reference 10.

7. Recognize potential emotional triggers for eating. Help families develop a list of healthful, nonfood strategies to cope with triggers such as boredom, anxiety, sadness, and anger.
8. Reinforce that healthy bodies come in all shapes and sizes.

Box 13-2. The Hunger Meter

Starving	Hungry	Neutral	Satisfied	Stuffed
1	2 Start eating here	3	4 Stop eating here	5
Very, very hungry - too hungry!! You may feel weak, your stomach may hurt, or you may have a headache	Your stomach feels empty and may be growling. You are ready to start to eat!	You are not hungry but not yet satisfied	You are not hungry and may feel uncomfortable if you ate more.	You feel a little too full and you feel uncomfortable

Children and adolescents can learn to recognize their body's signals of hunger and satiety and connect that to a number or rating on the meter. The aim is to eat when very hungry (stomach is beginning to growl, around a 2 on the hunger meter) and stop when comfortably full (around a 4 on the hunger meter). Clinicians may consider sharing this tool with patients and families to help them practice using hunger and satiety cues to guide intake. Clinicians can encourage patients to ask themselves "Am I hungry?" before eating. If the answer is no, clinicians can encourage patients to ask themselves follow-up questions such as "What prompted my desire to eat? Boredom, stress, availability of the food, social cues, … ?" If the answer is yes, clinicians can encourage patients to ask themselves "How hungry? Extremely, very, a little bit, … ?"

Hunger meter reproduced with permission from Zucker N, Craighead LW. *Children's Appetite Awareness Training*. Duke University Medical Center; 2003.

9. Encourage movement as a way to feel good and gain energy and strength.
10. Encourage families to follow an eating plan that promotes health and tastes good and that allows for favorite or highly enjoyable foods sometimes, even if those foods are not considered healthy by nutrition standards.

Strategies for Healthy Eating

Helping families take steps toward eating healthier or making a nutritional change in response to a health concern extends beyond providing education and increasing nutrition knowledge. Although there may not always be time or patient interest to deploy all the strategies, clinicians can support patients and their families in making changes that better align with the dietary guidelines by incorporating some of the following strategies for healthier eating into clinical practice.

Empowering Families to Cook

When families prepare meals at home, the nutritional value of the meal is likely to contain many more nutrients and less sugars and sodium than when eating out. Consequently, children are more likely to adhere more to the dietary guidelines and healthy eating plans described in chapters 11, Dietary Guidelines and Principles of Healthy Eating, and 12, Healthy Eating Plans. Clinicians should encourage families to eat more home-cooked meals. However, although home-cooked meals can be delicious, healthy, and easy to prepare, many families experience numerous barriers to home cooking, such as limited food preparation knowledge and skills, time, and financial resources. As such, clinicians may need to provide families with extra support to help increase a family's desire and self-efficacy to cook. Following are a few strategies that clinicians can deploy to offer this additional support:

- **Learn more about a patient and family's cultural and individual taste preferences, food values, and priorities.** Use this information to tailor nutrition recommendations to incorporate foods and routines that families are likely to enjoy. When available, connect families to community resources or programs that can help support them in making nutritional changes that align with their cultural practices and values.
- **Share recipes.** For patients who express an interest in cooking more meals at home but note that they do not know much about cooking, clinicians can start by sharing introductory recipes such as those included in Part 5, Frequently Asked Questions, Case Studies, and Recipes, most of which contain only a few ingredients and are easy to follow. Additionally, clinicians in many parts of the United States can refer to Share Our Strength's Cooking Matters or similar programs to teach nutrition, culinary, meal planning, and shopping skills for healthful foods at low cost to families with low income. Some of these programs involve parents and children together in learning culinary and nutrition skills. **Box 13-3** highlights culinary resources for families and clinicians.
- **Recommend substitutions.** Encourage families to steam, bake, grill, boil, broil, stir-fry, or microwave foods rather than fry, panfry, or sauté foods. In addition, using liquid fats such as olive, canola, or vegetable oil, rather than solid fats such as butter or margarine or tropical oils such as coconut or palm, helps decrease saturated fat intake. Families can reduce salt intake by seasoning foods with herbs, spices, lime or lemon juice, or vinegar instead of salt.
- **Share ideas of how to save time.** Many families perceive that they do not have time to make home-cooked meals on a daily or regular basis. A few strategies that can help save time include batch cooking, in which portions of the week's meals are prepared over the weekend and then frozen to easily reheat later in the week.
- **Encourage caregivers to involve children and adolescents in food selection and preparation.** When children help select and prepare foods, they are more likely to try and enjoy them. They also are more likely to learn how to recognize a balanced meal and become competent at home cooking as they grow older. Acknowledge that although teaching children to cook does not always save time at first, it can help save time in the long run, as children get older and can competently choose and prepare balanced family meals. Age-appropriate strategies to engage children and adolescents in meal preparation are highlighted in **Table 13-1**.

CLINICAL PRACTICE TIP

Box 13-3. Culinary Resources for Families and Clinicians

Resources for families	Resources for clinicians
Encourage families to visit Cooking Matters (https://cookingmatters.org) to access free cooking classes and digital resources, including healthy recipes and videos. Cooking Matters' aim is to help parents and other caregivers learn to choose and prepare healthful foods on a budget.	Clinicians can partner with Cooking Matters to bring its programs and resources to their community and can learn more at the campaign's website (https://cookingmatters.org/community-resources). Cooking Matters periodically offers various funding and grant opportunities.
Encourage families to visit ChopChop Family (www.chopchopfamily.org) for recipe ideas and tools to help children learn to cook.	Clinicians can visit the Tulane Goldring Center for Culinary Medicine website for continuing medical education opportunities, online cooking classes, and more (https://goldringcenter.tulane.edu).
Families can visit the Bonus Bites section of Raddish (www.raddishkids.com) for recipes, lesson plans for family use, and videos to help children learn basic cooking skills and prepare a wide variety of dishes.	Clinicians can find recipes, expert videos, and continuing education opportunities from the American College of Preventive Medicine at its website (https://members.acpm.org/page/culinarymedicine).
Visit HealthyChildren.org, the official American Academy of Pediatrics website for parents (www.healthychildren.org/recipes), for a variety of easy-to-make, child-friendly recipes.	Clinicians can enroll in a hands-on culinary continuing medical education experience by attending Healthy Kitchens, Healthy Lives, hosted by Harvard T.H. Chan School of Public Health and the Culinary Institute of America.

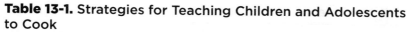

Table 13-1. Strategies for Teaching Children and Adolescents to Cook

Developmental stage	Kitchen tasks[a]
Toddler (ages 1–3)	• Sift dry contents • Stir ingredients • "Paint" pans/vegetables/chicken with oil with pastry brush • Play with dough and cookie cutters • Pick fresh herbs from garden or potted plant • Help arrange foods into interesting shapes and designs, such as smiley faces or stars
Preschool (ages 3–5)	• Rinse produce • Measure dry ingredients • Mix simple ingredients • Cut soft fruits or vegetables with a dull knife or dough scraper • Push the blender or food processor button to turn on the machine • Season foods with salt/pepper/herbs • Grease pan
School-aged (ages 5–11)	• Read recipe • Peel and chop vegetables • Crack egg • Clean lettuce for salad • Measure and mix dry and wet ingredients • Open cans
Adolescent (ages 12–18)	• Follow a simple recipe • Boil pasta • Chop vegetables • Plan balanced meals

[a] All tasks should be supervised by an adult.

Reproduced from reference 14.

Helping Families Plan Meals

Interventions that help families build desire and self-efficacy to eat more meals at home will positively influence nutrition and overall health. One way that clinicians can intervene is by encouraging families to create a meal plan that includes meals and snacks for the week. A healthy meal contains a balance of food groups to help provide for nutrient needs aligned with the dietary guidelines and MyPlate recommendations (refer to chapters 11, Dietary Guidelines and Principles of Healthy Eating, and 12, Healthy Eating Plans), and each snack includes 2 to 3 food groups, with at least 1 fruit or vegetable. A simple template for a meal plan is shown in **Table 13-2**. Patients can use this or a similar template to plan meals for the week. A sample completed meal plan and grocery

Table 13-2. Meal Planning Worksheet

Day	Breakfast	Lunch	Dinner	Snacks	Grocery list
Monday					
Tuesday					
Wednesday					
Thursday					
Friday					
Saturday					
Sunday					

list using mostly recipes included in Part 5, Frequently Asked Questions, Case Studies, and Recipes, is shown in **Table 13-3**. Although it may not be possible to always follow the meal plan, having a plan and considering in advance what to eat for the week helps decrease the frequency of eating out at restaurants or purchasing take-out food.

Sharing Tips for Healthier Food Selection and Storage

Efforts to help families improve their nutrition intake may sometimes include offering advice or suggestions on how to select or prepare foods. This section offers some key guidance that clinicians may consider sharing with patients and their families.

Food Selection Tips

Children are most likely to eat what is readily available in their home. As such, care-givers can significantly influence a child's eating habits by changing what foods are brought into the home. Sharing some of the following grocery shopping tips with families may help them adopt healthier nutrition habits. This information is best directed at the person or people in the family who are most often responsible for choosing and preparing meals, whether a parent, a grandparent, or other nutrition gatekeepers.

- Encourage families to create a grocery list that includes the ingredients needed for the week's meals and a detailed list of other snacks and beverages that the family may need for the week. Taking inventory of what is already available at home in the pantry, refrigerator, or freezer before selecting meals for the week or writing the grocery list can help save money and prevent food waste.
- Share the following tips for selecting affordable and high-quality ingredients:
  - **Meat, poultry, and seafood.** The leanest cuts of meat are the round and loin. The tenderest cuts of beef include the short loin and sirloin, as well as the very fatty ribs. The round is a medium tender cut. Poultry and fish are generally healthier than red meat and beef. Fish is very high in protein and essential nutrients, such as omega-3 polyunsaturated fats. Eating fish 2 times per week offers proven health benefits.[15]

Table 13-3. A Sample Weekly Meal Plan

Day	Breakfast	Lunch	Dinner	Snacks	Grocery list
Monday	Greek yogurt with berries and bananas	Whole Wheat Pita Veggie Pizzas[a]	Simple Baked Chicken Breast, Simple Roasted Vegetables[a]	Carrots and Cucumbers With Creamy Ranch Bean Dip[a]	Proteins ● Boneless, skinless chicken breasts ● Canned black beans ● Canned cannellini beans ● Canned tuna ● Eggs ● Ground turkey ● Nut butter (eg, peanut butter, almond butter)
Tuesday	Overnight Oats with fruit[a]	Chicken Whole Wheat Pita Wraps With Creamy Ranch Bean Dip[a]	Turkey-Spinach Meatballs With Spaghetti, Roasted Garlicky and Cheesy Broccoli[a]	Apple slices with nut butter	Dairy/dairy alternatives ● Milk (cow milk or plant-based variety) ● Shredded cheddar cheese ● Shredded mozzarella cheese ● Yogurt, Greek and/or plain, and vanilla or strawberry
Wednesday	Caramelized Banana Cinnamon Oatmeal[a]	Roasted Vegetable Grilled Cheese[a]	Turkey-bean chili with sweet potatoes (Refer to the variation of the Tofu-Bean Chili With Sweet Potatoes recipe.)[a]	Fruit kabobs	Grains ● Rice ● Old-fashioned rolled oats ● Whole grain spaghetti ● Whole wheat/whole grain bread ● Whole wheat pita bread
Thursday	Avocado toast, side of fruit	Tuna Melts With Whole Grain Bread[a]	Turkey and Vegetable Whole Wheat Chow Mein-style Noodles[a]	Half an avocado with salt and pepper	Produce ● Apples ● Avocados ● Baby spinach and frozen spinach ● Bananas ● Berries ● Broccoli
Friday	Toast with banana and nut butter	Creamy Broccoli and Cheese Soup[a]	Turkey white bean burgers with avocado (Refer to the variation of the Chicken Black Bean Burgers With Avocado recipe.)[a]	Frozen Yogurt Banana Pops[a]	

Continued

Table 13-3 (continued)

Day	Breakfast	Lunch	Dinner	Snacks	Grocery list
Saturday	Vegetable omelet	Tuna sandwiches, leftover Creamy Broccoli and Cheese Soup[a]	"All the Vegetables" Fried Rice[a]	Peppers with guacamole	Produce (continued) ● Carrots ● Cauliflower ● Celery ● Cucumbers ● Garlic ● Green onions ● Onions (white, yellow, or red) ● Peppers, red bell and green bell varieties ● Sweet potatoes ● Tomato Herbs/spices/condiments ● Broth, vegetable or chicken ● Dill pickles ● Dried dill weed ● Garlic powder ● Ground black pepper ● Ground cinnamon ● Ground cumin ● Honey ● Marinara sauce ● Mayonnaise, low-fat ● Olive oil ● Onion powder ● Salt ● Smoked paprika ● Soy sauce ● Tomato paste
Sunday	Veggie Frittata Muffins[a] (Use all leftover scraps of vegetables from the week.)	Leftovers Soup[a]	Baked Sweet Potatoes, leftover turkey-bean chili[a]	Banana split with yogurt and berries	

[a] Refer to Part 5, Frequently Asked Questions, Case Studies, and Recipes, for recipe.

— **Produce.** For the best taste (and smallest impact on the environment), patients might visit a local farmers market and choose produce that is locally grown and in season, whenever possible. Families who receive Supplemental Nutrition Assistance Program or Special Supplemental Nutrition Program for Women, Infants, and Children benefits may be able to use their benefit at select markets, and in some states, the Supplemental Nutrition Assistance Program value is doubled when spent at a farmers market. These purchases not only support the local farmer but also help ensure that the client gets the freshest produce available. That said, families do not need to choose fresh produce. The nutritional value of canned and frozen produce is essentially the same as that of fresh produce. In fact, canned and frozen produce can sometimes have even greater nutritional density. However, sometimes sugary syrup or juice is added to canned fruit, and salt is added to many canned vegetables. Clinicians may advise patients to choose fruit canned in its own juice and to review the Nutrition Facts label to choose canned vegetables with lower sodium or to rinse canned produce.

- Encourage patients to read and use nutrition labels to make healthier choices. Key points in interpreting the nutrition label are discussed in Chapter 1, Dietary Reference Intakes. Many food manufacturers participate in the voluntary Facts Up Front initiative of the Consumer Brands Association and the Food Marketing Institute in which information about key nutrients in a product, such as calories, saturated fat, sodium, and added sugars, are included in the front of the nutrition label. Some foods packages also include health claims that describe a relationship between a food substance and a reduced risk of a disease or health-related condition (eg, "Fiber decreases heart disease"). These are the most closely regulated front-of-package claims, requiring premarket review and FDA authorization. Structure/function claims (eg, "DHA promotes brain health" or "Calcium builds strong bones") sometimes appear on food packages and supplements. Although required to be truthful and not misleading, these claims do not require premarket review or FDA authorization.
- Advise families to buy groceries when not hungry and not rushed and to avoid purchasing unhealthful foods marketed at children.
- Share strategies that may help patients save money, such as cutting coupons, comparing unit prices listed on shelves and choosing the lower-cost item, buying generic and store brands, and purchasing frequently consumed items in bulk.
- Help families make informed decisions about whether to purchase non–genetically modified organism (GMO) products. A GMO is a plant, an animal, or a microorganism that has had its DNA changed through genetic engineering in which DNA is transferred from one organism to another to provide a desired trait, such as increased resistance to insects, drought tolerance, and improved nutritional value.
  - The reasons for genetic modification include higher crop yields, less crop loss, longer storage life, better appearance, better nutrition, or a combination of these qualities. Crops that may be derived from GMOs include soybeans, corn, potatoes, summer squash, apples, papayas, pineapple, sugar beets, and

ingredients derived from the crops, such as cornstarch, corn syrup, corn oil, soybean oil, canola oil, and granulated sugar. Most animal feed consists of GMO crops.

— Genetically modified organism foods have been available to consumers since the 1990s, but AquAdvantage Salmon, which is genetically engineered to grow faster than its nongenetically engineered Atlantic salmon counterpart, is the first GMO animal in the food supply.

— Genetically modified organism foods are closely regulated by the FDA, US Department of Agriculture, and Environmental Protection Agency and are safe for consumption.[16] Beginning in 2022, food makers, importers, and retailers are required to include whether the food or ingredients were derived from GMOs or bioengineered organisms. The food packaging must clearly state "bioengineered food," show the bioengineered food symbols, or include an electronic or digital link. Of note, restaurant foods and highly processed foods that no longer contain detectable amounts of the modified genetic material are exempt from the label requirement.

● Help families make informed decisions about whether to choose organic or conventional products. Many people believe that organic foods are superior to conventionally grown items. Knowing this belief, food manufacturers carefully promote and market their products to appeal to customers. The terminology can often be confusing or sometimes be misleading. **Table 13-4** includes several commonly used food marketing terms and the definition of each term. Researchers of studies evaluating the role of organic foods and health benefits over the past 60 years have concluded that there are insufficient data to determine whether organic foods are healthier than conventionally grown foods. Clinical trial data are based on short-term studies that have shown no differences between organic and conventionally grown produce and health outcomes. Some observational studies of varying quality showed an association with organic diet and reduced risk of metabolic syndrome, elevated body mass index, non-Hodgkin lymphoma, infertility, birth defects, allergic sensitization, otitis media, and preeclampsia.[18]

In its clinical report on organic foods, the American Academy of Pediatrics concludes that[17]

— The nutritional difference between organic and inorganic food seems minimal on the basis of the studies to date.

— Organic produce contains fewer pesticides than conventional produce. The health impacts of this difference are unclear.

— Organic animal husbandry that prohibits nontherapeutic antibiotics may reduce human disease caused by drug-resistant organisms.

— There is no clinically relevant difference between organic and conventional milk.

— Organic farming approaches are usually more expensive than conventional approaches.

— The price difference between organic and conventional food could be reduced or eliminated as organic farming techniques advance and the price of petroleum products increase.

Table 13-4. Commonly Used Food Product Marketing Terms

Term	Definition
100% organic	Must contain only organic ingredients (excluding water and salt)
Organic	Must consist of at least 95% organically produced ingredients (excluding water and salt). Any remaining product ingredients must consist of nonagricultural substances approved on the USDA National List of Allowed and Prohibited Substances.
Made with organic ingredients	Must contain at least 70% organic ingredients
Natural	Contains no artificial ingredients or added colors and is only minimally processed. The label must explain the use of the term.
Free range	Producers must demonstrate to the USDA that the animal has been allowed access to the outside.
No hormones (pork or poultry)	All poultry and pork sold in the United States must be hormone-free. Therefore, the phrase "no hormones added" cannot be used on the labels of pork or poultry unless followed by this statement: "Federal regulations prohibit the use of hormones."
No hormones (beef)	The phrase "no hormones administered" may be approved for use on the label of beef products if sufficient documentation is provided to the USDA by the producer showing that no hormones have been given to the animals, such as by injection or in their feed.
No antibiotics (red meat and poultry)	The phrase "no antibiotics added" may be used on labels for meat or poultry products if sufficient documentation is provided by the producer to the USDA demonstrating that the animals have not been given antibiotics.
Certified	*Certified* implies that the USDA Food Safety and Inspection Service and the Agriculture Marketing Service have officially evaluated a meat product.
Chemical-free	This term is not allowed to be used on a label.
Non-GMO	This term indicates that the food was produced without genetic engineering and the ingredients were not derived from GMOs. Organic foods are by definition non-GMO, but not all non-GMO foods are organic.

Abbreviations: GMO, genetically modified organism; USDA, US Department of Agriculture.
Adapted from reference 17.

— Organic farming reduces fossil fuel consumption and environmental contamination with pesticides and herbicides.

— Large prospective cohort studies may help enhance understanding of the relationship between pesticide exposure and consumption of hormone-treated animals and human disease.

Overall, organic foods are produced in ways that are more environmentally conscious and more costly than their conventionally grown counterparts. Thus, organic foods cost more than their conventionally grown counterparts, although the nutritional value is essentially equivalent. Although organic foods may contain lower amounts of pesticides, health implications of this difference are not well understood. In all, the American Academy of Pediatrics recommends that pediatricians advise patients and families as follows[17]:

— Encourage families to eat a diet rich in fruits, vegetables, whole grains, and dairy products.

— Share with families the previously listed conclusions, including nutrition, health, environmental, and cost issues.

— Share resources such as the Environmental Working Group Dirty Dozen and Clean Fifteen lists with families concerned about pesticide exposure (**Box 13-4**).

Food Storage Tips

In helping families minimize food waste and stretch their food budgets, clinicians may find occasion to offer the following food storage tips. The infographic in **Figure 13-1** shows recommended storage methods and locations for various products. Following these suggestions helps items last longer. This is especially important for produce because many families may be reluctant to purchase fresh fruits and vegetables if they feel the produce is unlikely to be eaten before it spoils. The FoodKeeper app, developed by the US Department of Agriculture, Cornell University, and the Food Marketing Institute, includes a complete guide for how long every food available in the United States keeps in the pantry, refrigerator, and freezer.

Additionally, **Figure 13-2** from the FDA shows how long different foods can be safely stored in the refrigerator and freezer.

Box 13-4. The Environmental Working Group Dirty Dozen and Clean Fifteen

The Environmental Working Group annually publishes a list of fruits and vegetables with levels of pesticides that are highest (the Dirty Dozen) and lowest (Clean Fifteen).

Dirty Dozen: It is recommended that families lower pesticide exposure by buying organically grown versions of these items when possible.

1. Strawberries
2. Spinach
3. Kale, collard, and mustard greens
4. Nectarines
5. Apples
6. Grapes
7. Bell and hot peppers
8. Cherries
9. Peaches
10. Pears
11. Celery
12. Tomatoes

Clean Fifteen: These produce items are low in pesticides; therefore, purchasing the organic versions of them is probably unnecessary.

1. Avocado
2. Sweet corn
3. Pineapple
4. Onions
5. Papaya
6. Sweet peas (frozen)
7. Asparagus
8. Honeydew melon
9. Kiwi
10. Cabbage
11. Mushrooms
12. Cantaloupe
13. Mangoes
14. Watermelon
15. Sweet potatoes

Lists reproduced from Environmental Working Group. EWG's 2022 Shopper's Guide to Pesticides in Produce. Accessed October 5, 2022. https://www.ewg.org/foodnews/summary.php.

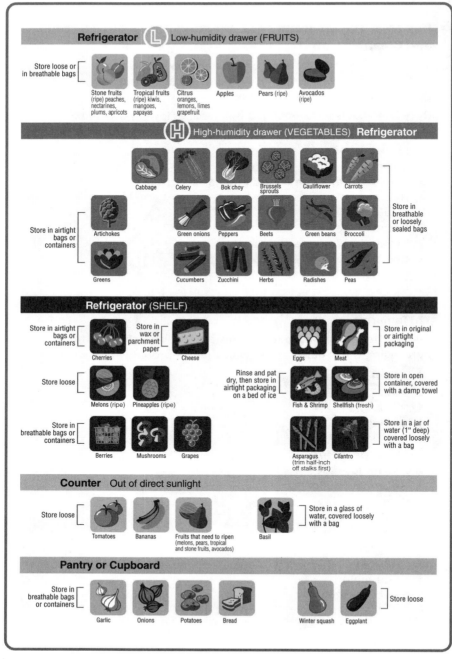

Figure 13-1. Food storage guide.

REFRIGERATOR & FREEZER STORAGE CHART

These short but safe time limits will help keep refrigerated food 40° F (4° C) from spoiling or becoming dangerous.
Since product dates aren't a guide for safe use of a product, consult this chart and follow these tips.
- Purchase the product before "sell-by" or expiration dates.
- Follow handling recommendations on product.
- Keep meat and poultry in its package until just before using.
- If freezing meat and poultry in its original package longer than 2 months, overwrap these packages with airtight heavy-duty foil, plastic wrap, or freezer paper; or place the package inside a plastic bag.

Because freezing 0° F (-18° C) keeps food safe indefinitely, the following recommended storage times are for quality only.

Product	Refrigerator	Freezer
Eggs		
Fresh, in shell	3 - 5 weeks	Don't freeze
Raw yolks, whites	2 - 4 days	1 year
Hard cooked	1 week	Don't freeze
Liquid pasteurized eggs or egg substitutes,		
opened	3 days	Don't freeze
unopened	10 days	1 year
TV Dinners, Frozen Casseroles		
Keep frozen until ready to heat		3 - 4 months
Deli & Vacuum-Packed Products		
Store-prepared (or homemade) egg, chicken, tuna, ham, macaroni salads	3 - 5 days	Don't freeze
Pre-stuffed pork & lamb chops, chicken breasts stuffed w/dressing	1 day	Don't freeze
Store-cooked convenience meals	3 - 4 days	Don't freeze
Commercial brand vacuum-packed dinners with USDA seal, unopened	2 weeks	Don't freeze
Raw Hamburger, Ground & Stew Meat		
Hamburger & stew meats	1 - 2 days	3 - 4 months
Ground turkey, veal, pork, lamb	1 - 2 days	3 - 4 months
Ham, Corned Beef		
Corned beef in pouch with pickling juices	5 - 7 days	Drained, 1 month
Ham, canned, labeled "Keep Refrigerated," unopened	6 - 9 months	Don't freeze
opened	3 - 5 days	1 - 2 months
Ham, fully cooked, whole	7 days	1 - 2 months
Ham, fully cooked, half	3 - 5 days	1 - 2 months
Ham, fully cooked, slices	3 - 4 days	1 - 2 months
Hot Dogs & Lunch Meats (in freezer wrap)		
Hot dogs,		
opened package	1 week	1 - 2 months
unopened package	2 weeks	1 - 2 months
Lunch meats,		
opened package	3 - 5 days	1 - 2 months
unopened package	2 weeks	1 - 2 months

Product	Refrigerator	Freezer
Soups & Stews		
Vegetable or meat-added & mixtures of them	3 - 4 days	2 - 3 months
Bacon & Sausage		
Bacon	7 days	1 month
Sausage, raw from pork, beef, chicken or turkey	1 - 2 days	1 - 2 months
Smoked breakfast links, patties	7 days	1 - 2 months
Fresh Meat (Beef, Veal, Lamb, & Pork)		
Steaks	3 - 5 days	6 - 12 months
Chops	3 - 5 days	4 - 6 months
Roasts	3 - 5 days	4 - 12 months
Variety meats (tongue, kidneys, liver, heart, chitterlings)	1 - 2 days	3 - 4 months
Meat Leftovers		
Cooked meat & meat dishes	3 - 4 days	2 - 3 months
Gravy & meat broth	1 - 2 days	2 - 3 months
Fresh Poultry		
Chicken or turkey, whole	1 - 2 days	1 year
Chicken or turkey, parts	1 - 2 days	9 months
Giblets	1 - 2 days	3 - 4 months
Cooked Poultry, Leftover		
Fried chicken	3 - 4 days	4 months
Cooked poultry dishes	3 - 4 days	4 - 6 months
Pieces, plain	3 - 4 days	4 months
Pieces covered with broth, gravy	3 - 4 days	6 months
Chicken nuggets, patties	3 - 4 days	1 - 3 months
Fish & Shellfish		
Lean fish	1 - 2 days	6 - 8 months
Fatty fish	1 - 2 days	2 - 3 months
Cooked fish	3 - 4 days	4 - 6 months
Smoked fish	14 days	2 months
Fresh shrimp, scallops, crawfish, squid	1 - 2 days	3 - 6 months
Canned seafood (Pantry, 5 years)	after opening 3 - 4 days	out of can 2 months

Figure 13-2. US Food and Drug Administration refrigerator and freezer storage chart.

Abbreviation: USDA, US Department of Agriculture.

Reproduced from US Food and Drug Administration. Food facts. 2019. Accessed October 5, 2022. https://www.fda.gov/media/101389/download.

In Sum

- Culinary medicine combines the art of cooking with the science of medicine. Its goal is to provide hands-on education about the influence of food on health and disease through cooking classes that teach the why and how of healthy eating patterns and low-cost, convenient, health-promoting, delicious home-cooked meals. Although primary care clinicians may not have the time, resources, or interest to offer cooking classes, sharing some key points may help families improve their overall nutrition intake while continuing to enjoy eating a wide variety of foods.

- Taste is a strong predictor of intake, especially for children. Humans evolved with a preference for sweet and salty foods and a dislike for bitter and sour foods. However, with repeated exposures, children can come to like a previously rejected food. Offering visually appealing meals, serving foods at their ideal temperature, and using flavor enhancers can help increase a child's desire to try a food and help increase their liking of a food.

- Nonnutritive sweeteners are readily available in the food supply and offer a strategy to increase sweetness of foods without the use of sugar and excess calories; however, their safety and utility for children are uncertain.

- Teaching child and adolescent patients to practice mindful and intuitive eating can help improve enjoyment of food and a healthy relationship with food while helping improve overall nutrition intake and avoid overeating or undereating.

- Helping patients and families learn to cook and meal plan can help improve nutrition intake and close the gap between the dietary guidelines and typical dietary intake. Additionally, offering patients strategies for food selection and storage to help stretch their food budget while being able to incorporate nutrient-dense foods such as fruits and vegetables can help translate recommendations into behavior changes. This includes strategies such as choosing frozen or canned produce when more economical, because their nutritional value is equivalent to fresh produce; choosing conventionally grown rather than organic foods most of the time; and storing foods and produce in such a way as to extend shelf life and maintain flavor and nutritional value.

- Overall, helping families increase skills in choosing, storing, and preparing food and adopt a more intuitive and mindful approach to eating is likely to help them move closer to their goals and improve overall nutrition, health, and well-being, while enjoying a wider diversity of tastes and food experiences.

References

1. Podzimek Š, Dušková M, Broukal Z, Rácz B, Stárka L, Dušková J. The evolution of taste and perinatal programming of taste preferences. *Physiol Res.* 2018;67(suppl 3):S421–S429 PMID: 30484669 doi: 10.33549/physiolres.934026

2. Breslin PAS. An evolutionary perspective on food and human taste. *Curr Biol.* 2013;23(9): R409–R418 PMID: 23660364 doi: 10.1016/j.cub.2013.04.010

3. Feeney E, O'Brien S, Scannell A, Markey A, Gibney ER. Genetic variation in taste perception: does it have a role in healthy eating? *Proc Nutr Soc.* 2011;70(1):135–143 PMID: 21092367 doi: 10.1017/S0029665110003976

4. Owen D. The science of delicious. *Natl Geogr Mag.* 2015;228(6):60–81. Accessed October 5, 2022. https://www.nationalgeographic.com/magazine/article/food-science-of-taste

5. Nekitsing C, Blundell-Birtill P, Cockroft JE, Hetherington MM. Systematic review and meta-analysis of strategies to increase vegetable consumption in preschool children aged 2-5 years. *Appetite.* 2018;127:138–154 PMID: 29702128 doi: 10.1016/j.appet.2018.04.019

6. Spill MK, Johns K, Callahan EH, et al. Repeated exposure to food and food acceptability in infants and toddlers: a systematic review. *Am J Clin Nutr.* 2019;109(suppl 1):978S–989S PMID: 30982874 doi: 10.1093/ajcn/nqy308

7. Memarian S, Moradi A, Hasani J, Mullan B. Can sweet food-specific inhibitory control training via a mobile application improve eating behavior in children with obesity? *Br J Health Psychol.* 2021;bjhp.12566 PMID: 34676624 doi: 10.1111/bjhp.12566

8. Falbe J, Thompson HR, Patel A, Madsen KA. Potentially addictive properties of sugar-sweetened beverages among adolescents. *Appetite.* 2019;133:130–137 PMID: 30385262 doi: 10.1016/j.appet.2018.10.032

9. Baker-Smith CM, de Ferranti SD, Cochran WJ, et al; American Academy of Pediatrics Committee on Nutrition and Section on Gastroenterology, Hepatology, and Nutrition. The use of nonnutritive sweeteners in children. *Pediatrics.* 2019;144(5):e20192765 PMID: 31659005 doi: 10.1542/peds.2019-2765

10. Nelson JB. Mindful eating: the art of presence while you eat. *Diabetes Spectr.* 2017;30(3):171–174 PMID: 28848310 doi: 10.2337/ds17-0015

11. Van Dyke N, Drinkwater EJ. Relationships between intuitive eating and health indicators: literature review. *Public Health Nutr.* 2014;17(8):1757–1766 PMID: 23962472 doi: 10.1017/S1368980013002139

12. Grider HS, Douglas SM, Raynor HA. The influence of mindful eating and/or intuitive eating approaches on dietary intake: a systematic review. *J Acad Nutr Diet.* 2021;121(4):709–727.e1 PMID: 33279464 doi: 10.1016/j.jand.2020.10.019

13. Njardvik U, Gunnarsdottir T, Olafsdottir AS, Craighead LW, Boles RE, Bjarnason R. Incorporating appetite awareness training within family-based behavioral treatment of pediatric obesity: a randomized controlled pilot study. *J Pediatr Psychol.* 2018;43(9):1017–1027 PMID: 30010923 doi: 10.1093/jpepsy/jsy055

14. Muth ND, Sampson S. *The Picky Eater Project: 6 Weeks to Happier, Healthier Family Mealtimes.* American Academy of Pediatrics; 2017

15. US Department of Health and Human Services, US Department of Agriculture. *Dietary Guidelines for Americans, 2020–2025.* 9th ed. 2020. Accessed October 5, 2022. https://www.dietaryguidelines.gov/sites/default/files/2020-12/Dietary_Guidelines_for_Americans_2020-2025.pdf

16. US Food and Drug Administration. GMO crops, animal food, and beyond. 2020. Accessed October 5, 2022. https://www.fda.gov/food/agricultural-biotechnology/gmo-crops-animal-food-and-beyond

17. Forman J, Silverstein J, Bhatia JJS, et al; American Academy of Pediatrics Committee on Nutrition and Council on Environmental Health. Organic foods: health and environmental advantages and disadvantages. *Pediatrics.* 2012;130(5):e1406–e1415 PMID: 23090335 doi: 10.1542/peds.2012-2579

18. Vigar V, Myers S, Oliver C, Arellano J, Robinson S, Leifert C. A systematic review of organic versus conventional food consumption: is there a measurable benefit on human health? *Nutrients.* 2019;12(1):7 PMID: 31861431 doi: 10.3390/nu12010007

CHAPTER 14

Theories of Behavior Change and Motivational Interviewing

The *Dietary Guidelines for Americans* highlight the disconnect between what children and adolescents are advised to eat to support optimal nutrition and their actual intakes.[1] Following are examples of this disconnect:

- The dietary guidelines advise that children 2 years and younger consume no added sugars. The average child 2 years or younger consumes 104 kcal or 6.5 tsp (27.7 g) of added sugar per day.
- The dietary guidelines advise that children and adolescents 2 years and older consume less than 10% of calories from added sugars. The scientific report leading to the guidelines advised an even lower marker, of less than 6% of calories from added sugars, for optimal health.[2] Nearly 80% of children and adolescents exceed the limit advised by the dietary guidelines.
- The dietary guidelines advise that children younger than 9 years consume no more than 1,500 mg/d of sodium and children and adolescents 9 years and older consume no more than 2,300 mg/d. Approximately 97% of children of all ages and sexes exceed this recommendation, other than adolescent girls, 77% of whom exceed the recommendation.
- Consistent with the dietary guidelines, pediatricians often advise children and adolescents to consume at least 5 servings of fruits and vegetables per day. The typical child and adolescent consumes less than 1 serving of fruit and 1 serving of vegetable per day.
- Very few children of any age meet whole grain and seafood recommendations.

The same disconnect exists between the *Physical Activity Guidelines for Americans* and the amount of physical activity that children and adolescents actually obtain. The physical activity guidelines advise that children and adolescents obtain at least 60 minutes of physical activity per day and at least 3 days of bone- and muscle-strengthening exercises per week. Few children and even fewer adolescents meet these recommendations. Adolescent girls in particular tend to exhibit very low rates of physical activity.[3]

Pediatricians can be an important source of credible nutrition information and should continue to share the recommendations and provide advice to eat better and move more. However, it is often not lack of knowledge or information that prevents children and adolescents from eating and moving optimally for the best physical and mental health. Efforts to help children, adolescents, and their families improve health habits are most impactful when tailored to their unique situation, accounting for social determinants of health, environmental factors, and readiness to change. Efforts to support behavior change are most effective when clinicians use coaching tools proven to help people change.

Behavior Change Theories

Understanding how to most effectively support people in making behavior changes has been an area of active research, leading to several theories of behavior change. Details of the best studied and most relevant behavior change theories are highlighted in **Table 14-1**. Familiarity with these theories can help clinicians decide on an approach when offering patient coaching, guidance, or advice to make a nutritional change. As described in the following section, the transtheoretical model (stages of change) is of particular utility in primary care.

The Transtheoretical Model (Stages of Change)

One of the best studied and most useful behavior change theories to help guide coaching strategies within primary care is the transtheoretical model of behavior change, also referred to as the *stages of change*. This model was first described by James Prochaska in studies evaluating the effectiveness of smoking cessation programs.[5] The stages of change construct recognizes behavior change as a process during which people pass through 6 well-defined stages. A patient may progress through the stages linearly, waver between stages, or progress and then relapse. Tailored strategies to help patients and their families move through the 6 stages of change are highlighted in **Table 14-2**. **Table 14-2** also describes relapse, which is not a stage in and of itself but an expected part of changing a behavior that is addressed in the transtheoretical model.

Processes of Change

The transtheoretical model includes many *processes of change*, techniques used to help people progress through the 6 stages of change.[8] **Table 14-3** highlights a few of the best studied and most applicable processes for pediatricians to use when supporting patients in making nutritional or physical activity changes.

A Primer on Motivational Interviewing

Motivational interviewing is a communication approach that can help clinicians support families and adolescent patients in making behavior changes. Motivational interviewing has been shown through thousands of studies to be a highly effective communication approach to help people who are ambivalent about making a change. People ambivalent about change are generally in the contemplation stage of the transtheoretical model and recognize both reasons to make a change and reasons not to do so. More than 25,000 scientific papers and 200 randomized controlled trials have been published since motivational interviewing was first described in the treatment of alcohol addiction in the 1980s.[9] Researchers found more than 130 review articles and meta-analyses published between 2000 and 2018 evaluating motivational interviewing and its role in stopping or preventing unhealthy behaviors (eg, substance use, gambling), promoting healthy behaviors (eg, oral health, nutrition, exercise, weight management, medication adherence), and changing the behavior for multiple health-related problems (eg, excess drinking, smoking, physical inactivity).[10] Although most of these studies were conducted with a focus on adults, several pediatric-focused studies have also

Table 14-1. An Overview of Behavior Change Theories

Theory/model	Premise	Key concepts	Example	Level of change
Classic learning theories	A new behavior develops from a series of small changes and extrinsic rewards. It is maintained through environmental cues and intrinsic rewards.	Reinforcement Cues Shaping	Parents applaud their toddler every time he takes a step when learning to walk. Eventually, he learns that walking is faster than crawling to reach his toys.	Individual
Health belief model	Health-related behavior depends on individual perception of risks and benefits. A person's confidence that they can continue a behavior (self-efficacy) predicts adherence.	Perceived susceptibility to disease Perceived severity of disease Perceived benefit of nutritional change Perceived barrier to nutritional change Cues to action Self-efficacy	A teen whose parent has diabetes is diagnosed with prediabetes and encouraged to be more active and eat more vegetables and fruits to help prevent type 2 diabetes. The teen enjoys playing with her dog and decides to take her dog for a walk each day to increase activity. She also likes cooking and decides to find some tasty vegetable recipes.	Individual
Transtheoretical model (stages of change; **Table 14-2**)	A person will change a behavior when they are ready. Readiness follows a nonlinear series of stages. Adherence is highest in action and maintenance stages.	Precontemplation Contemplation Preparation Action Maintenance Termination	A parent did not think their family needed to make any dietary changes until their child's low-density-lipoprotein cholesterol levels were very high. The parent then decided to try to have their family follow the Mediterranean-style eating plan, in particular by preparing fish 2 times per week. The parent purchased several Mediterranean-style cookbooks and ingredients to prepare several of the recipes.	Individual

Continued

Table 14-1 (*continued*)

Theory/model	Premise	Key concepts	Example	Level of change
Social cognitive theory	Behavior change and adherence are affected by environmental influences, personal factors, and attributes of the behavior. High self-efficacy and perceived benefit to making behavior change are critical for adherence.	Reciprocal determinism: Behavior influences and is influenced by personal factors and the social environment. Behavioral capability: The person has the knowledge and skills to perform the behavior. Self-efficacy Outcome expectations Observational learning Reinforcement	A pediatrician refers an interested family for a healthy cooking class to show them easy ways to incorporate more fruits and vegetables into mealtimes.	Interpersonal

| Theory of planned behavior | Behavior and adherence are determined by intention, which includes belief about outcome of the behavior and influence of the social environment, including what others think the person should do. This also includes perceived behavioral control, or perception of the ability to make the change (self-efficacy). | Attitude toward the nutritional change

Outcome expectations

Value of outcome expectations

Subjective norms

Beliefs of others

Motivation to comply with others

Perceived behavioral control | A teen decides to start exercising and starts to notice improved mood and fitness. She invites her sister to join her. Her sister notices this positive change and accepts the invitation. She would like to start exercising as well. | Interpersonal |
| Social support | Provision of several types of support helps improve adoption and adherence to new behavior. | Instrumental support: A social contact provides help to make change.

Informational support: A social contact provides information and resources to make change.

Emotional support: A social contact provides follow-up, feedback, and reinforcements. | A teen wants to learn to cook to make healthy eating easier. Her mother gives her a ride to cooking classes (instrumental support), helps her develop meal plans based on federal nutrition guidelines (informational support), and tells her how much she likes the meals the teen has made (emotional support). | Interpersonal |

Continued

Table 14-1 (*continued*)

Theory/model	Premise	Key concepts	Example	Level of change
Social ecological model	Effective interventions occur on multiple levels of influence, demonstrating the importance of environmental factors in influencing individual behaviors. The most effective interventions include multiple levels in multiple settings.	Multiple levels of influence ● Intrapersonal ● Interpersonal ● Group ● Institutional ● Community ● Public policy Multiple settings of influence ● Schools ● Workplaces ● Health care institutions ● Communities	A community-wide campaign is underway to reduce sugary drink consumption. The community schools, major workplaces, and health care institutions have all adopted the Centers for Disease Control and Prevention messaging "rethink your drink" to promote water. The local government is preparing to tax sugary drinks. Grocery stores are promoting sparkling water.	Environmental
Relapse prevention	Identifying high-risk situations and coming up with solutions before their occurrence can reduce lapses. Differentiating between lapse (short-term nonadherence) and relapse (long-term nonadherence) improves overall adherence.	Skills training Cognitive restructuring: The person monitors their thoughts and tries to change them to be more helpful. Lifestyle change in areas of exercise, stress management, and healthy eating	A teen who has tried to minimize desserts is going on a weeklong vacation to his grandmother's house. She tends to show him love by baking him many desserts every time he visits. He is preparing to ask her whether they can do something different this time.	Individual

Derived from reference 4 and National Center for Chronic Disease Prevention and Health Promotion, Centers for Disease Control and Prevention. *Understanding and promoting physical activity. Physical Activity and Health: A Report of the Surgeon General.* US Dept of Health and Human Services; 1996. Accessed October 28, 2022. https://www.cdc.gov/nccdphp/sgr/pdf/chap6.pdf.

Table 14-2. The Transtheoretical Model (Stages of Change)

Stage	Patient-clinician goals	Clinician strategies	Clinician sample statements
Precontemplation The patient does not believe there is a problem and does not recognize a need to change. The patient makes statements like • "I don't want to eat vegetables, and you can't make me." • "I don't think my diet needs to change." • "My nutrition is perfect the way it is."	Increase awareness of the risk of the status quo and the benefits of the change.	Validate that there is lack of readiness to change and that this decision is the patient's. Encourage reevaluation of current behavior and self-exploration without making any change. Provide information and resources to increase awareness, with the patient and family's permission.	"I understand that you don't think it will provide any benefit to make any changes to the way you eat right now. Would it be OK if I gave your mom a recipe that a lot of my patients love, just to have on hand—in case you change your mind or want to try it?"
Contemplation The patient believes that change is necessary and plans to act within the next 6 mo. The patient may remain in this stage for months to years. The patient makes statements like • "I know I need to exercise, but I just don't like it." • "I might be willing to try a vegetable." • "You can tell me more about what you I think I should be doing."	Recognize that the benefits of change outweigh the risks.	Encourage evaluation of the pros and cons of making change.	• "What might be some reasons to change nutrition habits at this time?" • "What things have helped you eat differently in the past?" • "What would help you this time?"

Continued

Table 14-2 (*continued*)

Stage	Patient-clinician goals	Clinician strategies	Clinician sample statements
Preparation The patient intends to make changes within the next month. The patient makes statements like ● "I know I need to change." ● "I've already started going for a walk every now and then." ● "I tried drinking water instead of soda when we went out to dinner last week."	Develop a structured plan for change (SMART goals and action plans are discussed in Chapter 15).	Verify that the patient has the skills needed to make behavior change, and encourage small steps to build self-efficacy. Identify and solve obstacles. Help identify social supports and set goals.	● "What steps have you already taken to get ready to make this change?" ● "What kinds of problems might you experience as you start to make this change? How will you overcome them?"
Action The patient has made and maintained substantial lifestyle changes within the past 6 mo. A patient in the action stage often struggles to make a permanent change, with adherence progressively decreasing over the first several months. This is typical of all types of behavioral changes and explains why many nutrition and activity programs are short-lived. The patient makes statements like ● "I joined a rec team and have been working out every day." ● "We've been cooking at home at least 3 times per week for the past 2 months." ● "I eat fruit at breakfast every day now."	Begin to make change.	Use behavioral modification strategies to support and sustain change, such as accountability partners, rewards, or pairing with other habits. Provide continual feedback on progress. Emphasize long-term benefits of adherence. Help patients plan for possible lapses and how to get back on track if and when they occur.	● "What do you think made you take this particular step to change?" ● "It must feel great to have started to make such an important change." ● "How are you celebrating your successes?"

Maintenance The patient has maintained a healthful change for >6 mo. Relapses occur less frequently, although it is not until change has been maintained for 5 y that the risk of relapse falls below 7%. The patient has high self-efficacy that they can maintain change and relies less frequently on processes of change than patients in the earlier stages of change. The patient makes statements like ● "We always have family dinners." ● "We have been going for a walk after dinner most nights of the week for the past year."	Maintain change.	Celebrate successes. Anticipate potential triggers for lapses. Make plans to prevent relapse.	● "How has your life changed since making this change?" ● "How confident do you feel you will be able to maintain this change in the long term?" ● "What are your high-risk temptations?"
Termination The final stage of change, when there is no temptation or risk of relapse. The patient experiences 100% self-efficacy and success with the behavior change. This stage is often left out of the transtheoretical model because it is difficult to attain.	Permanently adopt the habit.	None, because the patient has already adopted the behavior change	None, because the patient has already adopted the behavior change

Continued

Table 14-2 (*continued*)

Stage	Patient-clinician goals	Clinician strategies	Clinician sample statements
Relapse The patient has planned for or made a change but then lapsed to a previous behavior or mindset. This is an expected part of behavior change and generally occurs in the action and maintenance stages. The patient makes statements like • "We were doing great, but then we got off track during vacation." • "We had an illness that got in the way of exercise, and now it's hard to get started again."	Recognize triggers for lapses and prevent them.	Acknowledge that lapses are an expected part of behavior change. Incorporate relapse management activities such as role-playing difficult situations and purposefully avoiding situations that trigger unwanted behavior.	• "What did you do that helped you make the change for a while?" • "What did you learn from this experience that will help you when you give it another try?"

Derived from references 5–7.

Table 14-3. The Processes of Change

Process of change	Description	Example for pediatricians
Consciousness raising	Awareness is increased of the pros of making a change and the cons of keeping the status quo.	Share a handout on the benefits of drinking water and health effects of sugary drinks, or ask a patient to create their own version of a handout on the benefits of drinking water.
Dramatic relief	Emotionally moving testimony, documentary, or role-playing is used to increase motivation to make change.	Encourage a patient to watch a food-related documentary.
Self-reevaluation	The patient envisions themselves both with and without the unhealthy behavior.	Ask a patient to envision what might be different if they adopted a more physically active lifestyle.
Environmental reevaluation	The patient considers how their behaviors affect the people around them.	Ask an adolescent with picky eating habits how they think their eating habits affect other family members' food choices.
Helpful relationships or social support	The patient develops strong social networks to support healthful change.	Ask a patient who, among their family and friends, most supports their making a change.
Contingency management	Rewards are given for making planned behavior changes.	Help a patient develop a list of ways to celebrate or reward themselves when a goal is attained.
Self-liberation (willpower)	The patient commits to making a change. A verbal or public commitment increases adherence. However, an overreliance on willpower can make adherence to behavior change difficult.	Support a patient in telling their friends or family that they are making a nutritional change or pursuing a specific goal.
Counterconditioning (behavioral substitution)	Less healthy behaviors are replaced with healthy behaviors.	Help a patient develop a substitution plan. For example, a patient who always drinks a regular soda when he gets home from school might replace it with a glass of lemon water or unsweetened iced tea.

Continued

Table 14-3 (*continued*)

Process of change	Description	Example for pediatricians
Stimulus control	Cues for undesirable behavior are reduced, and cues for desirable behavior are increased.	Help a patient trying to lose weight develop a strategy to decrease exposure to the unwanted behavior. For example, a patient might make a plan together with their parents or other caregivers to avoid having junk food in the house.
Social liberation	Policy, peer influence, and societal norms are changed to promote individual behavior change.	Support an excise tax on sugary drinks to help reduce sugary drink intake among adolescents in locales where it is adopted.

Derived from reference 7.

shown benefit, especially when working with adolescents and adult caregivers.[11,12] The utility of motivational interviewing with younger children as the interviewees is not yet well established.

A mini training in motivational interviewing follows in the next section of this chapter.[6,13] It highlights the essentials of motivational interviewing along with suggested practice strategies to develop and improve motivational interviewing skills when working with pediatric patients and their families.

What Is Motivational Interviewing?

Motivational interviewing is described by its founders, psychologists William Miller and Stephen Rollnick, as a "collaborative conversation style for strengthening a person's own motivation and commitment to change."[9] In other words, it helps a person "talk themselves into change, based on their own values and interests."[9] Motivational interviewing relies on a *guiding style* of talking about change. With this approach, the clinician is more of a coach who helps guide the patient as they consider changing a health behavior. This is in contrast to a *directing style* of talking about change, in which the clinician tells a patient what to do and the patient is expected to (but often does not) follow through on the directive. It is also in contrast to a *following style* of talking about change, in which the patient leads with little input or guidance from the clinician. Motivational interviewing is most effective with adolescents and parents or other caregivers who are ambivalent about changing a behavior.

The Spirit of Motivational Interviewing

Although the method of motivational interviewing has been refined over time, the spirit of the approach remains unchanged: "[Motivational interviewing] involves a collaborative partnership with patients, a respectful evoking of their own motivation and wisdom, and a radical acceptance recognizing that ultimately whether change happens is each person's own choice, an autonomy that cannot be taken away no matter how much one might wish to at times."[9] The 4 pillars of the spirit of motivational interviewing ground the patient-clinician relationship. They are

- **Collaboration.** Collaboration describes a partnership between the patient and clinician.
- **Acceptance.** A motivational interviewing-centric clinician demonstrates "unconditional positive regard" for the patient, rooted in respect, trust, and empathy.
- **Compassion.** Motivational interviewing is used for the benefit of the patient, not the clinician.
- **Evocation.** The patient is the expert on themselves and their family. The role of the clinician is to "call forth the strength and wisdom from the patient."[9]

The 4 Processes of Motivational Interviewing

Motivational interviewing helps a person who is ambivalent about change "talk themselves" into changing a behavior. To help guide them toward this change, it is important to proceed stepwise through the following 4 processes, with the most emphasis on the third process: evoking. Only once a person has expressed that they are ready to change and are no longer ambivalent should the clinician proceed to the planning process.

- **Engaging** is the first process of the patient-clinician relationship, during which the clinician and patient build rapport and trust.
- **Focusing** helps the clinician and patient develop a shared agenda for the coaching sessions.
- **Evoking** is the heart of motivational interviewing, when the clinician helps the patient explore the patient's motivation to change and eventually resolve ambivalence about whether to move forward with a change. Much of the power of motivational interviewing lies in the art and science of evoking.
- **Planning** occurs once the patient has resolved to change and is ready to develop and implement an action plan. This occurs when the patient is "thinking and talking more about when and how to change and less about whether and why."[9]

Communication Tools

Motivational interviewing prompts a person to change the way they think—and feel—about change. A motivational interviewing conversation guides a patient toward *change talk,* statements that come from the patient arguing for why a change is needed and for their own capacity to change. Unlike the counterproductive effect that occurs when a clinician tries to convince a patient to change, when a patient talks themselves into change, they are much more likely to turn intention into action and then behavior change. As Miller and Rollnick state in their book *Motivational Interviewing: Helping People Change,* "If you are arguing for change and the patient is arguing against it, you've got it exactly backward."[9]

Motivational interviewing uses several communication tools to evoke change talk. They can be best remembered with the following mnemonic, OARS:

- **Open-ended questions.** These questions cannot be answered with a simple yes or no. Open-ended questions often start with how, what, why, and what if. For instance, instead of asking a patient who would like to eat healthier "Do you like fruits and vegetables?" ask "What fruits and vegetables do you enjoy the most?"
- **Affirmations.** Affirmations acknowledge a patient's strengths, abilities, and positive behaviors. They focus on what is going right more than what is going "wrong." Affirmations help a patient build confidence and self-efficacy for change. For example, a statement such as "You went for a walk even though you didn't feel like it at first" is much more likely to lead to continued positive change than a remark such as "Your walk was only 5 minutes instead of the 30 you had planned."
- **Reflective statements.** Reflective statements are a "best guess" at identifying the underlying meaning or intention of what a patient has said. Their purpose is to help a patient think more deeply about how they feel and the motivations behind their actions. If the reflective statement is inconsistent with what the patient intended, they will correct the clinician and likely elaborate. Reflective statements help a patient work through ambivalence and build confidence and commitment to making a change. For example, a response to a patient who says "I don't have time to exercise" might be "You would be more active if there were more minutes in the day." The patient is likely to respond with "Yeah, I think so." It is important that the spirit of motivational interviewing is maintained when providing reflective statements, so they are stated in a compassionate and warm manner and not in a tone that could come across as judgmental. Mastery of the use of reflective statements is essential to build fluency in motivational interviewing.
- **Summarizing statements.** Summarizing statements help pull together a patient's thoughts or offer a recapitulation of what the patient has said based on the clinician's understanding. Summarizing statements often come at the end of a coaching session and help ensure that the clinician and patient are on the same page and set the direction for next steps. For example, a clinician might summarize key points from a conversation with an adolescent about drinking more water and fewer sugary drinks by saying "You tend to drink sugary drinks a few times per day because you like how they taste and they are easily available in your house, but your health is really important to you and you are open to thinking about drinking more water."

How to Incorporate Motivational Interviewing Into Pediatric Practice

When implemented in practice, the following 10 strategies help increase skill in motivational interviewing. To begin, clinicians may choose a strategy from the list, practice it to near mastery, and then work on another strategy to mastery—and so on. Motivational interviewing is a skill that develops over time with patience and practice.

- **Talk less.** This coaching strategy is not unique to motivational interviewing, but it is critical to a successful motivational interviewing conversation. Engage with a patient and build a partnership by allowing the patient to do 50% or more of the talking.

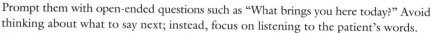

Prompt them with open-ended questions such as "What brings you here today?" Avoid thinking about what to say next; instead, focus on listening to the patient's words.

- **Listen for ambivalence about change.** A patient who responds "I am here because my mom told me I need to see you to get to a healthier weight" or in a similar manner may be ambivalent about change. In this example, the patient is present, which shows some degree of readiness to change, but it seems as if she came to the clinician appointment only because her mother made her, not out of her own desire. Motivational interviewing is the ideal communication approach for patients who are ambivalent, because it helps the patient move from considering change to becoming ready to change.

- **Recognize and evoke change talk.** The crux of motivational interviewing is responding effectively to change talk, or the patient's stated reasons why changing a health behavior is beneficial. Generally, change talk comes in the form of "desire, ability, reasons, and need" statements—referred to as *DARN*. The most impactful way to respond to change talk is with reflections (refer to the "Speak in reflections" item later in this list).

- Examples of DARN statements include
  — *Desire:* "I want to be able to run a 5K with my mom."
  — *Ability:* "I know that I could eat more fruits and vegetables if I really put my mind to it."
  — *Reasons:* "If I am able to avoid getting diabetes, I know that my quality of life will be so much better."
  — *Need:* "I need to be more active, but I'm just not sure how to fit that in my day."

- If a patient is not offering change talk during the natural course of a conversation, clinicians can consider using the following motivational interviewing strategies to evoke it:
  — *Query extremes.* Ask the patient what the worst-case scenario would be if a change were not made and what the best-case scenario would be if a change were made.
  — *Look back.* Ask the patient to think back to a time when they did not have the problem behavior and what life was like then.
  — *Look forward.* Ask the patient to envision and describe what life would be like if they made the change.
  — *Explore goals and values.* Ask the patient to share what things in life are most important to them and what life goals they hope to achieve in the long term.

- **Acknowledge sustain talk.** Recognizing *sustain talk,* or a patient's expressed reasons not to change, is important to reframe and deemphasize these statements. Clinicians should avoid falling into a trap of prompting more sustain talk, which then helps a patient move away from, rather than toward, making a change. Examples of sustain talk include discussion of barriers, challenges, or reasons why a change is not feasible or possible at the current time. Clinicians can try the following strategies to effectively respond to sustain talk. Oftentimes, these strategies will break a cycle of sustain talk and evoke change talk.
  — *Emphasize autonomy.* A clinician acknowledges that change is the decision of the patient. For example, a clinician might say "Only you can control whether you make a change."

- *Reframe.* The clinician offers a different meaning or perspective on the patient's statement. For example, if a patient says "I have tried and failed at losing weight so many times. I don't think I can do it this time either," the clinician might respond with an affirmation: "You have been persistent in trying to find the strategy that will work for you. Losing weight must be very important to you."

- *Agree, with a twist.* The clinician starts with a reflective statement to agree with the patient but follows it with a reframing statement. For example, the clinician may respond to a patient who says "I don't have time to cook healthy meals" with "Cooking healthy meals takes time. You have other ways to spend your time that are of higher priority."

- *Running head start.* The clinician prompts a patient to list the reasons not to change followed by reasons to change. This is similar to a listing of pros and cons. Of note, the listing of reasons not to change can reinforce the status quo. As such, this strategy should be used only when a patient has expressed little to no change talk.

- *Coming alongside.* Agree with a patient who has offered little or no change talk and an abundance of sustain talk that "perhaps, for now, it is better to stay as you are." Oftentimes, a comment such as this prompts a patient to respond with a statement containing some change talk (eg, "Oh no, I am not perfect. I can probably do something to improve"). Otherwise, if a patient does not truly wish to make any change, this comment can help preserve the relationship while avoiding spending a large amount of time and energy to help the patient change when they are not truly ready.

- **Speak in reflections.** Rather than ask numerous questions or provide a great deal of advice and instruction, clinicians should speak primarily in reflections—statements that repeat back to a patient what the clinician heard them say, including a best guess at the meaning of the statement. Most of the time, clinicians should reflect on change talk more so than sustain talk. Reflections come in many forms.
  - *Simple reflections:* Simple reflections repeat or restate what a patient said. For example, if a patient says "I want to lose weight," a simple reflection will be "Losing weight is important to you."
  - *Complex reflections:* A complex reflection is a statement aiming to discern the underlying meaning or feeling behind what a patient has said. For example, if a patient says "I love dessert, but I definitely don't want to get diabetes," an example of a complex reflection will be "You are afraid that if you keep eating the way you are eating, you are going to develop diabetes."
  - *Straight reflection:* A straight reflection is a simple or complex reflection in response to a patient's sustain talk. For example, if a patient says "I've already tried vegetables a million times, and I just don't like them," a clinician may respond with "You've already made a lot of effort to try to like vegetables, but it didn't work, and you can't see yourself ever liking them." Often, change talk follows a straight reflection.
  - *Amplified reflection:* An amplified reflection is an overstatement in response to sustain talk. It should be delivered with empathy and no sign of sarcasm

or frustration; otherwise, it could prompt a defensive or hostile reaction. An example may be a teen who states "I am only here because my mom made me come." An amplified reflection might be "Your mom is worrying needlessly about your health."

— *Double-sided reflection:* A double-sided reflection combines 2 reflections, one regarding a patient's sustain talk followed by another regarding a patient's change talk. For example, in response to a caregiver who expresses that it is really hard to find time to cook but she sees the importance of doing so, a double-sided reflection might be "You don't have time to cook, *and* when you do cook, you feel better and save money."

As a pediatrician learns the language of motivational interviewing, many statements will be simple reflections. With practice, more statements may be complex reflections, which help further prompt behavior change.

- **Use the confidence ruler.** The *confidence ruler* is a tool that helps a patient state the reasons for change and the best next steps for starting to plan for change. Clinicians can facilitate a patient's readiness for change, and help the patient transition from the evoking process to the planning process of motivational interviewing, by using the confidence ruler as follows:

1. Ask the patient the following question: "On a scale from 1 to 10, with 1 being very and 10 being not, how confident are you that you could make this change if you decided to do so?"

2. Next, ask a follow-up question: "Why are you an $[x]$ and not an $[x-2]$?" For instance, if a patient says they are a 5, a clinician might ask "Why are you a 5 and not a 3?" The patient will almost always answer this question with change talk. However, if the clinician asks "Why are you a 3 and not a 5?" sustain talk will ensue. For example, if a patient says they are a 5 in their confidence that they can eat a fruit at breakfast each day, a clinician should follow up with "Tell me why you chose 5 and not 3." The patient will likely respond with something like "Well, I know that eating fruit is good for me" or "It's pretty easy to grab a banana on my way to school." On the other hand, if a clinician asks "Why a 5 and not a 7?" a patient might respond with "Well, it's hard for me to remember to eat in the morning" or "I don't like to eat breakfast very much."

3. Respond with a reflective statement. For instance, in the previous example, a clinician might respond with "Being healthy is important to you" or "You could get into the habit of eating fruit in the morning if it were easy to eat on the run."

4. Finally, ask the following question: "What would it take to get from an $[x]$ to an $[x+2]$?" This helps a patient start to identify a change plan. For example, in the previous scenario, a clinician might ask "What would it take to get from a 5 to a 7?" The patient is likely to respond with a statement like "If we had a lot of fruit in the house, it'd be easier for me to eat it." This can help lead to the fourth process of motivational interviewing: planning. This occurs when goals and action plans are developed, as discussed in Chapter 15, SMART Goals and Action Plans.

- **Resist the righting reflex.** Miller and Rollnick refer to the tendency to give advice, push recommendations, and offer solutions as *the righting reflex.*[9] They refer to this as a reflex because it is nearly automatic for health care professionals to do it. Although well-meaning, the clinician's eagerness to promote the positive change in a patient ambivalent about change can invoke the patient's instinct to "defend" the status quo, making a sustained behavior change less likely. When tempted to provide advice or recommendations to a patient ambivalent about change, clinicians should first pause and then make a reflective statement to help prompt the patient to supply their own solutions. For example, in response to a patient who shares that she skips breakfast because she does not have time in the morning, instead of jumping into a discussion of possible ways that she can find time to eat breakfast, the clinician can offer a reflection. For example, the clinician can say "If there were more time in the morning, it would be easier to eat a healthy breakfast." The patient might respond with something like "Yes, if only I had just a little bit more time." Then, rather than immediately offer advice, such as suggesting that the patient go to bed and wake up earlier, the clinician can offer a statement to make it more likely that the patient will think of her own solution and thus be more likely to implement it. For example, "I wonder whether there might be a way to have more time in the morning." At this point, the patient might offer some ideas of ways to make more time in the morning, such as getting up earlier.

- **Recognize and reflect on CAT statements.** As patients begin to express statements indicating **C**ommitment, **A**ctivation, and **T**aking steps (CAT statements), also described as *mobilizing change talk,* clinicians should recognize that the patient has worked through ambivalence and is likely ready to begin planning for change. Commitment statements are versions of stating "I will change." Activation statements include "I am ready to change" or "I am prepared to change." Taking steps indicates that the patient has already begun to make a change. This strategy is parallel to the preparation stage in the transtheoretical model of behavior change. CAT statements are a cue that a patient may be ready to move into the planning process of motivational interviewing.

- **Inform and advise with permission.** In some cases, it is appropriate to offer a patient health education or advice. For example, once the patient is ready to begin planning, the patient may ask for help in coming up with meal plans or exercise programs. Clinicians should offer information and advice only if a patient specifically asks for these or only after explicitly asking for permission, which the patient has granted. Clinicians should ensure that the patient recognizes they are free to agree or disagree and the information should be used in the context of their own plan for change. Finally, in providing advice, clinicians should offer a "menu of options," or several possible solutions a patient could choose from, rather than one "best" plan.

- **Elicit-provide-elicit.** When providing information and advice, clinicians should follow the sequence of elicit-provide-elicit. "Elicit" uses open-ended questions to identify the patient's baseline level of knowledge about the topic. "Provide" offers information with permission, building off the patient's baseline knowledge. "Elicit" assesses the patient's understanding of the information offered.

Elicit-provide-elicit also allows for offering information in an autonomy-supporting way, which improves the therapeutic alliance.

Learning motivational interviewing is like learning a second language: it takes time, practice, and many mistakes to develop proficiency and grace. Clinicians can practice motivational interviewing by using Miller and Rollnick's 5 steps for beginners (**Box 14-1**) or the American Academy of Pediatrics and Kognito Change Talk app (**Box 14-2**). Additionally, the text *Motivational Interviewing in Health Care: Helping Patients Change Behavior* by Rollnick, Miller, and Butler is a helpful study guide (Guilford Press, 2022). Clinicians can assess their mastery of the use of OARS by recording a coaching session, with a patient's permission, and tallying responses with the tool in **Box 14-3**.

CLINICAL PRACTICE TIP

Box 14-1. Motivational Interviewing for Beginners: Miller and Rollnick's 5 Open-ended Questions

Miller and Rollnick suggest beginning practice of motivational interviewing with these 5 open-ended questions.[9] Clinicians should then follow a patient's response to each question with 2–3 reflective statements.

1. Why do you want to make this change?
2. How might you go about making this change?
3. What are the 3 best reasons for you to make this change?
4. How important is it for you to make this change? Why?
5. What do you think you'll do?

CLINICAL PRACTICE TIP

Box 14-2. Change Talk App

Clinicians can take time to practice conversations with virtual families and learn to apply motivational interviewing to drive positive change in their health behaviors by using the Change Talk app, developed by American Academy of Pediatrics Institute for Healthy Childhood Weight and Kognito (https://go.kognito.com/changetalk).

CLINICAL PRACTICE TIP

Box 14-3. OARS Self-assessment

Clinicians can record a change conversation with a patient, with the patient's permission, and then assess themselves by replaying the conversation and listening for OARS. On hearing an example of OARS, clinicians can place a hash mark in the appropriate row and note examples of each type of OARS response heard. Clinicians should aim for a 2:1 ratio of reflective statements to open-ended questions.

Clinician response	Count	Examples
Open-ended questions		
Affirmations		
Reflective statements		
Summaries		

In Sum

- Patients and families are more likely to make nutritional changes when they are motivated and ready to change. One of the best studied and most useful behavior change theories to help guide coaching strategies within primary care is the trans-theoretical model of behavior change, also referred to as *the stages of change*. This construct recognizes behavior change as a process during which people pass through 6 well-defined stages: precontemplation, contemplation, preparation, action, maintenance, and relapse. A patient may progress through the stages linearly, waver between stages, or progress and then relapse. Clinicians can focus their approach on helping families make changes by assessing a patient and family's stage of change.
- Motivational interviewing is a communication approach that facilitates partnership and enhanced communication with patients and families. Although it is particularly helpful when working with patients and families who are in the contemplation stage of change and are ambivalent about whether to make a change, motivational interviewing is good practice for communicating with and coaching all patients. Motivational interviewing includes 4 processes: engaging, focusing, evoking, and planning. Engaging is the process of building rapport and establishing a trusting relationship. Focusing is the process of shared agenda setting between the clinician and patient or family in deciding the goal for behavior change. Evoking is the process of bringing about a person's own motivation and desire to change through the clinician's use of open-ended questions, affirmations, reflective statements, and summarizing statements. The planning process occurs after a person has committed to making a change, and the clinician helps them move to the next stage of goal setting and developing action plans, the focus of Chapter 15, SMART Goals and Action Plans.

References

1. US Department of Health and Human Services, US Department of Agriculture. *Dietary Guidelines for Americans, 2020–2025*. 9th ed. 2020. Accessed October 6, 2022. https://www.dietaryguidelines.gov/sites/default/files/2020-12/Dietary_Guidelines_for_Americans_2020-2025.pdf

2. Dietary Guidelines Advisory Committee. *Scientific Report of the 2020 Dietary Guidelines Advisory Committee: Advisory Report to the Secretary of Agriculture and the Secretary of Health and Human Services*. Agricultural Research Services, US Dept of Agriculture; 2020

3. US Department of Health and Human Services. *Physical Activity Guidelines for Americans*. 2nd ed. US Dept of Health and Human Services; 2018

4. Sears SR, Brehm BA, Bell K. Understanding behavior change: theoretical models. In: Brehm BA, ed. *Psychology of Health and Fitness*. FA Davis Co; 2014:117–144

5. Prochaska JO. *Systems of Psychotherapy: A Transtheoretical Analysis*. Dorsey Press; 1979

6. Muth ND, Green D. *Coaching Behavior Change*. American Council on Exercise; 2014

7. Muth ND. *ACE Fitness Nutrition Manual*. American Council on Exercise; 2013

8. Prochaska JO, DiClemente CC. Stages and processes of self-change of smoking: toward an integrative model of change. *J Consult Clin Psychol*. 1983;51(3):390–395 PMID: 6863699 doi: 10.1037/0022-006X.51.3.390

9. Miller WR, Rollnick S. *Motivational Interviewing: Helping People Change*. 3rd ed. Guilford Press; 2013

10. Frost H, Campbell P, Maxwell M, et al. Effectiveness of motivational interviewing on adult behaviour change in health and social care settings: a systematic review of reviews. *PLoS One*. 2018;13(10):e0204890 PMID: 30335780 doi: 10.1371/journal.pone.0204890

11. Desai N. The role of motivational interviewing in children and adolescents in pediatric care. *Pediatr Ann*. 2019;48(9):e376–e379 PMID: 31505012 doi: 10.3928/19382359-20190816-01

12. Resnicow K, McMaster F, Bocian A, et al. Motivational interviewing and dietary counseling for obesity in primary care: an RCT. *Pediatrics*. 2015;135(4):649–657 PMID: 25825539 doi: 10.1542/peds.2014-1880

13. Muth ND. *An Introduction to Motivational Interviewing*. IDEA Fitness Journal; 2015

CHAPTER 15

SMART Goals and Action Plans

After families become ready to make behavior changes, the critical next step is for clinicians to help families identify and use the skills, tools, and resources needed to move from intention to action. Many families understand what they should eat for good health and want to eat in a healthful way, but often it is difficult for patients and families to translate nutrition knowledge to dietary changes. Helping patients and their families set SMART goals, create action plans, and develop skills to support changes, overcome barriers to change, and ensure accountability can help turn intentions to eat healthier into new nutrition habits.

SMART Goals

SMART is an acronym to describe goals that are Specific, Measurable, Attainable, Relevant, and Time bound (**Box 15-1**).

SMART goals help patients and families close the gap between nutrition recommendations and daily habits. For example, the *Dietary Guidelines for Americans* may advise that an adolescent consume 5 servings of vegetables and fruits per day, but the adolescent may eat only 1 serving of fruit and no vegetables most days. An initial SMART goal might be to eat at least 1 serving of fruit and 1 serving of vegetable each day for the next 2 weeks. Importantly, a patient will be most likely to achieve the goal if they are the one who selects it.

Choosing Positive Goals

For best results, clinicians should help patients choose either a positive behavior–focused goal or an approach goal, through which a patient tries to add a new behavior or skill—rather than a negative or avoidance goal, through which a patient tries to avoid a behavior. For example, a patient may have a goal to drink only water or

Box 15-1. SMART Goals

SPECIFIC	MEASURABLE	ATTAINABLE	RELEVANT	TIME-BOUND
What	How much	A stretch but not out of reach	Worthwhile	By when the goal will be accomplished
When	How many		Fits with short- and long-term vision or aims	
Where	How accomplishment of the goal will be determined			
Why				

milk at meals and snacks for the next month, which is more likely to lead to a behavior change than a goal to avoid soda for the next month. The increased water and milk consumption is likely to displace the soda, leading to the same goal outcome; however, focusing on the positive behavior is generally more motivating to the person making the change.[1]

Choosing Mastery Goals

Mastery goals are process centered and are focused on learning new skills (eg, learning to cook), whereas performance goals are outcome centered and are focused on achieving a specific outcome (eg, losing weight). Clinicians should aim to help patients set mastery, process-centered goals, especially as patients first start making changes. The patient has more direct control over whether process-centered goals are attained, making it more likely that they will achieve the goal. This approach builds confidence and self-efficacy to continue the change.[1]

Choosing Goals Within Patient Control

The ability to attain a goal needs to be within the control of the person who is setting the goal. For example, a parent may be tempted to set a goal that their child eats vegetables at each meal. Although a parent may be able to beg or bribe their child to eat a vegetable, ultimately it is up to their child whether they will eat the food. It is better if parents set goals within their own control to achieve. In this example, the parent's goal might be to serve a vegetable at dinner or include a vegetable tray with dip as a snack after school. This step of making vegetables readily available to their child makes it more likely that their child will choose to eat them.

Action Plans

Action plans outline concrete steps that a patient will take to achieve a goal. Action plans should indicate when, where, and how the action is to be carried out.[1] Action plans can also help address or resolve barriers that might impede a patient's progress toward a goal and help identify what information, knowledge, and skills a patient or parent needs to make a dietary change. Action plans should also include a plan for accountability and how the family will monitor goal progress and attainment.

For example, a parent may have a SMART goal to offer dinners each night that are consistent with MyPlate recommendations. However, this might be difficult accomplish if this parent is like those involved in a study of fifth graders and their adult caregivers that showed that one of the biggest barriers for adults trying to follow the dietary guidelines is lack of skills in preparing meals and recipes.[2]

This parent's action plan might be as follows:

- Identify and prepare 3 dinner recipes that follow the MyPlate guidelines.
- Plan dinners for the week ahead of time.
- Write and follow a grocery list.
- Keep track of home-cooked meals on a monthly calendar. Celebrate at the end of the month if at least 12 nights had MyPlate meals.

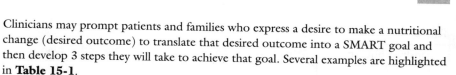

Clinicians may prompt patients and families who express a desire to make a nutritional change (desired outcome) to translate that desired outcome into a SMART goal and then develop 3 steps they will take to achieve that goal. Several examples are highlighted in **Table 15-1**.

Table 15-1. Sample SMART Goals and Action Plans

Desired outcome	SMART goal example	Possible action plan
An adolescent would like to eat more fruits and vegetables.	Eat at least 3 servings of fruits and vegetables per day for the next 2 wk.	• Include a piece of fruit at each breakfast. • Pack carrots, cucumbers, or celery sticks with lunch each day. • Make a salad to eat with dinner each night.
A parent would like their school-aged child to increase dairy intake.	Offer the child at least 3 servings of dairy per day for the next 2 wk.	• Offer plain yogurt with berries at breakfast each day. • Include a string cheese with lunch. • Serve a glass of milk at dinner each night.
A child and parent would like to work together to increase the child's fiber intake.	Eat at least 3 servings of whole grains each day for the next 2 wk.	• Eat a sandwich with 2 slices of whole grain bread at lunch. • For dinner, include a whole grain such as brown rice, whole wheat pasta, or quinoa. • Purchase whole grain crackers for a snack.
A parent would like their 12-year-old to decrease sugary drinks and juice. The 12-year-old agrees to try.	Drink only water or milk for the next 2 wk.	• Purchase sparkling water rather than soda at the grocery store. • Replace morning orange juice with a whole orange. • Drink water with the after-school snack.
An adolescent would like to decrease snacking.	Make a schedule for meals and snacks and eat only during those times for the next 2 wk.	• Write a schedule of mealtimes and snack times. • Drink water when feeling a need to eat outside planned times. • Savor meals and snacks by sitting at the kitchen table without distractions when it is time to eat.

Continued

Table 15-1 (*continued*)

Desired outcome	SMART goal example	Possible action plan
A family would like to all work together to decrease portion sizes.	Eat recommended portion sizes of all foods for the next 2 wk.	• Measure food portions to learn to visualize what a recommended serving looks like. • Use smaller plates and utensils at mealtimes.
An adolescent wants to decrease their sugar intake.	Consume on average < 25 g/d of added sugar for the next 2 wk.	• Read the Nutrition Facts label for all packaged products to identify added sugars content. • Eat dessert ≤ 2 d/wk. • Drink water instead of soda.
A mother-child dyad would like to increase their physical activity.	Engage in physical activity for at least 30 min/d for the next 2 wk.	• Go for a walk around the block after dinner every night. • Track steps each day.
A mother of a newborn would like to breastfeed her baby exclusively for the first 6 mo after birth and continue until her baby is at least 2 y of age.	Establish an initial goal to feed the newborn breast milk exclusively on demand for the first 2 wk after birth.	• Connect with a local lactation consultant. • Join a breastfeeding support group. • Learn about common breastfeeding challenges and how to overcome them. • Track feedings and number of wet and dirty diapers. • Drink a glass of water with each breastfeeding session.

Self-monitoring

In general, a patient is most likely to achieve a nutrition goal if they monitor their progress.[3] Nutrition logs can help increase a school-aged child's or adolescent's awareness of their dietary intake. However, on some occasions, self-monitoring is inadvisable, such as in the case of a restrictive eating disorder (eg, anorexia nervosa) or mental health concern (eg, obsessive-compulsive disorder). Like the 3-day food record described in Chapter 10, Dietary History, Social History, and Food Insecurity Screening, the nutrition log should include the time of day of consumption, the food eaten, and the portion size. Other factors may also be included to help raise awareness of potential cues for eating, such as the location, the presence of other people, the potential emotional triggers for eating, and the potential distractions during eating. In the case of self-monitoring to identify potential food triggers for physiological symptoms such as abdominal pain, relation of symptoms to dietary intake may also be included. Many online programs and apps are available for food tracking, including photo logs, which include pictures taken by a patient of their food and drink intake over a 24-hour period. Self-monitoring of behavior changes helps build in accountability. Clinicians should encourage patients to monitor goal progress and take time to celebrate and reward themselves (with nonfood rewards) once they have attained a goal.

The 5 A's of Behavior Change Counseling

The 5 A's, originally described for tobacco cessation programs, are a useful tool for pediatric primary care clinicians to help guide behavior change counseling.[4,5] The 5 A's have been described in various ways, including *assess, advise, agree, assist,* and *arrange* and *ask, advise, assess, assist/agree,* and *arrange.* A clinic visit using the latter 5 A's, adapted slightly to *assess* before *advising,* might proceed as follows:

- **Ask:** The clinician introduces themselves. The clinician asks open-ended questions to help establish a focus and set the agenda and then asks permission before providing advice and information.
- **Assess:** The clinician assesses a patient's readiness to change. The clinician uses **O**pen-ended questions, **A**ffirmations, **R**eflective statements, and **S**ummarizing statements (OARS) to explore ambivalence and prompt change talk (refer to Chapter 14, Theories of Behavior Change and Motivational Interviewing, for a full description of OARS).
- **Advise:** The clinician uses the elicit-provide-elicit approach to elucidate a patient and family's current understanding of their health situation or nutritional status, add information to help support the identified behavior change, and elicit the patient and family's understanding and thoughts in response to the information added.
- **Assist/agree:** If a patient is ready to make changes, the clinician then assists them in developing a SMART goal and action plans. The clinician and patient agree on next steps, including how to celebrate success each time an action plan is implemented and once the goal is attained.
- **Arrange:** Together, the patient and clinician establish a plan for follow-up. During follow-up, clinicians can appreciate the patient's time and engagement, affirm any positive changes already made, and voice confidence in their ability to succeed in making the change. Follow-up visits may help a patient improve adherence by increasing their sense of accountability.[6]

Improving Adherence

The World Health Organization defines adherence as "the extent to which a person's behavior—taking medication, following a diet, and/or executing lifestyle changes—corresponds with agreed recommendations from a health care provider."[7] Factors that influence a patient's or family's adherence to a nutritional change can be classified as person, condition, treatment, relationship with health care professional, and environment (**Table 15-2**).

Planning for lapses and incorporating relapse prevention and problem-solving skills training into conversations about behavior change can help improve long-term adherence to a nutritional change. The following 5-step approach may help patients and their families build problem-solving skills[9]:

1. **Identify potential challenges.** Clinicians can help patients and their families consider what types of challenges might arise and how to handle them. For example, ask "What is the most difficult part about maintaining this nutritional change?"

Table 15-2. Factors That Influence Adherence to Nutrition Recommendations

Factors that influence adherence	Example(s)
Person	• Individual beliefs about nutrition • Expectations of what would occur with a change • Home environment • Behavior patterns • Nutrition knowledge • Skill in translating knowledge into daily behaviors
Condition	• Severity or chronicity of a disease that is being treated or prevented through nutritional changes • Importance to the patient of outcome that is being pursued, such as weight loss or improved sports performance
Treatment	• Perceived difficulty, complexity, and extent of nutritional changes that are required to best prevent or treat a condition. If a patient perceives the eating plan to be easy to understand and follow, they are more likely to make the recommended changes. If they perceive it to be complex and hard to follow, adherence to the recommendation is unlikely.
Relationship with health care professional	• How well the patient and clinician connect, including factors such as engagement, trust, respect, and understanding. • The clinician-patient relationship can help increase adherence through a patient's increased sense of being held accountable.[6]
Environment	• Home, school, work, and other community settings. The beliefs and culture around food and eating in these settings play an important role in determining nutrition intake and adherence. • Other factors include food pricing, media and marketing, food access, and food policies.

Derived from reference 8 and Sirur R, Richardson J, Wishart L, Hanna S. The role of theory in increasing adherence to prescribed practice. *Physiother Can*. 2009;61(2):68–77.

2. **Explore possible solutions.** Clinicians can ask questions such as "Can you tell me about a time in the past when you had this challenge and overcame it?" "What might make it easier to continue this nutritional change?" or "How might you address this challenge?"

3. **Make a plan.** Clinicians can discuss with patients and their families the pros and cons of each potential solution and choose 1 or 2 strategies to use when the challenge

arises. For example, clinicians may ask the patient "What are some advantages of each solution we discussed? What are potential downsides?" After discussion, the clinician might ask "What of these potential solutions do you want to test out when the challenge comes up?"

4. **Implement the plan.** When the challenge is experienced, the patient responds with one or more of the solutions discussed in the plan.

5. **Evaluate the plan.** Clinicians can then work together with patients to assess how well the solution helped address the challenge. If the solution was ineffective, the clinician can start again at step 2, exploring other possible solutions.

The Role of the Family

The family is a powerful force in supporting, or opposing, positive health behavior changes. This is especially the case when working with children and adolescents. This section explores 7 strategies that pediatricians can use to help strengthen family relationships and supports to improve the likelihood of a successful behavior change.[10]

- **Offer guidance on children's typical nutritional and physical preferences and abilities by age and stage.** As children develop, opportunities emerge at different times to promote healthful nutrition and activity. Parents who understand typical childhood development are better able to guide their children toward healthier choices.

- **Help parents hone their parenting approach.** There are 4 major types of parenting approaches: authoritarian, authoritative (responsive), permissive, and neglectful. These approaches are classified across 2 domains: warmth and responsiveness and control and/or demandingness. Research clearly supports that an authoritative (responsive) approach, when a parent is high in both domains, is most productive and leads to the best outcomes[11] (**Figure 15-1**). The value and importance of responsive parenting and feeding approaches are described in Chapter 11, Dietary Guidelines and Principles of Healthy Eating. An important aspect of nutritional coaching is helping parents develop strategies to adopt a more responsive style.

- **Help parents assess and change their perceptions of both their own current and ideal behaviors and their children's.** Studies suggest that many parents underestimate their child's weight and overestimate the nutritional quality of their child's diet and level of physical activity.[11] The best way to gauge current status is to help parents self-monitor both their own nutrition and physical activity, and, to the extent possible, their child's. Pediatricians may then review this information and the child's growth chart and nutritional assessment to help families establish goal nutrition and activity behaviors, which should be based on dietary and activity guidelines but tailored to the individual family.

- **Emphasize the power of modeling.** Parents are potent role models for their children. Studies support that children model how to eat, portion control, table manners, eating rituals, social interactions during mealtime, and timing of meals after their parents. Making family meals a priority not only provides parents an opportunity for positive role modeling but also is associated with health, educational, and social benefits for children, as well as decreased risk-taking behavior in teens.[11] Children and teens also model their parents' physical activity (and sedentary) behaviors.

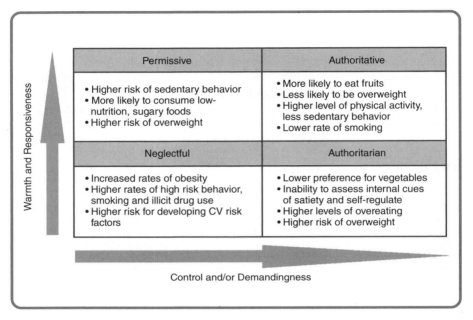

Figure 15-1. Parenting style and health effects.

Abbreviation: CV, cardiovascular.
Reproduced with permission from reference 11.

Having at least 1 physically active parent increases the odds that the children will be active. At the same time, high levels of parental television viewing and sedentary behavior predict child television viewing and sedentary behavior.[11]

- **Help parents create an environment that makes the healthy, active choice the easy choice.** Parents and their children share the home environment. If it is a healthy, active environment, by default the family members will be healthy and active. High availability of healthful foods and low availability of unhealthful foods helps make healthful food choices easier for everyone. Eating at home more often and cooking most meals support increased nutritional status, as does minimizing snacks and consumption of processed foods. Providing many opportunities for physical activity, and assistance (eg, transportation) to participate in activities, leads to more active families. In addition to the physical environment, family members share a behavioral environment, which includes self-efficacy for change, self-regulation, role modeling, and feeding practices. By using some of the coaching strategies described in this chapter, pediatricians can help families develop a plan to make changes feasibly and successfully.

- **Emphasize activities that promote quality time in addition to health benefits.** In the stresses of daily life, it is often difficult for families to take the time and energy needed to support strong bonds and family cohesion. Pediatricians can help parents identify opportunities to spend quality time with their children to grow and nurture those bonds. Whether doing baby massage for an infant, reading to a young child, taking a family walk, ensuring a parent date night, taking a trip to the farmers market, enrolling in an exercise class with a middle school–aged child, taking a one-on-one camping trip with a teen, or doing any other activity, small or large, the quality time together engaged in healthful activities yields big gains, because social support is a critical factor in sustaining any type of behavior change. In addition to helping build home and family support for behavior changes, pediatricians might encourage patients to recruit friends or family to make changes with them.

- **Help families practice coping with stress in productive ways.** In families, significant stress is a risk factor for unhealthy behaviors. For example, a parent who responds to stress with eating may have difficulty helping a child change a similar behavior. Financial stresses can affect meal planning, physical activities, family communication, and parenting quality. Clinicians should help patients identify stressors, their current response to those stressors, how the response may be affecting the family, and possible strategies to reduce or eliminate the stressors.
- **Help parents recognize and celebrate their successes.** Encourage families to notice even the smallest positive steps they make towards adopting healthier nutrition habits. Encourage them to monitor their goals and take the time to savor and celebrate once they have attained them.

In Sum

- Once a patient has moved to the planning process of motivational interviewing or the preparation stage of the transtheoretical model, they are ready to begin goal setting. The most effective goals are Specific, Measurable, Attainable, Relevant, and Time bound (SMART). Additionally, goals that are process centered, positive, and chosen by the patient to achieve are most likely to be achieved. Action plans are concrete steps that a patient plans to take to achieve the goal.
- Once a patient has begun to make a nutritional change, many factors influence adherence to the change. These factors can be classified as person, condition, treatment, relationship with health care professional, and environment. Helping patients build problem-solving skills and plan for lapses and relapses can help improve long-term adherence to a behavior change.
- Families play an important role in supporting a child's nutritional change. Parents who adopt an authoritative parenting style are more likely to have children that achieve and maintain their nutrition goals. Families can also support children and adolescents in making nutritional changes by having age-appropriate and developmentally appropriate expectations, serving as positive role models, creating a home environment that supports the nutritional change, spending quality time with the child or adolescent, and building skills to effectively manage stress.

References

1. Mann T, de Ridder D, Fujita K. Self-regulation of health behavior: social psychological approaches to goal setting and goal striving. *Health Psychol.* 2013;32(5):487–498 PMID: 23646832 doi: 10.1037/a0028533

2. Nicklas TA, Jahns L, Bogle ML, et al. Barriers and facilitators for consumer adherence to the *Dietary Guidelines for Americans:* the HEALTH study. *J Acad Nutr Diet.* 2013; 113(10):1317–1331 PMID: 23871110 doi: 10.1016/j.jand.2013.05.004

3. Harkin B, Webb TL, Chang BP, et al. Does monitoring goal progress promote goal attainment? a meta-analysis of the experimental evidence. *Psychol Bull.* 2016;142(2):198–229 PMID: 26479070 doi: 10.1037/bul0000025

4. Fiore MC, Bailey WC, Cohen SJ, et al. *Treating Tobacco Use and Dependence: Clinical Practice Guideline.* Public Health Service, US Dept of Health and Human Services; 2000

5. Whitlock EP, Orleans CT, Pender N, Allan J. Evaluating primary care behavioral counseling interventions: an evidence-based approach. *Am J Prev Med.* 2002;22(4):267–284 PMID: 11988383 doi: 10.1016/S0749-3797(02)00415-4

6. Oussedik E, Cline A, Su JJ, et al. Accountability in patient adherence. *Patient Prefer Adherence.* 2019;13:1511–1517 PMID: 31564838 doi: 10.2147/PPA.S213113

7. World Health Organization. *Adherence to Long-term Therapies: Evidence for Action.* World Health Organization; 2003:3

8. Desroches S, Lapointe A, Ratté S, Gravel K, Légaré F, Turcotte S. Interventions to enhance adherence to dietary advice for preventing and managing chronic diseases in adults. *Cochrane Database Syst Rev.* 2013;(2):CD008722

9. Middleton KR, Anton SD, Perri MG. Long-term adherence to health behavior change. *Am J Lifestyle Med.* 2013;7(6):395–404 PMID: 27547170 doi: 10.1177/1559827613488867

10. Muth ND. *Coaching the Whole Family.* IDEA Fitness Journal; 2016

11. Vedanthan R, Bansilal S, Soto AV, et al. Family-based approaches to cardiovascular health promotion. *J Am Coll Cardiol.* 2016;67(14):1725–1737 PMID: 27056780 doi: 10.1016/j.jacc.2016.01.036

Nutrition Prescription

Part 4, Nutrition Prescription, details nutrition prescription and guidance for special populations, including advice tailored to age and stage of development and to many of the most common conditions and chronic diseases. Chapter 16, Nutrition in Infancy, outlines how to advise families to optimize nutrition for preterm and full-term infants. Chapter 17, Nutrition in Childhood and Adolescence, provides tailored nutrition information for early childhood, middle childhood, and adolescence, including how to coach parents through the expected picky eating of toddlerhood, the more stable nutritional preferences in the school-age years, and the emerging independence and nutritional inadequacies associated with adolescence. Chapter 18, Sports and Athletic Performance, provides an overview of key sports nutrition principles and how to counsel patients to eat to optimize athletic performance while ensuring good health. Chapter 19, Mental Health, Behavioral, and Developmental Conditions, details nutrition principles for several common behavioral and developmental conditions, including depression and anxiety, attention-deficit/hyperactivity disorder, autism spectrum disorder, eating disorders, and special health care needs, and Chapter 20, Obesity and Related Health Conditions, details the nutritional management for children with obesity and related health conditions, such as hypercholesterolemia, hypertension, prediabetes and type 2 diabetes, and fatty liver. Chapter 21, Nutrition for Common Gastrointestinal, Autoimmune, and Inflammatory Conditions, provides an overview and nutrition strategies used in the treatment of some of the most common pediatric gastrointestinal and immune conditions, including constipation, irritable bowel syndrome, inflammatory bowel disease, gastroesophageal reflux disease, celiac disease, food allergies and intolerances, and type 1 diabetes.

CHAPTER 16

Nutrition in Infancy

A child's nutritional exposures and feeding experiences in infancy influence long-term health outcomes and shape taste preferences and food choices later in life. Parents rely heavily on nutritional advice from pediatricians, especially during this stage of development, offering an important opportunity for clinicians to provide support and guidance that can help parents raise healthy eaters.

Nutrition in the first 1,000 days after birth is critical in ensuring optimal neurological development and brain function. As stated in the American Academy of Pediatrics (AAP) policy statement advocating for improved nutrition in the first 1,000 days, "in the presence of a supportive environment, an attached primary caregiver, and a healthy diet, the brain typically thrives."[1]

Feeding Volume and Caloric Needs

For the first 6 months after birth, babies meet all caloric, nutrient, and fluid needs from appropriate intake of human (breast) milk or formula. In the first few days after birth, newborns consume small volumes of colostrum or formula and may lose up to 10% of their birth weight. However, in the second week after birth, breast milk or formula intake increases, and most newborns regain weight to birth weight by 2 weeks of age. Newborns and infants aged 0 to 6 months require about 23 fl oz (700 mL) per day.[2] Given that standard formula and breast milk contain about 20 kcal/fl oz, this is the equivalent of about 450 Cal/d, or about 90 kcal/kg of body weight (when the reference body weight is 11 lb [5 kg]).

Individual caloric needs can be estimated with the following equations by using the newborn's or infant's current weight[3]:

- Age 0 to 3 months: $(89 \times \text{weight [kg]} - 100) + 175$ kcal
- Age 4 to 6 months: $(89 \times \text{weight [kg]} - 100) + 56$ kcal

There are 30 mL in 1 fl oz and 2.2 lb in 1 kg. For most babies, this equation breaks needs down to typical intakes shown in **Table 16-1**.

A baby's volume and caloric needs increase rapidly in the first year after birth to support rapid growth. Typically, babies double their birth weight by 4 to 6 months of age (gaining about 4–7 oz [113–198 g] per week) and triple their birth weight by 1 year of age (gaining about 2–5 oz [57–142 g] per week from 6–12 months of age). Babies grow about 1 inch (2 cm) per month from birth to 6 months of age and then half an inch (1 cm) per month from 6 to 12 months of age, increasing their length by about 50% in the first year.[5]

For most healthy full-term infants, it is unnecessary to calculate fluid and caloric intake because infants are generally able to use internal feelings of hunger, thirst, and fullness to show signs of hunger and satiety. If parents respond to these signs, infants will generally

Table 16-1. Typical Volume and Caloric Intakes and Weight Gain in Newborns and Infants 0 to 12 Months of Age

Age (mo)	Volume (mL/kg/d)	Calories (kcal/kg of body weight)	Weight gain (g/d)
0-3	140-200	90-135	25-30
3-6	100	80	15-20
6-12	100; if weight > 10 kg, then 1,000 mL + 50 mL/kg for every 1 kg > 10 kg	80	10-15

Derived from reference 4.

receive the appropriate amounts of calories and fluids. Although pediatricians advise parents that their newborn eat at least 8 to 12 times per day to ensure sufficient intake for weight regain, once a newborn has regained weight to birth weight, clinicians may counsel parents to focus on responsive feeding and identified cues for hunger and fullness, to feed on demand, and to allow a healthy full-term newborn to sleep for longer stretches at night if the newborn does not awaken on their own for a feeding every 2 to 3 hours. Newborns and infants will generally meet nutritional needs over 24 hours, so if babies sleep for longer stretches at night, they will likely feed more frequently during the day.

Breastfeeding

The AAP recommends exclusive breastfeeding for about 6 months after birth and "supports continued breastfeeding, along with appropriate complementary foods introduced at about 6 months, as long as mutually desired by mother and child for 2 years or beyond."[6] Infants who are ever breastfed are less likely to experience acute otitis media, gastroenteritis, severe lower respiratory tract infections, necrotizing enterocolitis, overweight and obesity, type 1 diabetes, asthma, eczema, sudden infant death syndrome, and overall infant mortality than infants who are never breastfed. Longer duration of breastfeeding is associated with further decreased risk of type 1 diabetes and asthma.[7] Maternal benefits of breastfeeding include less postpartum bleeding, delayed ovulation, decreased incidence of postpartum depression, and lower rates of several diseases, such as hypertension, diabetes, cardiovascular disease, and some cancers.[7] Pediatricians are encouraged to refer to the AAP policy statement (https://doi.org/10.1542/peds.2022-057988) and technical report (https://doi.org/10.1542/peds.2022-057989) on breastfeeding and the use of human milk for more detailed information and guidance to support breastfeeding.

Nutritional Composition of Colostrum, Transitional Milk, and Mature Milk

Colostrum is the initial form of breast milk, present in very small amounts in the newborn's first 24 hours after birth and highly concentrated in protein, fat-soluble vitamins (especially beta carotene), minerals, electrolytes, and antibodies. Colostrum's protein composition includes 70% to 80% whey protein and 20% to 30% casein. All hospitals should promote that the newborn breastfeed for the first time within the first hour after birth and ensure that the mother-newborn dyad receive a lactation consultation at the hospital, during the hospitalization.

Transitional milk develops approximately 5 to 14 days after delivery. Compared to colostrum, it has decreased immunoglobulins and protein and increased lactose, fat, and total calories (approximately 20 kcal/fl oz).

By the time a newborn is 2 weeks of age, most women are producing mature milk. This milk provides the ideal nutritional composition for infant feeding. Milk protein consists of casein, a substance that clots or curds, and whey, a liquid that digests easily. Breast milk is generally 40% to 80% whey, depending on the stage of breastfeeding, a significantly higher percentage than is present in most formulas and the reason that breast milk may be easier for infants to digest than formula. The carbohydrate in breast milk is primarily lactose. Breast milk also contains anti-infective and anti-inflammatory factors; oligosaccharides that promote a healthy gut microbiome; growth factors; cells such as neutrophils, leukocytes, and stem cells; and probiotics, including bifidobacterial and lactobacilli, which establish the gut microbiota. The nutritional composition of breast milk is highlighted in **Table 16-2**.

Breastfed babies should receive a 400-IU (10-mcg) supplement of vitamin D starting at birth and continuing until the infant is weaned to vitamin D–fortified whole milk at 1 year of age. Maternal iron stores can ensure that a breastfed baby receives adequate iron until approximately 4 months of age. The AAP recommends that breastfed infants receive an iron supplement of 1 mg/kg/d beginning at 4 months of age and continuing until the infant consumes an adequate amount of iron-rich complementary foods (eg, meat, iron-rich vegetables) to meet the Dietary Reference Intake of 11 mg/d of iron.

How to Ensure Adequate Intake

Many breastfeeding mothers express concern that it is difficult to know whether their infant is receiving enough milk to ensure adequate growth and weight gain. In addition to tracking weight gain between clinic visits, as part of the newborn and 2- to 4-week health supervision visits for breastfeeding newborns, pediatricians can assess the newborn's milk intake by asking mothers about indicators of adequate intake, including type and number of stools and urinations, and by measuring newborn weights before and after a feeding with the same scale. If weight gain is inadequate, clinicians should further investigate the cause. They should obtain a detailed history of the mother and newborn, including the mother's medical, surgical, obstetric, and previous and present lactation and newborn feeding. Clinicians may also assess newborn latch and milk transfer during lactation sessions, with the breastfeeding mother's permission. Clinicians may encourage breastfeeding mothers to increase the frequency of feedings and increase the milk expression between feedings, which may help increase supply and newborn weight gain. Signs of insufficient milk intake, caused by either lack of supply or poor transfer, include delayed gut motility, fewer bowel movements, decreased urinary output, early jaundice, hunger, lethargy, and greater than 7% loss of body weight.

Table 16-2. Representative Values for Constituents of Human Milk

Constituent (per liter)	Mature milk (after 2 weeks' lactation)
Energy (kcal)	650–700
Macronutrients	
Lactose (g)	67–70
Oligosaccharides (g)	12–14
Total nitrogen (g)	1.9
Nonprotein nitrogen (% total nitrogen)	23
Protein nitrogen (% total nitrogen)	77
Total protein (g)	9
Total lipids (g)	35
Triglyceride (% total lipids)	97–98
Cholesterol (% total lipids)	0.4–0.5
Phospholipids (% total lipids)	0.6–0.8
Water-soluble vitamins	
Ascorbic acid (mg)	100
Thiamin (μg)	200
Riboflavin (μg)	400–600
Niacin (mg)	1.8–6.0
Vitamin B_6 (mg)	0.09–0.31
Folate (μg)	80–140
Vitamin B_{12} (μg)	0.5–1.0
Pantothenic acid (mg)	2–2.5
Biotin (μg)	5–9
Fat-soluble vitamins	
Retinol (mg)	0.3–0.6
Carotenoids (mg)	0.2–0.6
Vitamin K (μg)	2–3
Vitamin D (μg)	0.33
Vitamin E (mg)	3–8

Table 16-2 (*continued*)

Constituent (per liter)	Mature milk (after 2 weeks' lactation)
Fat-soluble vitamins (*continued*)	
Calcium (mg)	200–250
Magnesium (mg)	30–35
Phosphorus (mg)	120–140
Sodium (mg)	120–250
Potassium (mg)	400–550
Chloride (mg)	400–450
Trace elements	
Iron (mg)	0.3–0.9
Zinc (mg)	1–3
Copper (mg)	0.2–0.4
Manganese (µg)	3
Selenium (µg)	7–33
Iodine (µg)	150
Fluoride (µg)	4–15

Reproduced from American Academy of Pediatrics, American College of Obstetricians and Gynecologists. Composition of human milk. In: Schanler RJ, Krebs NF, Mass SB, eds. *Breastfeeding Handbook for Physicians.* 2nd ed. American Academy of Pediatrics, American College of Obstetricians and Gynecologists; 2014:41–52.

Clinicians should encourage parents to aim for approximately 10 to 45 minutes per feeding and should advise parents to ensure that feedings do not last more than 1 hour. However, the important factor is not the duration of feeding but whether the infant is receiving adequate intake.

Common Breastfeeding Challenges

Pediatricians can also help breastfeeding mothers address common breastfeeding challenges, including

- Nipple pain. This usually results from poor positioning, improper latch, or trauma from suckling on the nipple rather than the areola. Clinicians may advise mothers to lubricate and cover nipple wounds to promote healing. Continuing breastfeeding with a good latch promotes healing.
- Engorgement. Engorgement is caused by infrequent feedings or ineffective milk removal. It is most common between days 3 and 5 postpartum with the onset of lactogenesis. Engorgement is relieved by breastfeeding or manual pumping or expression before feedings.

- Clogged duct. Clogged ducts occur when the breast is not fully emptied. Treatment includes gentle massage to the duct and increased breastfeeding.
- Mastitis. Mastitis manifests as warmth, tenderness, edema, and erythema of the breast, along with fever, fatigue, and intense breast pain. Treatment includes breastfeeding, rest, analgesics, and antibiotics.

Freshly pumped breast milk can safely remain at room temperature for up to 4 hours or in the refrigerator for up to 4 days stored in a glass or hard plastic container and as an individual feeding. It can be frozen for 6 to 12 months.

Formula Feeding

Many babies are not exclusively breastfed for the first 6 months after birth, whether because of difficult milk production or latch, other feeding problems, baby or maternal health considerations, parental or caregiver preference, or other factors. In these cases, caregivers have the choice of more than 50 different infant formulas, which is an overwhelming number of options for many families. Although many formulas are marketed to provide infants with superior nutrition across a range of considerations or concerns, in many cases the nutritional composition across formula brands and formulations is similar. For example, most formulas include fats from docosahexaenoic acid and arachidonic acid. There is no evidence that organic formulas provide greater nutritional or health benefits than nonorganic formula. Many popular formula add-ons, such as probiotics and prebiotics, are appealing to parents, but studies to date have not shown clear benefit. Generally, generic brand formulas are nutritionally equivalent to brand name formulas.

Key differences between formulas include the composition of the protein and carbohydrates. Some formulas contain lactose in similar levels to those in breast milk, whereas others contain less or no lactose and instead include corn syrup, maltodextrin, or sucrose. Variations in protein and carbohydrate composition may benefit some babies with cow milk allergy or severe eczema.[8] Although specialty formulas are heavily marketed with purported benefits such as reduced gassiness, reflux, and colic, evidence of their efficacy for many of these claims is limited. In addition, a systematic review of the conduct and reporting of formula trials revealed that formula trials are generally unreliable because the formula industry is highly involved in these trials, findings are almost always reported as favorable, and transparency is limited regarding trial aims and reported trial results.[9] A more detailed overview of various formula options is shown in **Table 16-3**.

Parents may buy formula as ready-to-use liquid, concentrated liquid, or powder. When powdered formula is used, it is important for parents to carefully follow the instructions to ensure that the correct amount of water is added and electrolyte balance is maintained. Parents may choose to use filtered tap water or sterile water when preparing formula. Alkaline water is not advised.

Unconsumed prepared formula should be discarded within 1 hour after the infant feeding. If the formula has not been given to the infant, it can be stored in the refrigerator for up to 24 hours. An open container of ready-made formula should be covered, refrigerated, and discarded within 48 hours if not used.

Table 16-3. Formula Comparison

Formulation	Calories per ounce	Carbohydrate	Protein	Clinical considerations
Preterm discharge	22	Lactose	Cow milk, mostly whey	Increased caloric content supports growth in preterm infants.
Regular with docosahex-aenoic acid	20	Lactose	Whey and casein	Regular formula is appro-priate for most healthy full-term infants. Whether the addition of docosa-hexaenoic acid provides additional benefits (eg, improved visual func-tion and neural develop-ment) is an area of active investigation, with some studies showing benefit and others not.[10]
Soy protein isolate	20	Corn based Lactose-free	Soy	Recommended formula for galactosemia or lac-tase deficiency. Plant based, so may appeal to families who prefer vegetarian nutrient sources. Scientific evidence does not support claims of re-duced crying/fussiness/gas/poor sleep.
Reduced lactose	20	Corn based	Cow milk	There are few medical indications to reduce lactose. Parents often attribute crying/fussiness/gas/poor sleep to lactose in formula, but scientific evidence does not sup-port these claims.
Rice-starch thickener	20	Lactose and/or corn syrup solids and/or maltodextrin thickened with rice starch	Partially hydrolyzed casein or whey	Scientific evidence sup-ports that use of formula with rice-starch thickener contributes to modestly improved reflux.[11,12]

Continued

Table 16-3 (*continued*)

Formulation	Calories per ounce	Carbohydrate	Protein	Clinical considerations
Extensive milk protein hydrolysates	20	Corn or sucrose Lactose-free	Extensively hydrolyzed casein or whey	Recommended to use in cases of cow milk intolerance (5%–15% of infants) or allergy (2.0%–7.5% of infants) and high-risk atopic dermatitis or allergy.
Partial milk protein hydrolysates	20	Corn syrup or maltodextrin and lactose	Partially hydrolyzed casein or whey	Scientific evidence does not support claims of reduced crying/fussiness/gas/poor sleep. Very little scientific evidence supports that a 100% partially hydrolyzed whey-protein infant formula may reduce the risk of atopic dermatitis.[13]
Amino acid protein source	20	Corn syrup solids Lactose-free	Free amino acids	Recommended to use for infants with cow milk allergy with symptoms not improved while taking extensive hydrolysates. Other indications for use include ● Protein maldigestion ● Malabsorption ● Short bowel syndrome ● Food allergies ● Eosinophilic esophagitis ● High-risk atopic dermatitis or allergy
Toddler formula (follow-on or follow-up formula)	20	Corn syrup Lactose	Nonfat cow milk	Use is not recommended.

Derived from references 14 and 15.

The AAP and the Centers for Disease Control and Prevention recommend that parents choose formulas sold and marketed in the United States because these formulas are required to meet certain nutrition standards and safeguards (**Box 16-1**). The infant formula shortage crisis in 2022 prompted the US Food and Drug Administration to temporarily ease requirements for imported formulas in order to increase the supply of formula in the United States.

IN GREATER DEPTH

Box 16-1. Imported Formulas

Even before the 2022 formula shortage in the United States, many parents chose to purchase imported European formulas. These purchases were commonly made online through third-party vendors because the formulas are not registered with the US Food and Drug Administration (FDA). Parents often buy these formulas believing that they are healthier for their infant than US formulas because of stricter formula standards in Europe and use of higher-quality ingredients. For example, some European formulas are made with milk from goats or milk from pasture-raised cows. Some hypoallergenic European formulas contain lactose sugars rather than the corn sugar (maltodextrin or corn syrup) found in hypoallergenic US formulas. Nutritionally, US and European formulas are very similar, except for US formulas having slightly more iron and European formulas having more docosahexaenoic acid. The clinical significance of these differences is negligible. Purchasing European formulas through third-party vendors bypasses the safeguards put into place by the FDA to ensure that formula offers adequate nutrition for infants and includes manufacturing practices with specific controls to prevent contamination. Additionally, usual safety regulations in the country of origin may be bypassed, increasing risk of potential tampering and contamination for US consumers. The formulas also come at a steep price. For example, it can cost approximately $1.70 to make a 6–fl oz (177-mL) bottle of a European formula, whereas it costs about $0.50 to make a standard US formula.[16]

A study of 14 of the most popular imported European formulas showed that although the formulas were nutritionally similar to FDA-registered formulas, none met all the FDA labeling requirements, including 9 that did not have English labels. Without English labels, there is increased risk of improper formula preparation. European formula generally requires 1 fl oz (30 mL)

Continued

IN GREATER DEPTH

Box 16-1 (*continued*)

of water per 1 level scoop of powdered formula. US formulas generally require 1 unpacked level scoop per 2 fl oz (59 mL) of water. Improper mixing can lead to inadequate caloric intake, causing malnutrition. It also can lead to electrolyte imbalances in infants, which can potentially cause seizures. In addition, partially hydrolyzed European formulas can be labeled "hypoallergenic," which is inappropriate for infants with cow milk protein allergy.[17]

The Centers for Disease Control and Prevention notes, "There are some public claims that infant formulas sold in other countries and promoted as 'natural' or 'organic' are better for babies. However, there is no scientific evidence that these infant formulas are better for babies than commercial infant formulas sold in the United States. All infant formulas legally sold in the United States—whether made in the United States or imported from other countries—must be reviewed by FDA. The American Academy of Pediatrics warns against using illegally imported formulas, such as products ordered online from third-party distributors. FDA may not have reviewed these products. Illegally imported formulas also may not have been shipped and stored properly. FDA reviews all infant formulas sold legally in the United States to make sure they meet minimum nutritional and safety requirements. FDA also makes sure that the water used to make formulas meets safety standards set by the US Environmental Protection Agency."[18]

Clinicians should strongly discourage parents from preparing or purchasing homemade formula. A review of online parenting blogs revealed at least 59 blogs featuring 144 recipes for homemade infant formula, most of which advertised ingredients or recipe kits. The most commonly mentioned recipe ingredients were whole, raw cow milk; raw goat milk; and liver.[19] The potential negative effects associated with homemade formula include severe nutritional and electrolyte imbalances, serious health concerns, and death.[20]

Bottle-feeding

Whether with expressed breast milk or formula, many infants may feed by bottle at some point. Clinicians can share with parents the following best practices for bottle-feeding:

- Never prop the bottle; rather, hold it at an angle so the baby is not sucking in air. Alternatively, consider paced bottle-feeding with the bottle held flat and then tipped

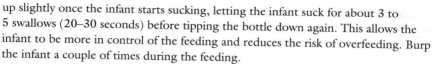

up slightly once the infant starts sucking, letting the infant suck for about 3 to 5 swallows (20–30 seconds) before tipping the bottle down again. This allows the infant to be more in control of the feeding and reduces the risk of overfeeding. Burp the infant a couple of times during the feeding.

- Make sure that the nipple hole is the right size and shape. A nipple that is too small may lead to frustration and fatigue in the infant, whereas a nipple that is too large may lead to gagging or fast gulping. Choosing the right nipple size is often a matter of trial and error. There are sizes for preterm infants, size 1 (generally for ages 0–6 months), and sizes 2–4 (most often preferred by older infants). Nipples also come in different shapes. The "best" shape is whichever one the baby prefers.
- Warm bottles by placing them into hot water for a few minutes. Never warm a bottle in the microwave.
- If a breastfeeding mother desires to introduce a bottle, introduce it 2 weeks or later after breastfeeding is well established. Breastfed babies often refuse bottles when offered by their mother, but not by other caregivers, because many may prefer to feed at the breast. However, a hungry baby will eventually eat and, if the mother is unavailable for breastfeeding, will eventually take a bottle from another caregiver.
- Avoid allowing the baby to fall asleep with the bottle because this causes early childhood caries for babies who have teeth. Wipe the baby's gums after feedings to prevent caries formation.
- Use a smaller bottle size when formula feeding younger infants. This helps prevent excessive intake and weight gain and may be an effective obesity prevention strategy.[21]

The Role of Infant Nutrition in Early Childhood Caries

Early childhood caries is defined as decayed, missing, or filled tooth surfaces in a child 72 months or younger. It results when the bacterium *Streptococcus mutans* or *Streptococcus sobrinus* interacts with the sugar sucrose, fructose, or glucose on the tooth surface. There, the bacterium metabolizes the sugar for energy, producing acetic acid, which breaks down the tooth enamel. Early childhood caries is often referred to as "baby bottle tooth decay" because of the high prevalence in infants given a bottle to go to bed or to be soothed.

Although dental caries, the most common chronic disease of childhood, most often develops in early childhood rather than infancy, the risk factors for dental caries start in infancy for many children, sometimes even before teeth erupt. Newly erupted teeth are more susceptible to caries because of immature enamel. The American Academy of Pediatric Dentistry notes that caries-promoting dietary practices are typically established by 12 months of age and tend to be maintained through early childhood.[22] Nutritional factors associated with the development and progression of caries, and anticipatory guidance to address the risk factors, are highlighted in **Table 16-4**.

The best way to optimize oral hygiene to prevent dental caries is brushing an infant's teeth 2 times per day with a rice-sized amount of fluoridated toothpaste once the infant has teeth. Additionally, consumption of fluoridated water after age 6 months helps prevent dental caries. Fluoride works by promoting enamel remineralization, reducing enamel demineralization, and inhibiting bacterial metabolism and acid production.

Table 16-4. Nutritional Factors Associated With Development and Progression of Dental Caries

Risk factor	Anticipatory guidance
Frequent nighttime bottle-feeding	Avoid putting babies to bed with a bottle containing human (breast) milk or formula.
Any nighttime bottle-feeding with juice	Avoid juice.
Repeated use of a sippy cup or no-spill cup	Use an open cup rather than a sippy cup. If a sippy cup is used, it should be used only for water without added juice for flavor. Wean the infant from the bottle at 12 mo of age.
Frequent between-meal consumption of sugary drinks (eg, juice, formula, soda) and sugary snacks	Avoid sugary drinks and snacks between meals.
Consumption of breast milk together with other carbohydrates	Avoid on demand breastfeeding once teeth erupt and other carbohydrates have been introduced into the diet.

Derived from American Academy of Pediatric Dentistry. Policy on early childhood caries (ECC): classifications, consequences, and preventive strategies. In: *The Reference Manual of Pediatric Dentistry*. American Academy of Pediatric Dentistry; 2020:79–81.

Excess fluoride during tooth development can lead to hypomineralization and subsequent discoloration of the teeth. Moderate and severe cases of fluorosis are very rare.[22] Parents can learn whether their water is fluoridated by accessing the water quality report or consumer confidence report on their local water utility's website or by accessing the Centers for Disease Control and Prevention website My Water's Fluoride (https://nccd.cdc.gov/doh_mwf/default/default.aspx).

Nutrition Considerations for Preterm Infants

Preterm infants have unique nutritional needs arising from a combination of the following risk factors for nutritional deficiency: (1) low stores of macronutrients, fat-soluble vitamins, and key minerals such as calcium, phosphorus, magnesium, iron, and trace minerals; (2) rapid growth, which further depletes stores; (3) an immature gastrointestinal system, which contributes to low concentrations of important digestive enzymes and delayed gastric emptying; (4) an immature renal system, which compromises fluid and electrolyte balance; and (5) increased risk of illnesses such as necrotizing enterocolitis, which further affect nutritional status. Very preterm or low birth weight infants generally require total parenteral nutrition that is then transitioned to enteral feedings. Given that this type of nutritional management is generally outside the scope of the primary care pediatrician, it is not discussed in depth in this chapter.

As a preterm infant grows and develops the strength, coordination, and skill to feed by mouth and transitions from the hospital-based neonatal intensive care to home-based care, the general pediatrician plays an important role in feeding monitoring and guidance. This is especially critical for infants with very low birth weight (VLBW) (<53 oz [1,500 g]). Infants with VLBW experience most of their catch-up growth after hospital discharge, and without careful attention to nutrition, they are at high risk of developing nutritional deficiencies that can contribute to poor neurodevelopmental outcomes.

When monitoring nutrition and growth for infants with VLBW, clinicians should consider the following guidance[23]:

- Encourage the feeding of fortified breast milk (preferred) or preterm formula (22–24 kcal/fl oz) for at least 12 weeks following hospital discharge, or until 4 months' corrected age. **Table 16-5** outlines one way to increase the caloric density of milk or standard formula by adding formula powder to prepared standard formula or breast milk. A mother may prefer to have some feedings be unfortified breast milk, so she can breastfeed, while fortifying the other feedings or giving formula for the other feedings. This preference should reflect shared decision-making by the mother and pediatrician. Sometimes, a mother may want to try to exclusively breastfeed for all feedings, which may be acceptable when the infant is breastfeeding well and has neither growth restriction nor evidence of protein or mineral insufficiency.[24]
- Recommend iron supplementation of 2 to 3 mg/kg/d until the infant is 6 to 12 months of age (uncorrected), depending on diet. Some infants who are fed preterm formula do not need additional supplementation; however, other preterm infants, such as infants who have VLBW or infants who have significant anemia of prematurity, may need additional supplementation up to 6 to 8 mg/kg/d. Monitor iron status of VLBW infants by following ferritin levels. If an infant's ferritin level is less than 35 ng/mL (35 mcg/L), iron supplementation should be increased. If an infant's ferritin level is greater than 300 ng/mL (300 mcg/L), supplementation should be stopped. Ferritin ranges between 35 and 300 ng/mL (35 and 300 mcg/L) are acceptable.[25]
- Recommend 400 IU (10 mcg) of vitamin D supplement per day for breastfed infants. Consider 200 to 400 IU (5–10 mcg) of vitamin D supplement per day for formula-fed preterm infants who receive formulas designed for full-term infants and who consume less than 27 fl oz (800 mL) of formula per day.[26]

Complementary Feeding

The AAP recommends introduction of complementary foods around 6 months of age, depending on an infant's developmental readiness for solid foods.[23] Solid foods should not be introduced before 4 months of age because of increased risk of obesity[26] and food allergies and should not be delayed beyond 6 months.[27]

Signs that an infant is ready for complementary foods include

- Fading of the extrusion reflex
- Elevation of the tongue to move pureed food forward and backward in the mouth
- Increase in demand for breastfeeding for several days
- Sitting with self-support by the arms
- Control of the head and neck

Refer to **Table 16-6** for an overview of infant intake and typical progression of feeding independence.

Table 16-5. An Example of How to Increase Caloric Density of Human Milk or Standard Infant Formula[a]

Goal (Cal/fl oz)[b]	Human milk or prepared standard formula (fl oz)	Amount of standard formula powder to be added to achieve goal
22	3	½ tsp
	4	½ tsp + ¼ tsp
	16	1 tbsp
24	2	½ tsp + ¼ tsp
	5	2 tsp
	8	1 tbsp

[a] Manufacturer information for standard formula powders (Cal/g, grams per scoop, grams per household measuring spoon) was used to calculate measurements that could be easily followed for fortification of breast milk. These measurements are reviewed regularly and adjusted based on changes in manufacturer data. Although changes in formula powder are typically minute and do not generally result in a need to change these measurements, significant future changes to manufacturer formulations could make this information obsolete. Please refer to the table source for the most up-to-date measurements.

[b] When using different formula brands, final calorie concentration may vary slightly. This is not generally clinically significant if a major US or generic formula is used. However, the information in this table should not be used with any European formulas or formulas not approved by the US Food and Drug Administration.

SI conversion factor: To convert fl oz to mL, multiply by 30.

Adapted with permission from Children's Minnesota Clinical Nutrition Team. Breast milk: fortified. Revised November 2020. Accessed October 25, 2022. https://www.childrensmn.org/references/pfs/nutr/breast-milk-fortified-(using-20-cal-oz-standard-formula).pdf.

First Foods

Adequate intake of key macronutrients (in particular, protein and long-chain polyunsaturated fatty acids) and micronutrients (in particular, zinc, copper, iodine, iron, folate, and choline) is critical for optimal brain development, especially during infancy.[1]

Sufficient intake of breast milk plus a vitamin D supplement or formula in the first 6 months after birth provides the macronutrients and micronutrients needed to support brain growth. Breastfeeding is associated with improved performance in intelligence tests, which persists after adjustments for maternal IQ. In addition, long-term follow-up studies suggest that breastfeeding influences school performance and adult income.[28] At 6 months of age, complementary foods should be introduced to provide adequate nutrition, especially for zinc, iron, vitamin D, and polyunsaturated fats.[1] Infants older than 6 months need about 11 g/d of iron. Parents can ensure that infants meet this recommendation by incorporating iron-rich foods into a daily meal plan.

Pediatricians previously recommended starting with rice cereal because of its high iron content (from fortification) and ease of offering. However, studies have shown that rice contains high levels of arsenic and should be minimized in an infant diet because of arsenic's harmful effect on neurological development. Infant oatmeal is an iron-fortified food and is a healthy alternative to rice cereal. However, it is not necessary that this food be introduced first. In fact, there is no "best" first food. Several healthful suggestions of first foods and how parents can prepare them are shown in **Table 16-7**.

Table 16-6. Infant Intake and Typical Progression of Feeding Independence

Age (mo)	Feeding skills	Physical skills	Oro-motor skills	Signs of hunger	Signs of fullness	No. of feedings per day	Fluid ounces per feeding (fl oz)[a]	Fluid ounces per day (fl oz/d)[a]
0–4	● Coordinated suck-swallow-breathe ● Able to swallow liquids and use tongue to suck	Brings hands to mouth around 3 mo	● Rooting reflex ● Sucking reflex ● Swallowing reflex ● Extrusion reflex	Early feeding cues: ● Increased alertness ● Rooting ● Lip smacking ● Opening the mouth	● Becoming fussy during feeding ● Falling asleep ● Pulling or turning away from the nipple, bottle, or spoon ● Extending or relaxing the arms	8–12	2–6	16–36
5	● Able to grasp objects voluntarily ● Learning to reach	● Good head control and able to sit with support ● Continues to grasp objects by using palmer grasp reflex	Disappearance of extrusion reflex	Late feeding cue: ● Crying and irritability		3–5	7–8	24–36

Continued

Table 16-6 (*continued*)

Age (mo)	Feeding skills	Physical skills	Oro-motor skills	Signs of hunger	Signs of fullness	No. of feedings per day	Fluid ounces per feeding (fl oz)[a]	Fluid ounces per day (fl oz/d)[a]
6	• Ready for high chair • Able to take spoonful of pureed or strained foods • Able to swallow without choking	Able to recognize spoon and holds mouth open when spoon approaches	• Transfers food from front of tongue to back • Closes lips around spoon • Able to hold and drink from a cup • Uses raking grasp to feed self	(*Refer to previous page.*)	(*Refer to previous page.*)	3–5	7–8	24–36

[a] These values are general guidance. Parents should be encouraged to use their infant's cues of hunger and fullness to determine infant intakes.

Table 16-7. Possible First Foods, Associated Rationales, and Preparation Tips for Parents

Food	Rationale for inclusion as a first food	Preparation tips to share with parents
Infant oatmeal	Infant oatmeal is a nutrient-rich alternative to rice cereal because it is high in fiber, and the infant variety has been fortified with essential nutrients, such as iron and vitamin E.	Single grain oatmeal cereal can be mixed with formula or human (breast) milk or added to vegetable or fruit purees.
Avocado	Easy to mash and feed, avocados are high in monounsaturated and polyunsaturated fats, vitamin K, and folate.	Cut the avocado in half, remove the seed, and mash the fruit with a fork. Soften with breast milk, formula, or a small amount of water.
Banana	Easy to mash and feed, bananas are high in potassium.	Peel and slice the banana, and mash the fruit with a fork to desired consistency.
Sweet potato	Sweet potatoes are high in iron and antioxidant vitamins A and C.	Pierce the flesh of the sweet potato multiple times, then microwave at 5-min intervals, checking for tenderness with a fork at each interval. The potato is cooked once it is tender and a fork passes easily into the flesh. or Roast whole or cubed sweet potatoes at 375 °F until fork tender (approximately 30 min if cubed or 45–60 min if whole).
Broccoli	High in iron and calcium, broccoli is also an excellent source of vitamins A, C, and B_6.	Steam broccoli until tender but still bright green, or roast it in the oven to bring out its natural sweetness. To roast broccoli, heat the oven to 450 °F and roast it for 15–20 min until slightly browned and crispy.

Continued

Table 16-7 (*continued*)

Food	Rationale for inclusion as a first food	Preparation tips to share with parents
Lentils	Lentils are an excellent form of plant-based protein. Lentils are also high in zinc and iron. Lentils contain phytates, which can interfere with iron absorption, but this interference can be countered by offering lentils with vitamin C–rich foods.	Lentils come in a wide variety: green, red, yellow, brown, and black. They are inexpensive and do not require any soaking, making them an easy and economical addition to a meal. Red, orange, and yellow lentils cook more quickly than other varieties. Once cooked, lentils are soft and mushy, making them an ideal first food. Simple red lentils: Add 2.5 c of water to a pot with 1 c of lentils. Bring water to a boil, then cover the pot with a lid and simmer the lentils for 30 min, or until tender.
Salmon	Salmon is high in B vitamins, choline, selenium, potassium, and iron. Additionally, salmon is perhaps best known for its omega-3 fatty acid content, particularly docosahexaenoic acid, which plays an important role in eye and brain development.	Salmon can be baked, poached, or steamed until firm and then blended with fruits and/or vegetables until smooth. Once an infant has tried each food individually, parents may try the following combinations: • Salmon, lentils, sweet potatoes • Salmon, avocado, oatmeal
Chicken	Chicken is high in choline, selenium, and iron. Choline is needed to produce acetylcholine, a neurotransmitter that helps regulate memory, mood, muscle control, and nervous system function. Selenium is essential for thyroid function.	Chicken can be poached or baked, but an even easier way to cook chicken is in a slow cooker. To increase acceptance, parents may offer chicken warmed slightly, pureed, and mixed with a food that their infant already likes. For example, once an infant has tried each food individually, parents may try the following combinations: • Chicken with butternut squash • Chicken with plums

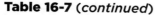

Table 16-7 (*continued*)

Food	Rationale for inclusion as a first food	Preparation tips to share with parents
Eggs	With 6 g of protein in 1 egg, eggs are a convenient and economical protein source. A good source of iron and rich in choline, folate, and selenium, eggs are also a good source of B vitamins.	Boil eggs until cooked through and firm. Remove the shells and cut eggs in half. Slice into small pieces or mash the yolks with a fork and then thin them with breast milk or formula or blend them with vegetable puree.
Peanuts and tree nuts	Nuts provide a source of protein and fatty acids. The wide variety of no-sugar nut butters and the ease in blending nuts to make a powder make it easy to introduce nuts early and often.	Because chunks of nut butter are a choking hazard, mix 1-2 tsp with cereal and breast milk or formula, or add nut flour to the infant's other foods.

Adapted with permission from Muth ND, Tanaka MS. *How to Raise Healthy Eaters: Starting Solids*. 2019.

Introduction of peanut and egg around 6 to 7 months of age helps reduce the risk of food allergy (**Box 16-2**). Evidence for protective effects of other foods, such as wheat, gluten, and shellfish, are less clear, although there is no evidence of a negative impact with early introduction.

Pediatricians typically advise starting with a single-ingredient food and waiting approximately 3 days before introducing the next food to make it easier to identify potential allergies. However, signs of allergy tend to occur immediately after ingestion, and it is not clear whether it is necessary to wait this long to trial new foods.[30] Most infants are accepting of new tastes, so the introduction of a variety of tastes and textures helps facilitate continued acceptance and reduced risk of pickiness later. Repeated exposure to rejected foods helps increase acceptance.

Historically, pediatricians have advised starting with pureed food and progressing according to developmental readiness as shown in **Table 16-8**, with advancement to finger foods and self-feeding occurring around 9 months of age. Baby foods are also categorized in this way, labeled by infant feeding "stage," with stage 1 being for infants new to complementary foods (6–7 months of age); stage 2, for developing eaters (7–8 months of age); and stage 3, for experienced eaters (9–12 months of age). Each stage includes an increased number of foods and textures, moving from full purees to chunky pieces. If parents choose to use jarred baby foods, they should be advised to portion out the food rather than feed their infant from the jar. Opened jars should be

IN GREATER DEPTH

Box 16-2. How to Lower Risk of Peanut Allergy: Findings From the LEAP Trial

The Learning Early About Peanut (LEAP) clinical trial showed that offering at least 6 g of peanut protein over ≥ 3 meals per week decreased the risk of peanut allergy. Only 3% of babies at high risk of peanut allergy who regularly consumed peanut developed an allergy by age 5 years, compared to 17% of babies who avoided peanut.[29] The following risk stratification based on the LEAP trial provides guidance on how to advise caregivers to introduce peanut:

- **Low risk factor (no eczema or other food allergy):** Caregivers may incorporate peanut protein into their infant's diet freely.
- **Moderate risk factor (mild to moderate eczema):** Caregivers may consider offering egg before peanut and, if their infant tolerates egg well, then offering peanut around 6 mo of age. No pediatrician evaluation is needed before offering peanut. If the infant has a reaction to egg, consider further testing before introducing peanut (refer to the following item, "Highest risk factor"). Peanut can be offered at approximately 6 mo of age.
- **Highest risk factor (severe eczema, egg allergy):** Consider requesting a blood test for peanut-specific immunoglobulin E. If the level is typical (<0.35 kU/L), peanut can be offered at home or in the pediatrician's office at 4–6 mo of age, after other first foods have been well tolerated. If the level is high (>0.35 kU/L), consider referral to an allergy specialist, and advise parents to wait to introduce peanut until after the allergy consultation and then proceed according to the specialist's recommendations.

Infants should consume at least 6–7 g/wk of peanut protein over at least 3 meals and snacks to optimally prevent future peanut allergy.

NOTE: Whole peanut is a choking hazard. The following strategies help parents introduce peanut protein safely:

- ½ tbsp of peanut butter (all natural, no added ingredients), creamy, thinned with human (breast) milk, formula, or water mixed with mashed bananas: 2 g of peanut protein
- ½ tbsp of peanut butter mixed with baby cereal: 2 g of peanut protein
- 1 tbsp of peanuts, finely crushed: 4 g of peanut protein
- 1 tbsp of peanut flour: 2 g of peanut protein

Derived from reference 29.

Table 16-8. Developmental Readiness for Advancing Solid Foods

Developmental milestone	Complementary food texture
Sits independently Grasps food with palms Sips from a small open cup	Thicker purees Soft, mashed foods without lumps
Crawls and pulls to a stand Uses jaw and tongue to mash food Plays with a spoon at mealtime Tries to hold a cup independently	Ground foods (eg, finely chopped meat or poultry) or soft, mashed foods with lumps (eg, mashed butternut squash or potatoes)
Puts objects into mouth Attempts to feed self Uses pincer grasp	Finger foods (any foods that dissolve easily, including crackers and dry cereal)

refrigerated, with any unused food consumed within 1 to 2 days. If the infant has been fed directly from the jar, the remaining food should be discarded after the feeding. Of note, repeated studies have shown many baby foods to be contaminated with arsenic, lead, cadmium, and mercury, posing potential risk to infant neurological development and long-term brain function. Ingredients that pose a particularly high risk of contamination include rice and ingredients such as cinnamon, amylase, an enzyme additive called *BAN 800,* and vitamin premix. Parents should avoid purchasing baby foods that contain any of these ingredients. Whenever possible, parents are encouraged to provide their infant with homemade baby food and appropriately sized and textured table foods.

Feeding Schedule

Parents frequently ask how many times per day to offer an infant solid foods and how to increase complementary feedings while decreasing breast milk or formula. Although there is no strict guideline or recommended best way to do this, the Pan American Health Organization and World Health Organization advise that complementary foods be offered approximately 2 to 3 times per day at 6 to 8 months of age and 3 to 4 times per day at 9 to 12 months of age, with healthy snacks 1 to 2 times per day, as desired.[31] Generally, by 12 months of age, most infants are eating 3 meals and 2 snacks consisting of solid foods. To help promote intake of solid foods, caregivers may consider offering solid foods or complementary foods first and then breast milk or formula. As complementary feedings are increased, infants gradually decrease the amount of breast milk and formula feedings (**Table 16-9**).

Baby-Led Weaning

In 2005, public health nurse Gillian Rapley promoted the idea of *baby-led weaning.* With baby-led weaning, from the onset of complementary feeding, infants are exposed to whole, textured foods rather than purees. The infant drives the feeding amount and

Table 16-9. Newborn and Infant Nutritional Needs

Need	Age		
	Birth–4 to 6 mo	**6–8 mo**	**9–12 mo**
Approximate total caloric needs[a]	450–650 Cal/d	50 kcal/lb (650–850 kcal/d)	
Approximate calories from solid foods (kcal/d)[a]	0	200	300
Human (breast) milk or formula	Approximately 4–6 fl oz per feeding	Breastfeed on demand. Formula-fed infants consume approximately 24–32 fl oz/d of formula, but parents should use the infant's cues rather than volume to determine how much to feed.	
Water	None	Approximately 4 fl oz; water can be offered in an open cup to help increase acceptance of water later and develop fine motor skills.	
Iron[b]	0.27 mg; breast milk and/or formula contains adequate amounts.	11 mg	
Zinc	2 mg; breast milk and/or formula contains adequate amounts.	3 mg	
Vitamin D	10 mcg; formula contains adequate amounts. Breastfed infants require supplementation.	10 mcg from formula or vitamin D supplement[c] Most foods do not contain vitamin D.	
Vegetables	Not applicable	4–8 tbsp	8–12 tbsp
Fruits		4–8 tbsp	8–12 tbsp
Protein-rich foods		2–4 tbsp	4–8 tbsp
Grains		2–4 tbsp	4–8 tbsp

SI conversion factor: To convert fl oz to mL, multiply by 30; mcg to IU, divide by 0.025.

[a] Calories are approximate. Clinicians should encourage caregivers to use their infant's cues of hunger and fullness to determine intake amounts.

[b] Routine iron supplementation in breastfed infants <9 mo of age does not seem to provide any positive effects and, in fact, may negatively affect growth.[7] However, infants with iron deficiency require increased iron intake from foods, fortified foods, or supplementation to prevent impaired neurobehavioral development.

[c] Vitamin D supplementation >10 mcg adds no known benefit.

Adapted with permission from Muth ND, Tanaka MS. *How to Raise Healthy Eaters: Starting Solids.* 2019. Based on data from US Department of Health and Human Services, US Department of Agriculture. *Dietary Guidelines for Americans, 2020-2025.* 9th ed. 2020. Accessed November 3, 2022. https://www.dietaryguidelines.gov/sites/default/files/2020-12/Dietary_Guidelines_for_Americans_2020-2025.pdf; Institute of Medicine. *Dietary Reference Intakes for Energy, Carbohydrate, Fiber, Fat, Fatty Acids, Cholesterol, Protein, and Amino Acids.* National Academies Press; 2005; and Pan American Health Organization (PAHO)/World Health Organization (WHO). *Guiding Principles for Complementary Feeding of the Breastfed Child.* PAHO/WHO; 2003.

is encouraged to self-feed all foods, thus eliminating purees because infants do not have the coordination to spoon-feed themselves. Overall, studies have shown that there is insufficient evidence currently available to draw conclusions about baby-led weaning.[32] Parents may choose to follow baby-led weaning, or a more traditional advancement of foods from purees to more textured table foods over time on the basis of developmental readiness.

Foods to Avoid in the First Year

Most infants are able to safely consume most foods after complementary feeding is introduced and tastes and textures are advanced. However, certain foods and drinks should be avoided before the infant's first birthday because of health and safety risks.

- Cow milk and other "milks." Cow milk can cause irritation and gastrointestinal bleeding in infants. Other milks, such as soy, almond, rice, and hemp milks, should also be avoided in the first year because they do not optimize nutrition for infants and some contain high levels of phytate, which can decrease the absorption of important minerals (eg, iron, zinc, calcium).
- Honey. Honey may contain botulism spores, which, when ingested, can release a toxin that may pose a life-threatening infection for an infant, causing muscle paralysis.
- Sugary foods and drinks, including 100% fruit juice. Sugary foods and drinks, including 100% fruit juice, provide unnecessary calories and may encourage a craving for sweet tastes.
- Salted foods. Infants need to learn to develop a taste for foods in their natural form. Salt provides unnecessary and excessive sodium intake. Also, infants are very likely to be willing to try new foods without needing any added flavor.
- Choking hazards. Foods that pose choking hazards include hot dogs, nuts, seeds, whole grapes, cherry tomatoes, raisins, raw carrots, apples, popcorn, hard candies, chunks of peanut butter, and hard or large chunks of any food.

Addressing Feeding Challenges

Parents and other caregivers may experience several challenges when introducing complementary foods. For example, some infants may have difficulty self-feeding or transitioning textures, whereas others may experience vomiting or gagging with feedings, constipation, taste refusal, or a food allergy. These challenges and the potential strategies to help address them are described in **Table 16-10**. Sometimes these challenges are associated with impaired weight gain, developmental delays, or health conditions that require further evaluation and intervention from other members of the health care team with expertise in infant feeding, such as an occupational therapist, a speech therapist, a developmental and behavioral pediatrician, a registered dietitian, or a psychologist.

Table 16-10. Common Infant Feeding Challenges

Common concern	Recommended plan
Difficulty self-feeding	Most infants start to self-feed finger foods by 9 mo of age. By 12 mo of age, an infant should be able to dip a spoon into food but will probably not spoon much food into their mouth. It is typical for some infants and toddlers to gain these skills earlier or later than these averages. If an infant is unable to achieve the skill required within a few months of these ages, the clinician can consider an occupational therapist consultation to assess feeding and help improve fine motor skills.
Difficulty transitioning to textures	Advise caregivers to start with their infant's preferred texture and slowly progress toward the refused consistency. For example, if an infant likes only purees, parents might start by making a puree only slightly thicker with less milk or water or, in the case of jarred food, adding a small amount of infant oatmeal to thicken the food. Caregivers should offer the gradually thickened texture repeatedly until their infant accepts it a few times. Then, parents may thicken the food a little bit more until achieving the initially refused texture. Alternatively, if an infant refuses purees but likes solid foods, parents may gradually make the texture of solid foods softer. In the case of textures not easily changed, parents should repeatedly offer the food in very small amounts.
Gagging, choking, or vomiting with feeding	For gagging, caregivers may thin the food's texture by adding a small amount of human (breast) milk, formula, or water to the food and offering a smaller amount. For spitting out, caregivers should take a break for a few days and then offer the food again. For spitting up, caregivers can thicken the food's texture by adding infant oatmeal or pureed fruit and then offer the food again in a few days. For vomiting, advise caregivers to be alert for signs of food allergy, such as forceful vomiting each time a specific food is offered, trouble breathing, or a rash. If any of these occurs, allergy is likely and should be evaluated further.
Constipation	Nearly all infants experience decreased stooling frequency when solid foods are first introduced. Concerning signs, such as blood in the stool, stomach hardness, or pain, may warrant further evaluation. In the absence of warning signs, reassurance and advice to offer more water, fiber, and stone fruits (eg, peaches, plums, nectarines, cherries, dates, prunes) may help.

Table 16-10 (*continued*)

Common concern	Recommended plan
Taste refusal	If a taste is rejected, advise caregivers to allow several days before offering it again. Caregivers can then offer the food again prepared in different developmentally appropriate ways (cooked or raw, soft or harder texture). Encourage caregivers to offer a food at least 10 times before concluding that a child does not like the taste. Advise caregivers to take a break for a month or two at that point and then offer the food again, because repeated exposures generally lead to increased acceptance.
Food allergy	Signs of a food allergy include hives, vomiting, or shortness of breath or wheezing shortly after consuming a food. If an infant shows signs of a food allergy, the potential inciting food should be avoided, and the patient should be referred to an allergist for further evaluation.

Derived from reference 5.

In Sum

- For about the first 6 months after birth, babies meet all caloric, nutrient, and fluid needs to support typical growth and development from appropriate intake of breast milk or formula. For most healthy full-term infants, it is unnecessary to calculate fluid and caloric intake because infants are generally able to use internal feelings of hunger, thirst, and fullness to show signs of hunger and satiety. If caregivers are responsive to these signs, infants will generally receive the appropriate amounts of calories and fluids.
- Breast milk is the preferred nutrition source for babies in the first 6 months after birth, with continued breastfeeding "as long as mutually desired by mother and child for 2 years or beyond."[6] That said, many babies are not exclusively breastfed or breast milk fed for the first 6 months after birth. In these cases, caregivers have more than 50 formulas from which to choose. Key differences between formulas include the composition of the protein and carbohydrates.
- Organic formulas; many popular formula add-ons, such as probiotics and prebiotics; and formulas marketing benefits for gassiness, colic, and sleeping difficulties appeal to parents, but studies to date have not shown clear benefit. Generally, generic brand formulas are nutritionally equivalent to brand name formulas. Many parents choose imported European formula for their infant; however, the AAP and the Centers for Disease Control and Prevention recommend that parents choose formulas sold and marketed in the United States because these formulas are required to meet certain nutrition standards and safeguards.
- Around 6 months of age, and no earlier than 4 months, infants should be introduced to complementary foods. First foods should be rich in iron, zinc, and

polyunsaturated fats to promote healthy neurocognitive development. Pediatricians typically advise starting with a single-ingredient food and waiting approximately 3 days before introducing the next food to make it easier to identify potential allergies. However, signs of allergy tend to occur immediately after ingestion, and it is not clear whether it is necessary to wait this long to trial new foods. Although pediatricians have historically recommended starting with pureed foods, providing more textured foods is acceptable as long as risk of choking is minimized.

- Infants should be exposed to a variety of tastes and textures. Early and frequent exposure to peanut and other common allergens may help reduce the risk of food allergy. Water should be introduced in an open cup around 6 months of age. To prevent dental caries, when caregivers are offering water from a sippy cup, cup, or container with a straw, no additional substances should be added. Certain foods and drinks should be avoided in the first year after birth because of potential health and safety risks. These include cow milk and plant-based "milks," honey, juice, sugary drinks and foods, salted foods, and foods that pose choking hazards.
- Ultimately, as infants progress from relying exclusively on breast milk or formula to meet nutritional needs to adding and advancing a variety of tastes and textures, pediatricians are presented with an important opportunity to provide nutritional guidance and help shape parent feeding practices that set the stage for healthful nutrition habits in childhood and beyond.

References

1. Schwarzenberg SJ, Georgieff MK, Daniels S, et al; American Academy of Pediatrics Committee on Nutrition. Advocacy for improving nutrition in the first 1000 days to support childhood development and adult health. *Pediatrics.* 2018;141(2):e20173716 PMID: 29358479 doi: 10.1542/peds.2017-3716
2. Institute of Medicine. *Dietary Reference Intakes for Energy, Carbohydrate, Fiber, Fat, Fatty Acids, Cholesterol, Protein, and Amino Acids.* National Academies Press; 2005
3. Institute of Medicine. *Dietary Reference Intakes: The Essential Guide to Nutrient Requirements.* National Academies Press; 2006
4. Holliday MA, Segar WE. The maintenance need for water in parenteral fluid therapy. *Pediatrics.* 1957;19(5):823–832 PMID: 13431307 doi: 10.1542/peds.19.5.823
5. Hagan JF Jr, Shaw JS, Duncan PM, eds. *Bright Futures: Guidelines for Health Supervision of Infants, Children, and Adolescents.* 4th ed. American Academy of Pediatrics; 2017 doi: 10.1542/9781610020237
6. Meek JY, Noble L. American Academy of Pediatrics Section on Breastfeeding. Breastfeeding and the use of human milk. *Pediatrics.* 2022;150(1):e2022057988 doi: 10.1542/peds.2022-057988
7. US Department of Health and Human Services, US Department of Agriculture. *Dietary Guidelines for Americans, 2020–2025.* 9th ed. 2020. Accessed October 25, 2022. https://www.dietaryguidelines.gov/sites/default/files/2020-12/Dietary_Guidelines_for_Americans_2020-2025.pdf
8. Osborn DA, Sinn JK, Jones LJ. Infant formulas containing hydrolysed protein for prevention of allergic disease. *Cochrane Database Syst Rev.* 2018;10(10):CD003664
9. Helfer B, Leonardi-Bee J, Mundell A, et al. Conduct and reporting of formula milk trials: systematic review. *BMJ.* 2021;375(2202):n2202 PMID: 34645600 doi: 10.1136/bmj.n2202

10. US Food and Drug Administration. Questions and answers for consumers concerning infant formula. Accessed October 25, 2022. https://www.fda.gov/food/people-risk-foodborne-illness/questions-answers-consumers-concerning-infant-formula

11. Kwok TC, Ojha S, Dorling J. Feed thickener for infants up to six months of age with gastro-oesophageal reflux. *Cochrane Database Syst Rev.* 2017;12(12):CD003211 PMID: 29207214 doi: 10.1002/14651858.CD003211.pub2

12. Horvath A, Dziechciarz P, Szajewska H. The effect of thickened-feed interventions on gastro-esophageal reflux in infants: systematic review and meta-analysis of randomized, controlled trials. *Pediatrics.* 2008;122(6):e1268–e1277 PMID: 19001038 doi: 10.1542/peds.2008-1900

13. Chung CS, Yamini S, Trumbo PR. FDA's health claim review: whey-protein partially hydrolyzed infant formula and atopic dermatitis. *Pediatrics.* 2012;130(2):e408–e414 PMID: 22778306 doi: 10.1542/peds.2012-0333

14. Green Corkins K, Shurley T. What's in the bottle? a review of infant formulas. *Nutr Clin Pract.* 2016;31(6):723–729 PMID: 27646861 doi: 10.1177/0884533616669362

15. Konek SH, Becker PJ. *Samour & King's Pediatric Nutrition in Clinical Care.* 5th ed. Jones & Bartlett; 2020

16. Szalinski C. Why US parents are choosing European baby formula. *New York Times.* March 12, 2021. Accessed October 25, 2022. https://www.nytimes.com/wirecutter/blog/us-parents-european-baby-formula

17. DiMaggio DM, Du N, Scherer C, et al. Comparison of imported European and US infant formulas: labeling, nutrient and safety concerns. *J Pediatr Gastroenterol Nutr.* 2019;69(4):480–486 PMID: 31107795 doi: 10.1097/MPG.0000000000002395

18. Centers for Disease Control and Prevention. Choosing an infant formula. Accessed October 25, 2022. https://www.cdc.gov/nutrition/infantandtoddlernutrition/formula-feeding/choosing-an-infant-formula.html

19. Davis SA, Knol LL, Crowe-White KM, Turner LW, McKinley E. Homemade infant formula recipes may contain harmful ingredients: a quantitative content analysis of blogs. *Public Health Nutr.* 2020;23(8):1334–1339 PMID: 32157977 doi: 10.1017/S136898001900421X

20. Vieira MA, Kube PK, van Helmond JL, et al. Recipe for disaster: homemade formula leading to severe complications in 2 infants. *Pediatrics.* 2021;148(3):e2021050947 PMID: 34446537 doi: 10.1542/peds.2021-050947

21. Wood CT, Skinner AC, Yin HS, et al. Bottle size and weight gain in formula-fed infants. *Pediatrics.* 2016;138(1):e20154538 PMID: 27273748 doi: 10.1542/peds.2015-4538

22. American Academy of Pediatric Dentistry. Policy on early childhood caries (ECC): classifications, consequences, and preventive strategies. In: *The Reference Manual of Pediatric Dentistry.* American Academy of Pediatric Dentistry; 2020:79–81

23. American Academy of Pediatrics Committee on Nutrition. *Pediatric Nutrition.* Kleinman RE, Greer FR, eds. 8th ed. American Academy of Pediatrics; 2020

24. O'Connor DL, Khan S, Weishuhn K, et al; Postdischarge Feeding Study Group. Growth and nutrient intakes of human milk-fed preterm infants provided with extra energy and nutrients after hospital discharge. *Pediatrics.* 2008;121(4):766–776 PMID: 18381542 doi: 10.1542/peds.2007-0054

25. American Academy of Pediatrics Committee on Nutrition. Nutritional needs of the preterm infant. In: Kleinman RE, Greer FR, eds. *Pediatric Nutrition.* 8th ed. American Academy of Pediatrics; 2020:113–162

26. Huh SY, Rifas-Shiman SL, Taveras EM, Oken E, Gillman MW. Timing of solid food introduction and risk of obesity in preschool-aged children. *Pediatrics.* 2011;127(3):e544–e551 PMID: 21300681 doi: 10.1542/peds.2010-0740

27. Abrams EM, Hildebrand K, Blair B, Chan ES. Timing of introduction of allergenic solids for infants at high risk. *Paediatr Child Health*. 2019;24(1):56–57 PMID: 30833823 doi: 10.1093/pch/pxy195

28. Horta BL, Loret de Mola C, Victora CG. Breastfeeding and intelligence: a systematic review and meta-analysis. *Acta Paediatr*. 2015;104(467):14–19 PMID: 26211556 doi: 10.1111/apa.13139

29. Du Toit G, Roberts G, Sayre PH, et al; LEAP Study Team. Randomized trial of peanut consumption in infants at risk for peanut allergy. *N Engl J Med*. 2015;372(9):803–813 PMID: 25705822 doi: 10.1056/NEJMoa1414850

30. Samady W, Campbell E, Aktas ON, et al. Recommendations on complementary food introduction among pediatric practitioners. *JAMA Netw Open*. 2020;3(8):e2013070 PMID: 32804213 doi: 10.1001/jamanetworkopen.2020.13070

31. Division of Health Promotion and Protection Food and Nutrition Program. *Guiding Principles for Complementary Feeding of the Breastfed Child*. Pan American Health Organization, World Health Organization; 2003

32. Brown A, Jones SW, Rowan H. Baby-led weaning: the evidence to date. *Curr Nutr Rep*. 2017;6(2):148–156 PMID: 28596930 doi: 10.1007/s13668-017-0201-2

CHAPTER 17

Nutrition in Childhood and Adolescence

The guidance and support that pediatricians provide to parents and children during childhood and adolescence can help shape overall nutritional status and health for decades into the future. This chapter provides an overview of recommended nutrition practices to promote optimal health from age 1 year through adolescence, based largely on the American Academy of Pediatrics (AAP) Bright Futures recommendations for promoting healthful nutrition[1] and the *2020–2025 Dietary Guidelines for Americans*[2] and its accompanying scientific report of the 2020 Dietary Guidelines Advisory Committee.[3]

Early Childhood (Ages 1–4 Years)

Healthful nutrition in early childhood helps increase the likelihood that a child will continue healthy habits throughout childhood and adolescence and into adulthood. However, this is also a stage of development that poses new nutritional challenges for parents and children, because toddlers exhibit an age-appropriate dislike of unfamiliar foods (neophobia), rejection of many bitter tastes (eg, green vegetables), and preference for sugary foods and drinks. Parents frequently rely on advice from pediatricians to navigate this stage and help their child develop healthful nutrition practices.

Developmental Expectations

Although the average infant is generally eager to try new tastes and textures, around 18 months to 2 years of age, it is typical for children to begin to exhibit selective eating habits, during which they refuse to eat certain foods, and *food jags,* during which they favor only 1 or 2 foods. It is typical for a toddler to be very hungry and eat a large amount on one day and to eat hardly anything on other days. Although toddler eating patterns can be very distressing because parents worry that their child will not grow well and will become malnourished, over the course of a week most toddlers tend to balance intake to meet nutrient needs when mostly nutritious foods are available.

Helping parents recognize that it is typical for appetite and intake to decrease and for growth to slow can minimize anxiety and prevent feeding practices that pressure a child to eat when not hungry. Monitoring a child's growth chart and recognizing early whether a child has started to notably increase or decrease in weight or weight-for-length (for children < 2 years of age) or body mass index percentile (for children ≥ 2 years) can help prompt a conversation about parent feeding practices and identify potential opportunities for changes to prevent later weight or obesity concerns.

Optimal Parent Feeding Practices

Caloric intake and the nutritional quality of a child's diet depend on what meals are eaten, how much time passes between each meal (meal timing), how much food is eaten at each meal (meal size), and the specific foods that are consumed (food selection). The recommended parenting approach is an authoritative, or responsive, parenting style in which parents play an important role in determining meal and snack timing—when meals and snacks are served and what food is offered. Children are allowed to control their meal size and food selection. This approach encourages and supports a child in using their own cues of hunger and satiety to decide how much to eat. Although schedules may vary among families, generally children aged 1 to 4 years should consume 3 meals and 2 snacks per day.

Recommended Nutrition Sources and Portion Sizes

Ideally, children eat in a way that is consistent with the dietary guidelines. As discussed in Chapter 11, Dietary Guidelines and Principles of Healthy Eating, the dietary guidelines advocate a diet high in fruits, vegetables, and whole grains and low in saturated fat, sugar, and salt. Protein needs can be met through animal-source foods such as meat, poultry, seafood, eggs, and dairy products, as well as through plant-based foods. The guidelines advise that children 2 years and younger consume no added sugars and that added sugars be less than 10% of total calories for children and adults 2 years and older.[2] Recommended amounts are shown in **Table 17-1**.

Standard portion sizes can be difficult to approximate, and parents often believe that children need much larger portions than what is recommended. Standard measurements as referenced throughout the dietary guidelines are shown in **Table 17-2**. In addition, clinicians can share with parents the simple method for estimating appropriate portion sizes for their young child described in **Box 17-1**.

When children consume a diet that resembles MyPlate and the dietary guidelines, supplementation with vitamin and minerals is generally unnecessary. However, many children may not be eating in an optimally nutritious way and may not be getting all the nutrients they need. For instance, despite the dietary guidelines' emphasis on fruit and vegetable consumption, the Feeding Infants and Toddlers Study showed that more than 20% of 0- to 2-year-olds ate no fruits or vegetables, although more than 1 in 3 consumed a sugary drink and half consumed juice on the day of recall.[4] Children aged 2 to 4 years had somewhat more nutritious intake: although 27% did not consume a vegetable on the day of recall, about 75% consumed at least 1 portion of fruit. Nearly all had a dessert, sugary drink, or sweet, and 45% specifically consumed a sugary drink. Nearly half had 100% fruit juice, and 81% consumed cow milk.[5] When a pediatrician suspects that a child may not be consuming sufficient vitamins and minerals, advising the use of a multivitamin may be warranted. Additionally, children who consume less than the recommended servings of dairy, or acceptable substitute (refer to the following section), should take a 400-IU (10-mcg) vitamin D supplement.

Table 17-1. Nutritional Needs in Early Childhood

Need	Age (y)			
	1	**2–3**	**4**	**5**
Approximate total caloric needs (Cal)[a]	800	1,000	1,200	1,400
Vegetables (c)	¾	1	1½	1½
Fruits (c)	¾	1	1½	1½
Protein-rich foods (oz)	2	2	3	4
Grains (oz)	2¼	3	4	5
Dairy (c)	1¾[b]	2	2½	2½
Water (c)	1–4	1–4	1–5	1.5–5.0
Added sugars	None	None	<10% total calories OR <25 g	<10% total calories OR <25 g
Sodium (mg)	<1,200	<1,200	<1,500	<1,500

[a] Calorie level ranges for ages 2-5 years: 1,000–1,400 Cal (girls); 1,000–1,600 Cal (boys).
[b] Human (breast) milk is a dairy equivalent.
Adapted from reference 2.

Milk and Plant-Based Milks

In early childhood, children tend to consume sufficient cow or soy milk, meeting calcium and vitamin D needs. Other products sold as "milk," such as almond milk, rice milk, or coconut milk, are generally lower in protein, often contain added sugars, and may have decreased calcium and vitamin D bioavailability. Although popular with many parents, non-soy plant-based "milks" have not been studied sufficiently to promote their use. Flavoring, such as chocolate or vanilla, may make cow or soy milk more palatable than white milk for some children but is high in added sugars (**Table 17-3**). Cow or soy milk without added sugars and water are the preferred drinks at this age and throughout childhood. Additionally, continued breastfeeding beyond 1 year of age, as mutually desired by the child and mother for 2 years or beyond, is also recommended. Transitional milk and toddler/follow-on formula are rarely, if ever, recommended.

Some toddlers overconsume milk, displacing other foods and nutrients. When children overconsume milk, they are at increased risk for iron deficiency because milk does not contain iron. For this reason, the AAP Bright Futures guidelines recommend screening hemoglobin level at this age in children with reported milk intakes greater than recommendations.[1]

Table 17-2. Standard Portions

Portion size	Equivalent options
1 c vegetables	1 c raw or cooked/canned vegetables 2 c leafy salad greens 1 c 100% vegetable juice
1 c fruit	1 c raw, frozen, or cooked/canned fruit ½ c dried fruit 1 c 100% fruit juice
1 oz protein	1 oz seafood, lean meat, or poultry 1 egg 1 tbsp peanut butter ¼ c cooked beans, peas, or lentils
1 oz grains	1 slice bread 1 oz ready-to-eat cereal ½ c cooked rice, pasta, or cereal
1 c dairy	1 c dairy milk or yogurt 1 c lactose-free dairy milk or yogurt 1 c fortified soy milk or yogurt 1½ oz natural cheese

---

CLINICAL PRACTICE TIP

Box 17-1. Portion Sizes Based on Tablespoon per Year of Age

Clinicians can help patients approximate portion size by following the general rule that an appropriate portion size for a young child is about a tablespoon per year of age, with more given on the basis of the child's appetite.

Establishing Meal Patterns

Encourage parents to offer young children 3 meals and 2 snacks per day, following a consistent schedule or routine to the extent possible to prevent grazing and to ensure hunger at mealtimes. Milk is best offered only with meals to prevent excess consumption and lower the risk of dental caries. Water is the preferred option between meals and snacks. The most nutritious snacks are whole foods such as fruits and vegetables or minimally processed snacks such as cheese sticks or whole grain crackers. Many parents

Table 17-3. Nutritional Content of Cow Milk and Plant-Based Milks

Milk or plant-based "milk" (per 8 fl oz)	Calories (Cal)	Saturated fat (g)	Protein (g)	Calcium (mg) % daily value	Vitamin D (IU) % daily value	Clinical considerations
Cow			8	280-300 29%	100-120 18%	• Skim or low-fat (1%) milk is recommended for children > 2 y of age (or >1 y with weight/length > 95th percentile). • Contains lactose, which may be a concern for children with lactose intolerance. • Organic milk is nutritionally equivalent to conventional milk. • Chocolate milk contains about 11 g of added sugars per 8 fl oz.
Skim	80	0				
1%	100	1.5				
2%	120	3.0				
Whole	150	4.6				
1% chocolate	150	2.0				
Soy (original)	110	0.5	8	450 30%	120 15%	• Nutritionally equivalent to cow milk, plus fortified with iron. • Plant compounds may help decrease cholesterol level in children with increased cholesterol level. • Flavored soy milk (eg, vanilla, chocolate) contains 8-14 g of added sugars per 8 fl oz.

Continued

Table 17-3 (*continued*)

Milk or plant-based "milk" (per 8 fl oz)	Calories (Cal)	Saturated fat (g)	Protein (g)	Calcium (mg) % daily value	Vitamin D (IU) % daily value	Clinical considerations
Pea protein (unsweetened original)	80	0.5	8	440 35%	240 30%	• Nutritionally equivalent to cow milk, although it may have lesser bioavailability of calcium and vitamin D. • Dairy-free. • More expensive than milk. • One popular brand makes a "kids" formulation, which includes 5 g of added sugars, prebiotics, and 50 mg of algal oil containing the omega-3 fatty acid docosahexaenoic acid.
Almond (original)	60	0	1	450 35%	200 25%	• High in sodium (180 mg per 8 fl oz) • Low in protein • Contains added sugars
Hemp (original)	140	1	4	270 20%	80 10%	• High in omega-3 fatty acids • Relatively low in protein • Contains added sugars
Oat	120	0	3	0	0	• Relatively low in protein • Contains added sugars • Does not contain calcium or vitamin D unless specially fortified

Coconut (unsweetened)	360	33	0	0	0	• High in calories • High in saturated fat • Does not contain protein • Does not contain calcium or vitamin D unless specially fortified
Rice	120	0	1	450 30%	200 25%	• Low in protein. • Rice products contain arsenic. • Usually fortified with calcium and vitamin D.

Conversion factor: To convert IU to mcg, multiply by 0.025.

like to offer their children vegetable pouches because children tend to like them and they are an easy way for children to consume a serving of vegetables. Although these pouches are convenient and contain mostly pureed fruits and vegetables, they should not be relied on as a substitute for offering vegetables with other meals and snacks. Repeated exposure to the taste and texture of a food increases liking, but the flavor and texture of vegetables are masked in pouches. Also, overconsumption of these pouches can lead to excess caloric intake and may impede oro-motor development because of limited chewing and increased sucking.

Mealtimes should be limited to 20 to 30 minutes, or for as long as a child can pay attention and maintain interest in eating. Family mealtimes offer young children many benefits, including teaching young children how to eat, building social skills, and increasing the likelihood that young children will try the foods the rest of their family is eating. Mealtimes should be free of distractions such as television, tablets, and other media so children have a chance to socialize with their family and pay attention to their food and eating. Parents should be advised to encourage child self-feeding and tolerate age-appropriate food exploration and messes whenever possible to help children build fine motor skills and increase familiarity with different foods and textures.

Foods and Drinks to Avoid

Foods that pose a choking hazard should be avoided, including peanuts and whole nuts, chewing gum, popcorn, chips, round slices of hot dogs or sausages, raw carrot sticks, whole grapes and cherries, large pieces of raw vegetables or fruit, whole cherry or grape tomatoes, tough meat, and hard candy. To further minimize choking risk, foods should be cut into very small pieces, and children should not be allowed to run, play, or lie down while eating. Parents should be encouraged to learn first aid for choking and cardiopulmonary resuscitation in case of choking.

Children have an innate preference for sweet and salty tastes and an unlearned dislike of bitter and sour tastes. Most processed snacks and many foods marketed to young children contain added salt or sugar. Young children may prefer or request these foods if they are readily available. The easiest way for parents to minimize sugar and salt consumption and promote vegetable and fruit intake in young children is to keep access to sugary, salty, and highly processed foods to a minimum. In fact, the dietary guidelines recommend that children younger than 2 years not consume any added sugars or more than 1,200 mg/d of sodium.[2]

Sugary drinks, including soda, sports drinks, fruit drinks, and other beverages with added sugars, should be avoided in early childhood. The AAP suggests that when a family does not have access to whole, frozen, or canned fruit to meet nutritional needs, no more than 4 fl oz (118 mL) of 100% juice per day be acceptable for children aged 1 to 3 years and no more than 4 to 6 fl oz (118–177 mL) per day be acceptable for children aged 4 to 6 years.[6] If a family does have access to whole, frozen, or canned fruits, the children should meet nutritional needs through these products and avoid 100% fruit juice. Highlights of the AAP statement on 100% fruit juice are included in **Box 17-2**.

IN GREATER DEPTH

Box 17-2. American Academy of Pediatrics Guidance on Juice

Parents often ask pediatricians whether juice is healthy and, if so, how much juice their child should drink. The American Academy of Pediatrics published the following guidance for pediatricians on how to advise families on consumption of 100% fruit juice:

1. Juice should not be introduced into the diet of infants before 12 mo of age unless clinically indicated, such as in the case of constipation. The intake of juice should be limited to, at most,
   - 4 fl oz (118 mL) per day for toddlers 1–3 y of age
   - 4–6 fl oz (118–177 mL) per day for children 4–6 y of age
   - 8 fl oz (237 mL) per day for children and adolescents 7–18 y of age
2. Toddlers should not be given juice from bottles or easily transportable covered cups that allow them to consume juice easily throughout the day. Toddlers should not be given juice at bedtime. These practices increase the risk of dental caries and caloric overconsumption.
3. Children should be encouraged to eat whole fruit to meet their recommended daily fruit intake and should be educated regarding the benefit of fiber intake and the longer time to consume the same kilocalories of whole fruit as of fruit juice.
4. Families should be educated that, to satisfy fluid requirements, human (breast) milk and/or infant formula is sufficient for infants and low-fat/nonfat milk and water are sufficient for older children.
5. Consumption of unpasteurized juice products should be strongly discouraged in infants, children, and adolescents.
6. Grapefruit juice should be avoided in any child taking medication metabolized by CYP3A4, such as acetaminophen.
7. In the evaluation of children with overnutrition and undernutrition, the pediatrician should determine the amount of juice being consumed.
8. In the evaluation of children with chronic diarrhea, excessive flatulence, abdominal pain, and bloating, the pediatrician should determine the amount of juice being consumed.
9. In the evaluation of the risk of dental caries, pediatricians should routinely discuss the relationship between fruit juice and dental decay and determine the amount and means of juice consumption.

Continued

IN GREATER DEPTH

Box 17-2 (*continued*)

10. Pediatricians should routinely discuss the use of fruit juice and fruit drinks and should educate older children, adolescents, and their parents about differences between the two.
11. Pediatricians should advocate for reduced fruit juice in the diets of young children and eliminated fruit juice in the diets of children with abnormal (poor or excessive) weight gain.
12. Pediatricians should support policies that seek to reduce the consumption of fruit juice and promote the consumption of whole fruit by toddlers and young children (eg, child care centers/preschools) already exposed to juices, including through the Special Supplemental Nutrition Program for Women, Infants, and Children.

Adapted from reference 6.

Strategies to Address Picky Eating

Young children often refuse new foods. In fact, neophobia is developmentally appropriate and expected between 18 months and 3 years of age. Clinicians may advise parents that this stage is developmentally appropriate and encourage parents to respond by using some of the feeding strategies described in **Table 17-4**. For children with severe picky eating (refer to Chapter 19, Mental Health, Behavioral, and Developmental Conditions), these strategies may be most successful with the help of a feeding specialist, such as an occupational therapist or a pediatric psychologist.

Other common nutritional challenges that parents experience at this stage of their child's development are shown in **Table 17-5**, along with possible solutions for clinicians to share with parents.

Middle Childhood (Ages 5–11 Years)

By middle childhood, many taste preferences and eating habits are well established. Most feeding and behavioral concerns from early childhood have been resolved for many children, although some food dislikes may persist. Although preferences may be established, children at this age develop increasing awareness of the role of food in promoting health and may be more willing to try new foods as a way to improve health.

Table 17-4. Feeding Strategies That May Help Children Accept New Foods and Reverse Picky Eating

Strategy	Description	Examples
Practice responsive feeding	Parents structure mealtimes and the food environment, and children are encouraged to listen to their body's cues of hunger and satiety in deciding how much to eat.	Parents practice division of responsibility in which they control what food is offered, when, and where, but their child chooses what foods to eat and how much. For instance, parents choose what times meals and snacks occur, require their child to be at the kitchen table without distractions while eating, and offer MyPlate-consistent meals, but they allow their child to choose what to eat from the foods offered and how much.
Create a home environment that supports healthful nutrition	Parents help increase the likelihood that a child will try a food by increasing accessibility and exposure, making the foods look and taste good, and parental modeling.	Parents take extra steps to make it easy for children to obtain fruits and vegetables by leaving a bowl of fruit on the counter, offering a colorful variety of vegetables and/or fruits at mealtimes, cooking at home whenever possible, incorporating healthful nutrition into their own eating plan, and more.
Anticipate food refusal	Parents expect children to refuse foods sometimes, or even often. They recognize that this is typical.	Rather than consider a food off-limits, parents reintroduce it 3-14 d later because they recognize that a child may be more willing to accept the food with repeated exposures. Parents avoid the urge to force or bribe their child to eat a food.

Continued

Table 17-4 (*continued*)

Strategy	Description	Examples
Bridging	Parents introduce new foods that are similar in taste or texture to a food the child already likes.	Parents help a child learn to like a new food by offering a food that is similar in taste or texture to an existing preferred food. For example, a child who likes pumpkin pie can eventually learn to like sweet potatoes, butternut squash, and carrots: pumpkin pie creates a bridge to sweet potato pie, which creates a bridge to mashed sweet potatoes, which creates a bridge to mashed butternut squash, which creates a bridge to mashed carrots, which creates a bridge to roasted carrots, which creates a bridge to raw carrots.
Fading	Parents gradually transition from a preferred food or texture to a new food or texture. There are several types of fading. *Simultaneous fading:* A small amount of new or non-preferred food is offered at the same time as or mixed with a preferred food. Initially, the new food is indiscernible, but the amount is gradually increased. *Stimulus fading:* The preferred food is paired with a small amount of non-preferred food. Over time, the quantity of the preferred food is decreased and the quantity of the non-preferred food is increased. *Size fading:* The child starts with a very small bite of a food. The child allows the food to touch their lips, touch their tongue, be placed into their mouth, and initially be chewed and spit out. Eventually, the child chews and swallows the food. The bite size is gradually increased with repeated exposures. *Texture fading:* The child starts with a preferred texture, such as pureed food, and then the texture is gradually changed, from pureed to finely chopped to chopped to bite-size.	1. Start with a fruit smoothie. 2. Add a small amount of spinach or kale for a "green smoothie" that tastes mostly the same but now has a different color. 3. Further increase the spinach or kale so the taste of it is somewhat recognizable. Initially preferred food: fruit smoothie New food: spinach or kale paired with sweet taste in green smoothie

Shaping	Behavior is broken down into small steps. Each step is positively reinforced with praise, attention, or another reward.	1. Prepare a food or meal that has an appealing smell. 2. Invite the child to help prepare the food or to smell the food. 3. Place the food onto the child's plate. Allow them time to examine the food. 4. Prompt the child to lick the food, but do not force or require this step. 5. If the child licks the food, prompt them to taste a small bite, but do not force this step. 6. If the child takes a small bite of the food, prompt them to take a bigger bite, but do not force this step. At each step, provide the child with positive attention and affirmations.
Pairing	Introduce a new food alongside a food a child already likes.	Pair bitter tastes with generally more preferred sweet or salty tastes. For example, pair broccoli with cheese.
Repeated exposure	Offer the child the same food repeatedly over time.	Introduce one new food at a time. Offer a small amount at the beginning of the meal. If the food is refused, offer it again in a similar or new way in 3–5 d.
Motivation to eat	Children will be most open to trying new foods if they are hungry.	Schedule meals and limit snacks to ensure that a child is hungry when a new food is introduced. Parents should introduce foods that they most want their child to try when their child is the hungriest.

Continued

Table 17-4 (*continued*)

Strategy	Description	Examples
Social modeling	The child witnesses another person they like or admire eating the food, such as a sibling, friend, or parent.	Parents model eating a variety of foods at mealtimes. Parents never ask their child to eat something they themselves will not eat. Parents help increase the impact of social modeling by avoiding distractions at mealtimes such as televisions and other media.
Differential reinforcement	Give positive attention and rewards for desired behaviors, and ignore undesired behaviors.	Meal "time-out" during which praise and positive attention are given when the child tries new foods and attention is withdrawn when the child is disruptive or nonadherent

Adapted from Muth ND, Sampson S. Troubleshooting. *The Picky Eater Project: 6 Weeks to Happier, Healthier Family Mealtimes.* American Academy of Pediatrics; 2016:199-222.

Table 17-5. Common Nutritional Challenges in Early Childhood and Possible Solutions

Common nutritional challenges	Possible solutions to share with parents
Refusal of fruits and/or vegetables	● Include a fruit and vegetable at every meal. When children are repeatedly exposed to foods, or help choose, prepare, or grow foods, they are often more willing to try them. ● Offer healthy snacks (eg, vegetables with dip) when children are most hungry. ● Offer vegetables with sauces and dips to increase acceptance of vegetables.
Refusal or underconsumption of milk	● Continue to offer milk. ● Offer cheese and yogurt. ● Offer an equivalent milk substitute (eg, soy milk).
Overconsumption of milk	● Limit milk to mealtimes. ● Offer water between meals. ● Wean from bottle to cup at 12 mo of age.
Refusal of water	● Continue to offer water. ● Try infusing water with sliced lemon, cucumbers, or fruit. ● Avoid offering juice or other sweet drinks.
Refusal of meats	● Offer bite-size pieces of moist, tender meat or poultry. ● Offer bone-free fish, such as canned tuna and salmon. ● Incorporate meat into prepared dishes, such as spaghetti with meat sauce or casseroles. ● Offer legumes, eggs, and cheese as alternative protein sources.
Overconsumption of sweets	● Avoid keeping sweets in the home. ● Schedule "dessert" days to decrease daily or habitual consumption while allowing sweets. ● Avoid using sweets as a reward or bribe. ● Choose low-sugar snack foods.
Consumption of large portions	● Offer food on a smaller plate. ● Use toddler-sized utensils. ● Minimize distractions during meals and snacks. ● Offer meals and snacks at scheduled times and locations. ● Encourage water consumption with meals and snacks to help increase satiety.

Nutritional Needs

Nutritional needs remain fairly stable during middle childhood, with boys and girls needing about the same number of calories and nutrients per day. Following an eating pattern that includes the food groups and amounts shown in **Table 17-6** helps children meet macronutrient and micronutrient Dietary Reference Intakes to support optimal growth and nutrition. Children are best able to meet the recommended intakes by consuming 3 balanced meals and 1 to 2 nutritious snacks per day.

Common Concerns

Despite recommendations for ample fruit and vegetable intake and at least 2½ c (0.6 L) of dairy or the equivalent per day to meet nutritional needs, and otherwise water to meet hydration needs, the nutrition intake for most school-aged children falls short. School-aged children consume less than recommended amounts of

Table 17-6. Nutritional Needs in Middle Childhood

Need	Age (y)		
	5	**6–8**	**9–11**
Approximate total caloric needs (Cal)	1,200	1,400	1,600
Vegetables (c)	1½	1½	2
Fruits (c)	1½	1½	1½
Protein-rich foods (oz)	3	4	5
Grains (oz)	4	5	5
Dairy (c)[a]	2½	2½	3
Water (c)[a]	4½	4½	7
Limit on calories from other sources (eg, added sugars, fats) (Cal)	80	90	150
Added sugars[b]	<10% total calories OR <25 g	<10% total calories OR <25 g	<10% total calories OR <25 g
Sodium (mg)	<1,200	<1,500	<1,800

[a] 1 c = 8 oz.

[b] 4 g = 1 tsp.

Derived from references 2 and 7.

vegetables, fruits, whole grains, and dairy and more than recommended amounts of processed grains, added sugars, saturated fat, and sodium, as shown in **figures 17-1** (ages 5–8 years) and **17-2** (ages 9–13 years). As discussed in Chapter 10, Dietary History, Social History, and Food Insecurity Screening, many complex social and environmental factors affect a child's nutrition intake and their likelihood of meeting dietary recommendations.

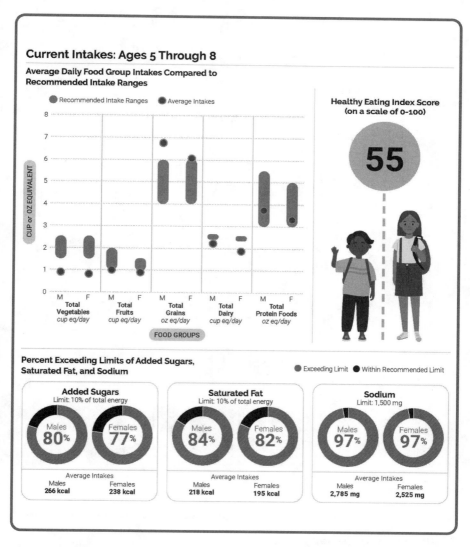

Figure 17-1. Current dietary intake of children aged 5–8 y.

Continued

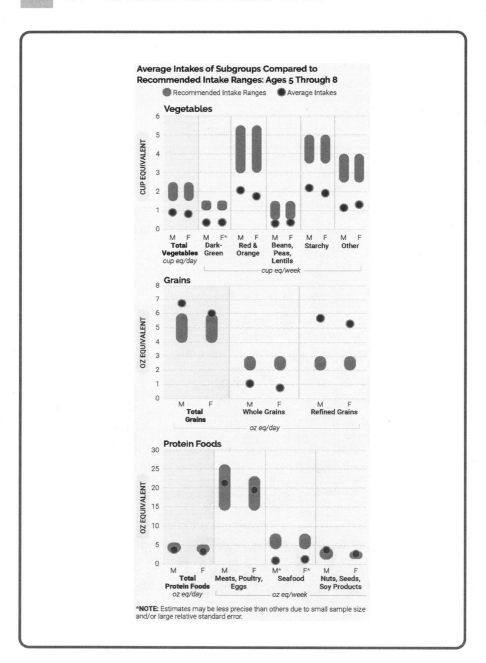

Figure 17-1 (*continued*)

Reproduced from reference 2.

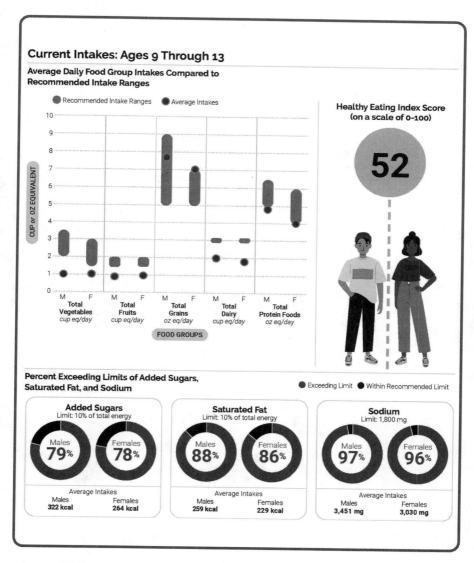

Figure 17-2. Current dietary intake of children and adolescents aged 9–13 y.

Continued

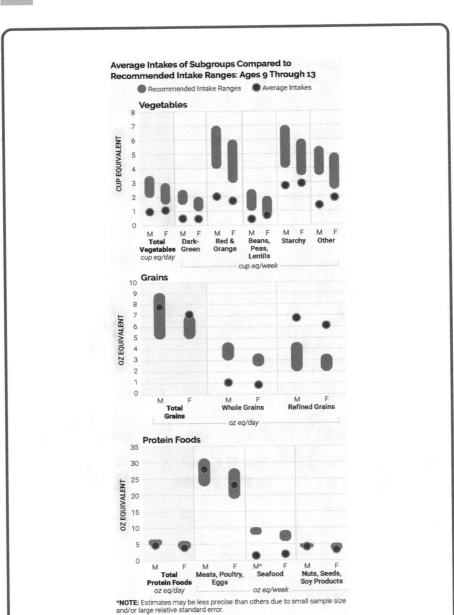

Figure 17-2 (*continued*)

Reproduced from reference 2.

Strategies to Promote Optimal Nutrition

Many of the strategies that help younger children adopt healthier nutrition habits also apply in middle childhood. For example, regular meals and snack times help promote balanced meals and minimize snacking throughout the day. Children who participate in family mealtimes tend to have parents who eat more nutritiously, and they benefit from the increased socialization and family connectedness that result from family mealtimes. Parents can play a particularly impactful role by modeling not only healthy eating and activity habits but also a healthy relationship with food and a healthy body image. Older siblings and peers also serve as powerful influences and role models at this age. Children enrolled in school meal programs benefit from food offerings aligned with the dietary guidelines and MyPlate recommendations for their ages (detailed in chapters 11, Dietary Guidelines and Principles of Healthy Eating, and 12, Healthy Eating Plans).

Addressing Common Nutritional Concerns

Common nutritional concerns that develop in middle childhood and possible solutions that clinicians can share with parents are outlined in **Table 17-7**.

Adolescence (Ages 12–17 Years)

The growing independence and physical, cognitive, social, and emotional changes that accompany adolescence offer an important opportunity to shape nutritional beliefs and choices. For most teens, a large percentage of nutrition decisions occur outside the home, in between structured activities, and under the influence of peers. Consequently, eating patterns tend to be more variable and erratic than for other stages of development. Many teens skip breakfast, and very few achieve recommended intakes of fruits, vegetables, and key nutrients. This is also a phase of development during which many mental health and body image concerns arise, alongside a higher prevalence of disordered eating and more severe obesity.

Nutritional Needs

Nutritional needs during adolescence are outlined in **Table 17-8**. Studies suggest that the adolescent diet is most likely to be lacking in fruits and vegetables, whole grains, and dairy products. In fact, a review of the National Health and Nutrition Examination Survey showed that 0% of the 4,673 adolescents surveyed had an ideal healthy diet score (defined as 4–5 of the components of the ideal healthy diet score measures), whereas 90% had a poor score (0–1 measures) and 10% had an intermediate score (2–3 measures).[8] Components of an ideal healthy diet score include consuming (1) more than 4½ c (675 g) of fruits and vegetables per day, (2) more than two 3½-oz (99-g) servings of fish per week, (3) more than three 1-oz (28-g) equivalent servings of fiber-rich whole grains per day (defined as > 1.1 g of fiber per 10 g of carbohydrate), (4) less than 1,500 mg/d of sodium, and (5) less than 450 kcal/wk of sugar-sweetened beverages. For adolescents, consuming less than 1 serving of fruit per day and/or less than 2 servings of vegetables per day is a nutritional risk factor for low intake of fiber,

Table 17-7. Common Nutritional Concerns in Middle Childhood and Possible Solutions

Common nutritional concerns	Possible solutions to share with parents
Low intake of fruits and vegetables	• Include a fruit and vegetable at every meal. • Keep fruits and vegetables accessible and readily available (eg, fruit bowl on the counter, cleaned and cut vegetables in the refrigerator). • Minimize access to alternative snacks.
Low intake of milk	• Offer milk at every meal. • Avoid purchase of alternative drinks such as juice and soda. • Offer other milk products, including yogurt and cheese and milk substitutes.
High intake of sugary drinks and processed snacks	• Have only water and milk available to drink at home. • Share health risks of sugar and amount of sugar that is contained in sugary drinks. • Offer water and milk at mealtimes. • Avoid purchasing sugary snacks. • Schedule 2-3 d/wk for dessert.
Consumption of large portions	• Reteach how to use feelings of hunger and satiety to guide intake. • Help identify triggers for eating. • Use smaller plates and utensils. • Practice slowing down while eating (eg, put fork down between bites, take sip of water between bites, have family meals and socialize more during mealtimes).
Obesity, eating disorder, or other weight concern	• Discuss concerns about weight sensitively, with the focus on health rather than weight. • Help establish small goals and small changes to progress toward goals. • Seek additional professional and community resources and supports as needed, such as a registered dietitian and/or a mental health professional.

Table 17-8. Adolescent Nutritional Needs

Need	Age (y) and Sex				
	12–13 (girls)	12 (boys) 14–17 (girls)	13–14 (boys)	15 (boys)	16–17 (boys)
Approximate total caloric needs (Cal)[a]	1,600	1,800	2,000	2,200	2,400
Vegetables (c)	2	2½	2½	3	3
Fruits (c)	1½	1½	2	2	2
Protein-rich foods (oz eq/d)	5	5	5½	6	6½
Grains (oz eq/d)	5	6	6	7	8
Dairy (c eq/d)[b]	3	3	3	3	3
Water (c)[b,c]	4	5	8	8	8
Limit on calories from other sources (eg, added sugars, fats) (Cal)	100	140	240	250	320
Added sugars[d]	<10% total calories OR <25 g	<10% total calories OR <25 g	<10% total calories OR <25 g	<10% total calories OR <25 g	<10% total calories OR <25 g
Sodium (mg)	<2,300	<2,300	<2,300	<2,300	<2,300

[a] Calorie levels are based on needs of a teen of average height and weight for that age. Needs vary on the basis of activity level, with an approximately additional 200 Cal/d for moderately active teens. For more detailed information, refer to the *2020–2025 Dietary Guidelines for Americans*.
[b] 1 c = 8 oz.
[c] Recommended water assumes that teens are meeting remainder of oral fluid needs from dairy intake of 3 c/d. Total recommended daily fluid intake from drinks = dairy (c) + water (c).
[d] 4 g = 1 tsp.
Derived from references 2 and 9.

vitamins, and minerals. Risk of inadequate fiber intake is also increased if adolescents consume less than 3 servings of whole grains per day, and risk of inadequate calcium and vitamin D intake is increased if adolescents consume less than 3 servings of dairy per day.

Additionally, adolescent girls are at increased risk of iron deficiency, especially if they experience heavy menstrual periods.[3] For most teens, added sugars, saturated fat, and sodium intakes far exceed recommended limits. High intakes of these nutrients are associated with increased risk of cardiovascular disease, obesity, and other health harms (refer to Chapter 20, Obesity and Related Health Conditions). Other common risk factors for nutritional inadequacy include skipping meals more than 2 times per week, dieting, and disordered eating. Significant weight loss or weight gain can be a sign of stress, depression, organic disease, eating disorders, or obesogenic behaviors or environment. Severe restriction and purging are associated with substance use, suicidal behaviors, and serious medical complications. These and other common nutritional concerns during adolescence are summarized in **Figure 17-3**

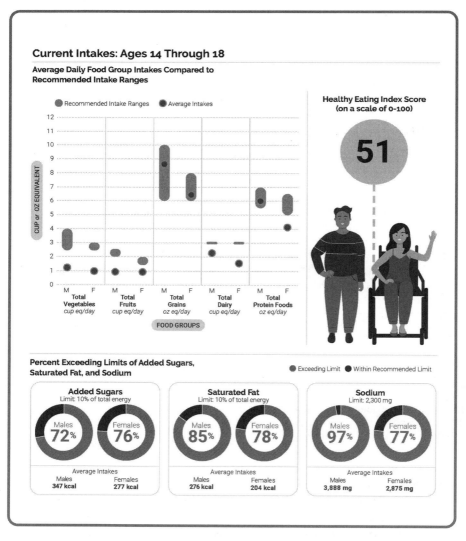

Figure 17-3. Current dietary intake of adolescents aged 14–18 y.

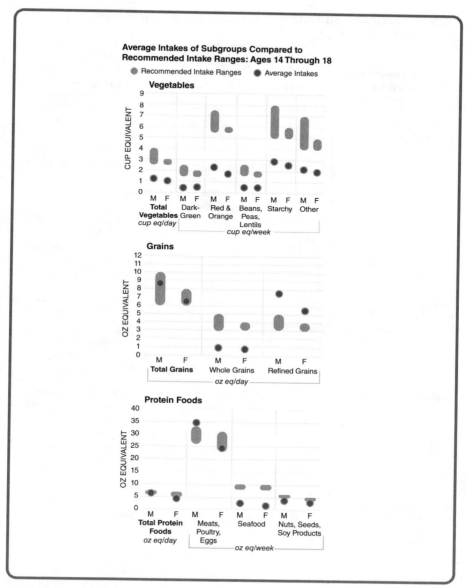

Figure 17-3 (*continued*)

Reproduced from reference 2.

and detailed more in Chapter 19, Mental Health, Behavioral, and Developmental Conditions. Potential strategies to address these nutritional concerns and the severe decrease in physical activity that occurs in adolescence (especially among girls) are discussed in **Table 17-9**.

Table 17-9. Common Nutritional Concerns in Adolescence and Possible Solutions

Common nutritional concerns	Guidance for clinicians	Possible solutions to share with parents and other caregivers
Insufficient intake of fruits and/or vegetables	• Assess a patient's interest and willingness to increase fruit and vegetable intake. • Encourage teens to plan and prepare their own balanced lunches and help with dinner and meal planning.	• Have balanced family meals as often as possible. • Make fruits and vegetables readily available in the home. • Model consumption of fruits and vegetables. • Help teens learn to cook. • Have meal nights that include traditional foods from other cultures, including fruits and vegetables.
Decreased consumption of milk and dairy	Share information about the benefits and importance of adequate calcium and vitamin D intake.	• Encourage milk with meals. • Incorporate low-sugar yogurt and cheeses into meals and snacks.
Carbohydrate restriction	• Affirm plans to limit processed carbohydrates but encourage whole grains. • Share health benefits of fiber, including increased satiety, regular bowel function, and improved cholesterol levels.	Encourage consumption of whole grains, fruits, and vegetables while limiting purchase of refined and highly processed carbohydrates.
High intake of sugary drinks	• Share the health risks of high intake of sugary drinks. • Share information about marketing tactics to try to increase teen consumption of sugary drinks. • Discuss options to make drinking water more fun and to enhance taste, such as sparkling and infused water.	• Avoid purchasing sugary drinks or storing them at home. • Offer milk and water with meals.

Table 17-9 (*continued*)

Common nutritional concerns	Guidance for clinicians	Possible solutions to share with parents and other caregivers
High intakes of added sugars, sodium, and saturated fats	• Discuss alternatives to foods and drinks high in added sugars and/or sodium. • Explore strategies to reduce processed food and drink intake.	• Avoid keeping sweets and heavily processed snacks in the home. • Schedule "dessert" days to decrease daily or habitual consumption while allowing sweets. • Minimize eating at fast-food restaurants, doing so as infrequently as possible and no more than 2 times per week.
Skipping of meals	Encourage a schedule and routine for meals and snacks.	• Schedule times for meals and snacks each day. • Prepare or plan meals the night before. • Educate adolescents on the benefits of balanced meals. • Ensure adequate food access. • Monitor for signs of unhealthy weight loss practice.
Significant weight loss or weight gain in the past 6 mo	• Interpret anthropometric measures and growth curves in context. • Use sensitive language to explore potential reasons for the change and best next steps. • Connect with community resources as needed.	• Address the concern in a sensitive manner. • Aim to identify cause of weight change. • Seek resources for further evaluation and treatment.

Continued

Table 17-9 (*continued*)

Common nutritional concerns	Guidance for clinicians	Possible solutions to share with parents and other caregivers
Signs of eating disorders, body image concerns, dieting, excessive physical activity, supplement use, and/or unsafe weight loss methods	• Remind patients that healthy body weight is based on genetically determined size and shape and is not a socially defined ideal. • Avoid stigmatizing language. • Emphasize health, and help set specific goals to improve or optimize health behaviors around nutrition and physical activity. • Ask adolescents about supplement use, and advise them of potential health harms. • Monitor for signs of an eating disorder. Seek outside supports, including a dietitian and a therapist, as indicated.	• Address the concern in a sensitive manner. • Seek resources for further evaluation and treatment.
Decreased physical activity	• Help adolescents identify fun ways to achieve 60 min/d of physical activity. • Share that physical activity also helps with a variety of potential mental health and behavioral concerns, such as depression and inattention. • Encourage teens to find ways to be active with their friends.	• Help teens explore potential physical activities that they may enjoy doing. • Help facilitate transportation and logistics for the physical activity when possible. • Offer to engage in physical activities together when feasible.

Table 17-9 (*continued*)

Common nutritional concerns	Guidance for clinicians	Possible solutions to share with parents and other caregivers
Food insecurity (Refer to Chapter 10, Dietary History, Social History, and Food Insecurity Screening, for more information.)	• Many resources are available to help access healthful foods, including the Supplemental Nutrition Assistance Program, food pantries, school breakfast and lunch programs, and mental health resources when appropriate. • Share resources that help families eat healthy on a budget. Several are available at MyPlate (www. myplate.gov).	• Connect with local resources in the community to help support access to healthful foods and to help increase knowledge and skill in choosing and preparing healthful foods on a budget (eg, 211 [call 211 or visit 211.org], Cooking Matters [https:// cookingmatters.org]).

In Sum

- Pediatricians and other clinicians who work with children, adolescents, and their families play an important role in providing developmentally tailored nutritional guidance to help promote healthful nutrition.
- Pediatricians can help parents anticipate typical changes to a child's appetite and feeding practices. For example, the average infant is generally eager to try new tastes and textures. Around 18 months to 2 years of age, it is typical for children to begin to exhibit picky eating habits, during which they refuse to eat certain foods, and food jags, during which they favor only 1 or 2 foods. Neophobia is typical and common at this age. As children get older, they are more likely to be willing to try new foods, although most school-aged children and adolescents consume lower than recommended amounts of fruits, vegetables, whole grains, and dairy products and higher than recommended amounts of added sugars, saturated fat, and sodium.
- The recommended parenting approach to help children and adolescents adopt healthier eating patterns is an authoritative, or responsive, parenting style in which parents play an important role in determining meal and snack timing—when meals and snacks are served and what food is offered. Children and adolescents are allowed to control their meal size and food selection. This approach encourages and supports a child in using their own cues of hunger and satiety to decide how much to eat.
- Many common nutritional concerns across childhood and adolescence can be addressed with repeated exposures to a variety of tastes and textures, increased accessibility to nutritious foods, and decreased accessibility to less nutritious foods that are high in added sugars and sodium.

References

1. Hagan JF Jr, Shaw JS, Duncan PM, eds. *Bright Futures: Guidelines for Health Supervision of Infants, Children, and Adolescents.* 4th ed. American Academy of Pediatrics; 2017 doi: 10.1542/9781610020237

2. US Department of Health and Human Services, US Department of Agriculture. *Dietary Guidelines for Americans, 2020–2025.* 9th ed. 2020. Accessed October 26, 2022. https://www.dietaryguidelines.gov/sites/default/files/2020-12/Dietary_Guidelines_for_Americans_2020-2025.pdf

3. Dietary Guidelines Advisory Committee. *Scientific Report of the 2020 Dietary Guidelines Advisory Committee: Advisory Report to the Secretary of Agriculture and the Secretary of Health and Human Services.* Agricultural Research Service, US Dept of Agriculture; 2020

4. Roess AA, Jacquier EF, Catellier DJ, et al. Food consumption patterns of infants and toddlers: findings from the Feeding Infants and Toddlers Study (FITS) 2016. *J Nutr.* 2018;148(suppl 3):1525S–1535S PMID: 30247583 doi: 10.1093/jn/nxy171

5. Welker EB, Jacquier EF, Catellier DJ, Anater AS, Story MT. Room for improvement remains in food consumption patterns of young children aged 2–4 years. *J Nutr.* 2018;148(9S)(suppl 3):1536S–1546S PMID: 29878237 doi: 10.1093/jn/nxx053

6. Heyman MB, Abrams SA, Heitlinger LA, et al; American Academy of Pediatrics Section on Gastroenterology, Hepatology, and Nutrition and Committee on Nutrition. Fruit juice in infants, children, and adolescents: current recommendations. *Pediatrics.* 2017;139(6):e20170967 PMID: 28562300 doi: 10.1542/peds.2017-0967

7. Johnson RK, Appel LJ, Brands M, et al; American Heart Association Nutrition Committee of the Council on Nutrition, Physical Activity, and Metabolism and the Council on Epidemiology and Prevention. Dietary sugars intake and cardiovascular health: a scientific statement from the American Heart Association. *Circulation.* 2009;120(11):1011–1020 PMID: 19704096 doi: 10.1161/CIRCULATIONAHA.109.192627

8. Shay CM, Ning H, Daniels SR, Rooks CR, Gidding SS, Lloyd-Jones DM. Status of cardiovascular health in US adolescents: prevalence estimates from the National Health and Nutrition Examination Surveys (NHANES) 2005–2010. *Circulation.* 2013;127(13):1369–1376 PMID: 23547177 doi: 10.1161/CIRCULATIONAHA.113.001559

9. Institute of Medicine. *Dietary Reference Intakes for Energy, Carbohydrate, Fiber, Fat, Fatty Acids, Cholesterol, Protein, and Amino Acids.* National Academies Press; 2005

CHAPTER 18

Sports and Athletic Performance

Beyond playing a role in promoting optimal health, well-planned nutrition intake can offer a strategic performance advantage for young athletes competing at the highest levels. At the same time, poorly planned nutrition intake in highly active youth can lead to negative performance and health risks. Eating in a way that supports optimal performance, growth, and health is particularly challenging for athletes, who often have demanding school, training, socializing, and work schedules; limited knowledge of nutrition principles in general and in sports; reliance on others to purchase and prepare foods; and unhealthy eating environments during training, competition, and travel.[1] Many athletes are motivated to make nutritional changes to improve their sports performance or attain fitness or strength gains, giving pediatricians an opportunity to provide nutrition information and counseling to help guide patients toward nutrition strategies to achieve their performance goals. Implementation of these strategies will not only improve an athlete's sports performance but also help improve the overall quality of their dietary intake.

Additionally, during conversations about sports nutrition and sports performance, pediatricians have an opportunity to assess for supplement use and steer patients toward safe, evidence-informed nutrition practices to improve sports performance. Because most children are not involved in competitive sports, this chapter also includes key nutrition and activity principles that apply across all levels of activity and that can be shared with patients and their families.

Energy Needs

Highly active children and adolescents have increased caloric needs to fuel strenuous exercise regimens and optimize growth and development. Typical energy needs for children and adolescents that are based on physical activity level are shown in Chapter 1, Dietary Reference Intakes (refer to **Table 1-1**). Clinicians can use the estimated energy requirement equation from the Appendix (refer to **tables A-6 and A-7**) to individualize recommendations more to patients. Increased caloric needs are best met primarily through increased intake of nutrient-dense whole grains, lean proteins, fruits, and vegetables.

Caloric intake must meet caloric needs to ensure sufficient energy availability. *Energy availability* refers to the energy requirements necessary for optimal health and function. Energy availability is calculated as dietary intake minus exercise energy expenditure normalized to fat-free mass, as follows:

$$\text{Energy availability} = (\text{Energy intake} - \text{Estimated energy expenditure})/ \text{Fat-free mass (kilograms)}.$$

To calculate energy availability, clinicians need to know a patient's typical daily energy intake, their number of calories expended from exercise (estimated energy expenditure), and their lean body mass (fat-free mass). Pediatricians rarely have the data needed to calculate a patient's energy availability, but sometimes a sports dietitian or sports medicine clinic has the tools to do so.

An energy availability of 45 kcal/kg of fat-free mass per day is associated with energy balance and optimal health. Insufficient energy availability negatively affects performance through decreased endurance and strength, increased injury risk, decreased training response, impaired judgment, decreased coordination and concentration, irritability, and depression. Chronically low energy availability (particularly consumption of < 30 kcal/kg of fat-free mass per day) results in *relative energy deficiency in sport* (RED-S). RED-S is associated with disruption in metabolism, menstruation, bone health, immunity, protein synthesis, growth, psychological health, and cardiovascular, gastrointestinal, endocrine, and hematologic functioning.[2,3] RED-S is an expanded concept of the female athlete triad (**Box 18-1**).

The Female Athlete Triad Coalition Consensus Panel developed a scoring rubric for level of participation and return-to-play medical risk stratification to help clinicians categorize athletes with RED-S and triad-related risk factors into low-, moderate-, or high-risk categories. Decisions regarding sports participation, level of participation permitted, and return to play are made on the basis of the athlete's risk category (**Table 18-1**). Risk category can be reassessed as the athlete progresses through treatment of RED-S (refer to Chapter 19, Mental Health, Behavioral, and Developmental Conditions, for discussion of treatment of eating disorders). These recommendations have been endorsed by the American Academy of Pediatrics (AAP).[5]

Following is a summary of AAP guidance for pediatricians that is based on the Triad Consensus Panel recommendations[5]:

1. Screen for signs of RED-S at the health supervision visit or sports preparticipation physical evaluation. If an athlete responds yes to any of the triad screening questions included in the preparticipation physical evaluation history, continue the screening with the remaining questions suggested by the Female Athlete Triad Coalition.
2. Treat functional hypothalamic amenorrhea resulting from low energy availability with restoration of optimal energy availability. Treatment with oral contraceptive pills is not first-line therapy.
3. Engage a multidisciplinary team in the management of RED-S, including a nutrition professional and a mental health professional, if needed.
4. Treatment goals may include reversal of weight loss (if present), return to a body weight associated with typical menses (which can take up to 1 y), attainment of a body mass index greater than 18.5 or greater than 85% of expected body weight, and a minimum caloric intake of 2,000 kcal/d. These goals can usually be met through a gradual increase of 200 to 600 kcal/d and reduction in training volume of 1 day per week.
5. Consider using a written treatment plan signed by the pediatrician, athlete, and parent that outlines and defines the treatment plan and expectations of all 3 parties.
6. Request dual-energy x-ray absorptiometry to measure bone mineral density in patients with amenorrhea lasting longer than 6 months or with a history of stress fractures.
7. Advise athletes to consume adequate intakes of calcium (1,300 mg/d) and vitamin D (600 IU/d) for optimal bone health, from food sources or from supplementation, if needed.

IN GREATER DEPTH

Box 18-1. Relative Energy Deficiency in Sport

As shown in the figure, *relative energy deficiency in sport* is a more comprehensive term than *female athlete triad,* which describes 3 entities of energy availability, menstrual function, and bone health in females, because the ill health effects of low energy availability not only extend beyond the triad but also affect males. In fact, male athletes with severe low energy availability may be at risk for *male athlete triad,* which consists of low energy availability and impaired gonadal function and bone health, although this construct is less well-defined than the female athlete triad.[4]

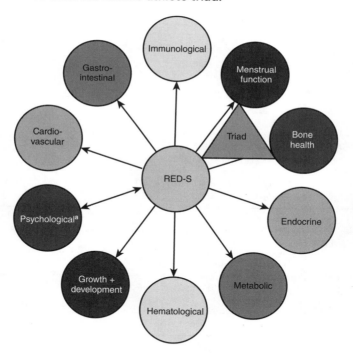

Figure. Health consequences of relative energy deficiency in sport (RED-S) showing an expanded concept of the female athlete triad to acknowledge a wider range of outcomes and the application to male athletes.

[a]Psychological consequences can either precede RED-S or be the result of RED-S.
Figure reproduced with permission from Mountjoy M, Sundgot-Borgen J, Burke L, et al. The IOC consensus statement: beyond the Female Athlete Triad—Relative Energy Deficiency in Sport (RED-S). *Br J Sports Med.* 2014;48(7):491–497.

Continued

IN GREATER DEPTH

Box 18-1 (*continued*)

The Triad Consensus Panel advises clinicians to screen for relative energy deficiency in sport as part of the sports PPE by asking the screening questions as shown in the following table:

Question	Included on the fourth-edition PPE form
1. Do you worry about your weight or body composition?	✓
2. Do you limit or carefully control the foods that you eat?	✓
3. Do you try to lose weight to meet weight or image/appearance requirements in your sport?	✓
4. Does your weight affect the way you feel about yourself?	—
5. Do you worry that you have lost control over how much you eat?	—
6. Do you make yourself vomit or use diuretics or laxatives after you eat?	—
7. Do you currently or have you ever had an eating disorder?	✓
8. Do you ever eat in secret?	—
9. What age was your first menstrual period?	✓
10. Do you have monthly menstrual cycles?	✓
11. How many menstrual cycles have you had in the past year?	✓
12. Have you ever had a stress fracture?	✓

Abbreviation: PPE, preparticipation physical evaluation.

Table adapted from reference 5.

Table 18-1. The Relative Energy Deficiency in Sport Risk Stratification for Sports Clearance

Risk factors	Magnitude of risk		
	Low risk = 0 points each	Moderate risk = 1 point each	High risk = 2 points each
Low EA with or without DE/ED	☐ No dietary restriction	☐ Some dietary restriction[a]; current/past history of DE	☐ Meets *DSM-V* criteria for ED[b]
Low BMI	☐ BMI ≥18.5 **or** ≥90% EW[c] **or** weight stable	☐ BMI 17.5 to <18.5 **or** <90% EW **or** 5 to <10% weight loss/month	☐ BMI ≤17.5 **or** <85% EW **or** ≥10% weight loss/month
Delayed menarche	☐ Menarche <15 years	☐ Menarche 15 to <16 years	☐ Menarche ≥16 years
Oligomenorrhea and/or amenorrhea	☐ > 9 menses in 12 months[b]	☐ 6-9 menses in 12 months[b]	☐ <6 menses in 12 months[b]
Low BMD	☐ Z score ≥-1.0	☐ Z score -1.0[d] to <-2.0	☐ Z score ≤-2.0
Stress reaction/fracture	☐ None	☐ 1	☐ ≥2; ≥1 high risk or of trabecular bone sites[e]
Cumulative risk (total each column, then add total for score)	_____ points +	_____ points +	_____ points = total score

Continued

Table 18-1 (*continued*)

	Cumulative risk score	Low risk	Moderate risk	High risk
Full clearance	0–1 point	☐		
Provisional/limited clearance	2–5 points		☐ Provisional clearance ☐ Limited clearance	
Restricted from training and competition	≥6 points			☐ Restricted from training/competition-provisional ☐ Disqualified

Abbreviations: BMD, bone mineral density; BMI, body mass index; DE, disordered eating, *DSM-V, Diagnostic and Statistical Manual of Mental Disorders, Fifth Edition*; EA, energy availability; ED, eating disorder; EW, expected weight; RTP, return to play.

[a] Some dietary restriction as evidenced by self-report or low/inadequate energy intake on diet logs.

[b] Currently experiencing or has a history.

[c] ≥90% EW; absolute BMI cutoffs should be not used for adolescents.

[d] Weight-bearing sport.

[e] High-risk skeletal sites associated with low BMD and delay in RTP in athletes with one or more components of the triad include stress reaction/fracture of trabecular sites (femoral neck, sacrum, and pelvis).

Clearance/RTP status for athletes at moderate-to-high risk for the triad: provisional clearance/RTP—clearance determined from risk stratification at the time of evaluation (with possibility for status to change over time depending on athlete's clinical progress); limited clearance/RTP—clearance/RTP granted but with modification in training as specified by a physician (with possibility for status to change depending on clinical progress and new information gathered); restricted from training/competition (provisional)—athlete not cleared or able to RTP at present time, with clearance status reevaluated by a physician and a multidisciplinary team with clinical progress; disqualified—not safe to participate at present time. Clearance status is to be determined in the future depending on clinical progress, if appropriate. It is the recommendation of the consensus panel that the athletes diagnosed with anorexia nervosa who have a BMI <16 kg · m^{-2} or with moderate-to-severe bulimia nervosa (purging >4 times per week) should be restricted from training and competition categorically. Future participation is dependent on treatment of their ED, including ascertainment of BMI >18.5 kg · m^{-2}, cessation of bingeing and purging, and close interval follow-up with the multidisciplinary team.

Reproduced with permission from reference 2.

Children and adolescents who engage in moderate levels of physical activity or those who are incorporating increased physical activity or exercise as part of a weight management program may not have notably increased caloric needs that are related to exercise. In these cases, the aim is to reinforce healthy eating patterns, including 3 meals and 1 to 2 snacks per day, with emphasis on fruits and vegetables, whole grains, and lean proteins. Additional caloric intake or strategic fueling and refueling is generally unnecessary.

Macronutrient Needs

Athletes require careful attention to macronutrient intake to optimize sports performance. Macronutrient needs vary on the basis of performance goals, sex, and age of a patient and frequency, intensity, time, and type of activity.

Carbohydrate

Carbohydrate intake is an important goal in sports nutrition for several reasons.
- Carbohydrate is the body's preferred energy source.
- Carbohydrates can be used as fuel over a wide range of exercise intensities, using both aerobic and anaerobic energy systems.
- Carbohydrates are stored in the body in relatively low supply in muscle and liver, but availability can be easily increased through dietary intake.
- High carbohydrate availability during exercise helps fuel exercise, maintain concentration, and reduce fatigue and perception of effort.
- Sufficient carbohydrate intake helps spare dietary protein and amino acids so they may be used for muscle building rather than as an energy source.
- Carbohydrate intake within 20 minutes of completion of a strenuous exercise session helps replenish glycogen stores.

Athletes should consume at least 50% of their daily calories from carbohydrates and at least meet the recommended dietary allowance of carbohydrate of 130 g/d. Some athletes may need higher carbohydrate intakes, ranging from 3 to 10 g/kg of body weight depending on multiple factors, including the athlete's total energy requirements, the fuel demands of their training and/or competition, and the balance between their performance goals and their body composition goals.[6]

Protein

Well-timed protein intake helps repair and remodel muscle tissue, support tendon and bone strength, and increase muscle mass. Most adolescent athletes need about 1.0 to 1.5 g/kg of body weight of protein.[5] Most athletes achieve this level of intake spontaneously. Protein intake should be spread throughout the day. However, to optimize muscle repair and strengthening, athletes should consume high-quality proteins within 1 hour following strenuous training.

Fat

Fat is in abundant supply in the body as an energy source, in the forms of plasma free fatty acids, intramuscular triglycerides, and adipose tissue. Athletes do not need more fat than nonathletes of the same age. Athletes are advised to consume no less than 20% of calories from fat to prevent fat-soluble vitamin and essential fatty acid deficiencies, and no more than 10% of calories should come from saturated fat.[6]

Nutrition Before, During, and After Exercise

Strategic fueling before, during, and after exercise can help athletes optimize sports performance and recovery. The goals of careful attention to the timing of nutrition intake around activity and competition are set to ensure optimal nutrient availability to support strenuous activity while delaying or preventing factors that negatively affect performance. Factors that can negatively affect performance include mental fatigue, dehydration, gastrointestinal discomfort, glycogen depletion, hypoglycemia, and acid-base imbalance.

Pre-exercise Nutrition

The goal of pre-exercise fueling is to ensure adequate carbohydrate availability to fuel exercise without causing gastrointestinal upset. To support this goal, pediatricians can advise young athletes to consider the following strategies for meals and snacks consumed before exercise:

- Eat carbohydrates. Carbohydrate intake before exercise helps maximize blood glucose availability to fuel sports performance. Specifically, in the 1 to 4 hours before exercise, athletes should eat 1 to 4 g/kg of body weight of carbohydrate.[6] For example, a 110-lb (50-kg) athlete should eat 50 to 200 g of carbohydrate in the 1 to 4 hours before exercise. The carbohydrates can be consumed as one meal or as one or more snacks. Low glycemic index choices may provide a more sustained source of energy when carbohydrates cannot be consumed during exercise. Endurance athletes may benefit from carbohydrate loading with carbohydrate intake of 10 to 12 g/kg of body weight per 24 hours in the 36 to 48 hours before an endurance event lasting longer than 90 minutes.[6] However, an important caveat is that carbohydrate loading has not been well studied in young athletes; therefore, there is insufficient evidence to recommend whether youth endurance athletes should engage in carbohydrate loading.
- Choose foods low in fat and fiber. High-fat and high-fiber foods eaten before exercise slow gastric emptying and can cause gastrointestinal discomfort such as abdominal pain, cramping, or the need to defecate.
- Trial foods before competition day. Athletes should experiment with their pre-exercise fueling plan before competition day to determine what foods and regimen they best tolerate. Although one regimen may work well in improving performance without adverse effects for a given athlete, it may not work well for a different athlete. Athletes should develop their own plan that is based on the preceding guidance to find a routine that works well for them.

Nutrition During Exercise

The goal of fueling during exercise is to provide the body with the essential nutrients needed by muscle cells to maintain optimal blood glucose levels. Pediatricians can offer young athletes the following advice to accomplish this goal:

- For exercise lasting less than 60 minutes, consume water. No additional carbohydrate intake is necessary. Assuming that the athlete is not in a sustained energy deficit, their body's existing glucose and glycogen stores provide adequate glucose availability. Any intake other than water provides no additional performance benefit and can be detrimental by causing gastrointestinal distress or unnecessary caloric intake.
- For exercise lasting longer than 60 minutes, consume 30 to 60 g of carbohydrate per hour of training to ensure adequate glucose availability and energy supply.[6] Carbohydrate consumption during prolonged exercise is especially important for athletes who exercise in extreme heat, cold, or high altitude; for athletes who did not consume adequate amounts of food or drink before the training session or competition; and for athletes who restricted energy intake for weight loss.
- Time carbohydrate consumption during prolonged exercise (>60 minutes) to begin shortly after the onset of the workout or competition. Aim for 30 to 60 g of carbohydrate per hour of exercise. Divide this up to consume 10 to 15 g of carbohydrate every 15 to 20 minutes.[6]

Post-exercise Nutrition

The main goals of post-exercise fueling are to replenish glycogen stores and facilitate muscle repair. Encourage patients to take the following steps to achieve these goals and support optimal recovery:

- Eat regularly scheduled meals and snacks. Most athletes do not need aggressive post-exercise replenishment because typical eating and drinking patterns following exercise support recovery within 20 to 48 hours.
- Eat or drink some form of carbohydrate within 30 minutes of completing an intensive exercise session or competition, to replace glycogen stores.
- Eat high-carbohydrate meals and snacks in the 4 hours after the intensive exercise session or competition if there is less than 8 hours' recovery between 2 demanding sessions, such as in the case of a tournament weekend. Studies show that athletes who consume 1.0 to 1.2 g/kg of body weight of carbohydrate or 0.8 g/kg of carbohydrate and 0.3 g/kg of protein per hour for 4 hours and then resume usual intake optimize glycogen repletion.[6]
- Consume 15 to 25 g of high-quality protein within 2 hours of a high-intensity muscle-conditioning program to optimize muscle protein synthesis.[6] Because exercise enhances the rate of muscle protein synthesis for up to 24 hours after completion, consumption of high-quality protein with meals and snacks helps build muscle mass. Dairy proteins seem to be the most effective at building muscle mass, given their high leucine content, although lean meat, soy, and egg may also be beneficial.[6]

Examples of nutrition before, during, and after exercise are shown in **Box 18-2**.

Box 18-2. Examples of Nutrition for Before, During, and After Exercise

Pre-exercise nutrition	Nutrition during exercise (activity > 60 min)	Post-exercise nutrition
Bowl of cereal Bagel with cream cheese or jam Banana	Carbohydrate mouth rinse Sports drink Orange slices Raisins	Granola bar Apple and peanut butter Toast and peanut butter Salted nuts and pretzels 8 fl oz chocolate milk Greek yogurt with granola Hummus and pita Fruit smoothie Trail mix Date Nut Butter Energy Bites[a]

SI conversion factor: To convert fl oz to mL, multiply by 30.
[a] Refer to Part 5, Frequently Asked Questions, Case Studies, and Recipes, for recipe.

Fluids and Hydration

Attention to hydration before, during, and after exercise can help improve athletic performance while preventing negative performance and health impacts that can occur with dehydration or overhydration. Pediatricians can provide athletes with the following information to help optimize hydration:

- **Before exercise.** To pre-hydrate for optimal performance, athletes should drink 5 to 10 mL/kg of body weight (2–4 mL/lb of body weight) in the 2 to 4 hours before exercise.
- **During exercise.** Most athletes need 1.7 to 3.4 c (0.4–0.8 L) of fluids per hour of exercise depending on intensity, duration, weather, altitude, and other factors. Fluid needs are higher during exercise, largely because of fluid losses from sweat. The goal is to avoid more than 2% of body weight loss between the start and completion of an exercise bout.
  - Fluid consumed should be water only for exercise lasting less than 60 minutes.
  - Carbohydrate-containing sports drinks may be an option for athletes engaging in exercise lasting longer than 60 minutes when rapid carbohydrate or electrolyte replenishment is needed. Sports drinks contain 2 to 19 g of carbohydrates (glucose and fructose forms) and 10 to 70 Cal per serving (8 fl oz [240 mL]). Intake should be limited to what is needed to fuel prolonged exercise.[7]

— Sodium should be consumed during exercise when large sweat losses occur, such as exercise lasting longer than 2 hours or exercise producing high sweat rates (eg, running in high heat or humidity).

— Cold fluids can reduce body heat and improve performance in hot temperatures.

— Athletes, in particular recreational athletes engaging in extended exercise bouts, such as older adolescents participating in long-distance events (eg, half-marathons, marathons), should be sure not to overconsume liquids, which can lead to a somewhat rare but very dangerous hyponatremia.

● **After exercise.** Athletes are advised to rehydrate at a rate of 5.3 to 6.3 c (1.25–1.50 L) of fluid per 1 kg of body weight loss during exercise. Including salt-containing foods or fluids helps retain consumed fluids.[6]

Table 18-2 summarizes the macronutrient and fluid recommendations at baseline and before, during, and after exercise.

Micronutrients Needs

Although most micronutrient needs do not increase with high levels of physical activity, some athletes are more likely to experience inadequate micronutrient intake. In particular, athletes who severely restrict caloric intake, eliminate one or more food groups from their diet, or consume poorly planned diets are at increased risk for insufficient micronutrient intake. Micronutrients of concern are highlighted in **Box 18-3**.

Supplements

The AAP advises against performance-enhancing supplement use in youth athletes.[8] However, because some adolescent athletes take perceived performance-enhancing supplements, it is important for pediatricians to be familiar with the most commonly used supplements to provide a well-informed rationale when advising patients to avoid their use. Patients most likely to try or routinely use supplements include older teens, boys, those who have body dissatisfaction, those who have a higher body mass index, those who train in a commercial gym, and those who use alcohol or drugs or engage in other risk-taking behaviors. Protein supplements, creatine, and caffeine (eg, energy drinks, coffee drinks and soda) are the most commonly used supplements in adolescents.[8] **Box 18-4** highlights an AAP resource that can help clinicians confidently discuss supplement use with adolescent patients.

Few supplements produce good evidence of a notable performance benefit. For example, vitamin and mineral supplements do not improve performance unless reversing a preexisting deficiency. Many sports drinks, bars, and gels offer a practical choice to meet sports nutrition goals, but they are more costly than whole foods. Some supplements, such as caffeine and creatine, may produce evidence of benefit in certain situations, but they are not recommended for children and adolescents.[6,8]

Table 18-2 Summary of Macronutrient and Fluid Needs for Athletes Engaging in High-Intensity Physical Activity

	Baseline	Pre-exercise	During exercise	Post-exercise
Carbohy-drate	3–12 g/kg of body weight per day, depending on intensity of exercise	36–48 h before exercise: >90 min: 10–12 g/kg of body weight per 24 h <90 min: 7–12 g/kg of body weight per 24 h 1–4 h before exercise: 1–4 g/kg of body weight	Exercise duration <45 min: none Exercise duration 45–75 min: Carbohydrate mouth rinse (swish for 10–15 s) 1.0–2.5 h: 30 g/h 2.5–3.0 h: up to 90 g/h	1.0–1.2 g/kg of body weight per hour for 4 h for quick recovery OR 0.8 g/kg of body weight per hour for 4 h combined with 0.4 g/kg of protein per hour
Protein	1.2–2.0 g/kg of body weight per day	No strategy needed	None needed unless engaging in heavy lifting	0.4 g/kg of body weight per hour for 4 h combined with 0.8 g/kg of carbohydrate per hour for quick recovery 15–25 g high-quality protein within 2 h 0.3 g/kg of body weight every 3–5 h up to 24 h after training to build muscle
Fat	No less than 20% of total calories from fat	No strategy needed	Minimal, to prevent gastro-intestinal distress	No strategy needed
Fluids	Dietary Reference Intakes suggest 2.7 L/d for girls and 3.7 L/d for boys.	2–4 h before exercise: 5–10 mL/kg of body weight	0.4–0.8 L/h of exercise Include sodium-containing fluids with exercise >2 h.	1.25–1.50 L/kg of body weight lost during exercise

Conversion factor: To convert L to c, multiply by 4.23.

Derived from reference 6.

Box 18-3. Micronutrients of Concern

Some athletes are more likely to experience low levels of the following key micronutrients:

Iron

- Inadequate iron intake in the diet in combination with iron losses from urine, sweat, and stool; gastrointestinal bleeding resulting from strenuous and prolonged exercise; and hemolysis from intense exercise result in low iron levels in many athletes.
- Low levels affect physical and mental performance and overall health.
- Athletes most likely to experience low levels: distance runners; swimmers; gymnasts; volleyball, basketball, and tennis players; vegetarians; and blood donors.

Vitamin D

- Low levels affect calcium and phosphorus absorption and metabolism and bone health.
- Athletes most likely to experience low levels live at a latitude > 35th parallel north (north of the southern border of Tennessee) or train and compete indoors, have dark complexion, have high body fat content, train in early morning and evening, and/or regularly use sunscreen that blocks UV-B exposure.

Calcium

- Low levels increase risk of bone health problems, including stress fractures.
- Athletes most likely to experience low levels: girls.

Antioxidants

- Exercise can increase oxygen consumption up to 10- to 15-fold, increasing release of oxidants.
- Athletes most likely to experience low levels restrict energy intake, follow a low-fat diet, and/or limit dietary intake of fruits, vegetables, and whole grains.

Derived from reference 6.

> ## CLINICAL PRACTICE TIP
> ### Box 18-4. *Artificial Perfection: Talking to Teens about Performance Enhancement*
> The American Academy of Pediatrics and Kognito partnered to produce *Artificial Perfection: Talking to Teens about Performance Enhancement,* which the American Academy of Pediatrics and Kognito describe as "a free, role-play simulation designed to prepare pediatricians and other child health professionals to lead real-life conversation with teens about appearance and performance-enhancing substances."[9] The simulation is available at Kognito (https://aap.kognito.com).

Supplement Regulations

The Dietary Supplement Health and Education Act of 1994 dictates supplement production, marketing, and safety guidelines. The act established that a dietary supplement is "a product (other than tobacco) that functions to supplement the diet and contains one or more of the following ingredients: (A) a vitamin; (B) a mineral; (C) an herb or other botanical; (D) an amino acid; (E) a dietary supplement used by man to supplement the diet by increasing the total dietary intake; or (F) a concentrate, metabolite, constituent, extract, or combination of any ingredient described in clause (A), (B), (C), (D), or (E)." Supplements must contain an ingredient label including the name and quantity of each dietary ingredient. The label must also identify the product as a "dietary supplement."[10]

Unlike with the approval process for new medicines, which involves extensive testing for safety and efficacy before the US Food and Drug Administration (FDA) approves their use, the FDA does not closely regulate supplements. Supplement manufacturers are required to notify the FDA 75 days before marketing a new product to the public. Manufacturers are asked to include, with the notification, a statement that the product is thought to be generally safe for the consumer. However, there is no guarantee that a supplement includes the ingredients in the amounts specified on the label, and in some cases, additional unlisted ingredients, such as heavy metals, stimulants, or banned substances, contaminate the supplement. Contamination typically occurs inadvertently because of poor manufacturing practices. Additionally, the FDA does not proactively ensure supplement safety once products are on the market; rather, it investigates the supplements that have raised high suspicion for health or safety threats.

Table 18-3 provides an overview of some of the supplements that pediatricians are most likely to encounter when working with athletes.

Table 18-3. Commonly Used Supplements

Supplement	Function	Safety	Clinical considerations
Sports bars, gels, and drinks	Convenient option to achieve recommended macronutrient and electrolyte goals during exercise	Safe as long as no caffeine or other nonnutritional supplements are added to the sports bars, gels, or drinks	More costly than whole foods. Unnecessary for most recreational athletes and may contribute to excess sugar and caloric intake
Specific micronutrient supplements (eg, iron, calcium, vitamin D, omega-3 fatty acids)	Can help reverse nutrient deficiencies	Potentially unsafe if nutrients are provided in excess of 100% of the recommended dietary allowance	Ineffective unless there is a specific nutrient deficiency
Caffeine	Stimulant that reduces perception of fatigue and can improve exercise performance	Chronic caffeine use contributes to high blood pressure, high blood glucose level, decreased bone density, agitation and anxiousness, sleeplessness, and, for many, withdrawal symptoms, including headache, irritability, increased fatigue, drowsiness, decreased alertness, difficulty concentrating, and decreased energy and activity levels. Dangerous at high doses.	The amount of caffeine in food and drinks is unregulated. The American Academy of Pediatrics advises that energy drinks containing stimulants never be consumed by children and adolescents.[8]

Continued

Table 18-3 (*continued*)

Supplement	Function	Safety	Clinical considerations
Whey protein supplement	Whey contains high levels of the amino acids that play an important role in muscle hypertrophy. It is also rapidly digested and absorbed and effectively stimulates muscle protein synthesis following a resistance-training workout.	Generally safe	Protein needs are best met through the intake of whole foods.
Casein protein supplement	Casein, which gives milk its white color, allows a sustained, slow release of amino acids into the bloodstream, sometimes lasting for hours.	Generally safe	Protein needs are easily and best met through the intake of whole foods.
Branched-chain amino acids (leucine, isoleucine, and valine)	Following exercise, the branched-chain amino acids, especially leucine, increase the rate of protein synthesis and decrease the rate of protein catabolism.	Ingestion of single amino acids could result in imbalance of other amino acids.	Protein needs are easily and best met through the intake of whole foods.
Creatine (sold as creatine monohydrate)	Effective in building muscle mass, especially when combined with intensive strength training. With creatine loading or supplementation, athletes increase muscle stores of the energy-containing compound, which can then be used to increase effort during a high-intensity weight-lifting session.	Has not been evaluated in pediatric populations, although there are limited known adverse effects in adults	The American Academy of Pediatrics advises against creatine use in children and adolescents.[8]

Derived from references 6 and 8.

A Team Approach

A general pediatrician can serve as an excellent source of basic sports nutrition information. For athletes at the elite level or those striving to achieve an aggressive performance goal, referral to a registered dietitian who is a certified specialist in sports dietetics (CSSD) can help patients develop individualized sports nutrition programs, which, when paired with a strategic fitness plan, can help them exceed their performance goals. Patients can find a sports dietitian by zip code and dietetics specialty at EatRight (www.eatright.org/find-a-nutrition-expert).

Physical Activity Benefits and Guidelines for Children and Adolescents

Few behaviors more significantly influence child health than physical activity. Although some children and adolescents are highly active and engage in sports at a high level that requires extra nutrition support to optimize their performance, most engage in insufficient levels of physical activity. Overall, youth physical activity levels have decreased over time. The 2019 Youth Risk Behavior Survey revealed that fewer than 1 in 4 adolescents reported levels of activity that were consistent with the AAP recommendation to engage in at least 60 minutes per day on all 7 days of the week, less than half had exercised to strengthen or tone their muscles on at least 3 days per week, and just 16.5% met both aerobic and muscle-strengthening guidelines. Just more than half of students had played on at least 1 sports team.[11]

Benefits of Physical Activity

Physical activity improves heart health, muscular fitness, and bone health. It also reduces risk of increased body weight and adiposity.[12] Physical activity also benefits academic and mental health. Studies support that an acute bout of physical activity and regular moderate to vigorous physical activity improve cognition, including memory, processing speed, attention, and academic performance, in children and adolescents aged 5 to 13 years. Physical activity also greatly improves behavior and sleep and reduces feelings of anxiety and depression.

2018 Physical Activity Guidelines for Youth

The 2018 *Physical Activity Guidelines for Americans*[12] recommend that children and adolescents aged 6 to 13 years attain the following goals:

- Cardiovascular exercise, most days, if not all. Children and adolescents should engage in at least 60 minutes of moderate to vigorous cardiovascular activity, such as brisk walking, jogging, skipping with a jump rope, biking, or movement portion of ball sports.
- Muscle-strengthening exercise, such as resistance training and calisthenics, at least 2 to 3 days per week. The AAP recommends that muscle training last 20 to 30 minutes and take place on nonconsecutive days, beginning with 1 to 2 sets of 8 to 12 repetitions of at least 1 exercise for each muscle group. Resistance-training intensity and

volume can be gradually increased as strength and resistance-training skill competency increase.[13]

- Bone-strengthening exercise, such as skipping with a jump rope and tumbling, at least 3 days per week.

The 2018 Physical Activity Guidelines Advisory Committee concluded that there is strong evidence that physical activity of children aged 3 to 5 years is associated with decreased risk of excessive weight gain and improved health of bone. Children in this age-group should aim to achieve at least the median level of physical activity for children of this age, which is 3 hours or more of physical activity per day.[14] Infants should be physically active several times per day, mostly through interactive floor-based play. For all children and adolescents, it is important that physical activity be appropriate for a child's age and be enjoyable and varied.

Helping Children and Adolescents Achieve Physical Activity Guidelines

There are many steps that pediatricians can take to help support children and adolescents in their communities in becoming more physically active. Several potential strategies are outlined in this section, and the AAP clinical report "Physical Activity Assessment and Counseling in Pediatric Clinical Settings" provides more detailed information for pediatricians[15] (https://pediatrics.aappublications.org/content/145/3/e20193992).

- **Pair physical activity and nutritional counseling.** While encouraging and supporting children to eat a healthy diet, pediatricians may also encourage families to engage in enjoyable physical activities, ideally for at least 60 minutes per day.
- **Tailor recommendations to age, stage, and ability. Table 18-4** highlights recommended frequency, intensity, time, and type (FITT) of physical activity for children by stage from ages 0 to 18.
- **Identify and focus on a child's interests.** Pediatricians can support families in increasing physical activity by asking questions that help identify a child's interests and can explore possible ways that a child might be able to participate in physical activities that they enjoy. Studies support that children and adolescents who participate in sports spend more time outdoors, are more likely to walk or ride their bike to and/or from school, and are most likely to meet physical activity guidelines.[16]
- **Identify and address barriers and lapses.** Families may experience barriers to beginning an activity program. It is important for clinicians to assess both a family's strengths and the family's opportunities to increase a child's activity levels, while assessing and addressing potential barriers. Common challenges to starting and continuing physical activity include
  — Income factors: Many youth activity programs require a parental financial investment. Many families of low income cannot afford to pay for these opportunities.
  — Safety: Access to safe play is limited for many children.
  — Time: Many working families do not have the availability to transport children to sports and other recreational activities. Many after-school and child care

Table 18-4. The FITT Principles for Youth Physical Activity From Infancy to Adolescence

	Age					
	Newborn or infant (0-12 mo)	Toddler (1-3 y)	Preschooler (3-5 y)	Elementary schooler (5-11 y)	Middle schooler (11-14 y)	High schooler (14-18 y)
Frequency		Any		Every day		
Intensity				Moderate to vigorous and vigorous		
Time	Throughout the day	180+ min/d			60+ min/d	
Type	Floor-based play, tummy time to help develop basic skills (sitting up, rolling, crawling, pulling to a stand, walking)	Outdoor free play Playground Any opportunity to develop gross motor skills (walking, running, climbing, jumping, throwing, kicking)	Outdoor free play Playground Any opportunity to develop fundamental movement skills (walking, running, swimming, tumbling, throwing, catching)	Cardiovascular, such as walking, jogging, running, biking, or swimming Muscle strengthening (resistance training after age 7-8, calisthenics, or gymnastics) at least 3 d/wk Bone strengthening with high-impact activities, such as gymnastics, basketball, skipping with a jump rope, or running	Cardiovascular, such as walking, jogging, running, biking, or swimming Muscle strengthening (resistance training, calisthenics, or gymnastics) at least 3 d/wk Bone strengthening with high-impact activities, such as gymnastics, basketball, skipping with a jump rope, or running	Cardiovascular, such as walking, jogging, running, biking, or swimming Muscle strengthening (resistance training, calisthenics, or gymnastics) at least 3 d/wk Bone strengthening with high-impact activities, such as gymnastics, basketball, skipping with a jump rope, or running

Continued

Table 18-4 (*continued*)

	Age					
	Newborn or infant (0–12 mo)	**Toddler (1–3 y)**	**Preschooler (3–5 y)**	**Elementary schooler (5–11 y)**	**Middle schooler (11–14 y)**	**High schooler (14–18 y)**
Type (*continued*)				Organized sports with flexible rules and short instruction time. Focus on enjoyment rather than competition	Activities that are enjoyable and encourage socialization and competition, when appropriate	Activities that are enjoyable and encourage socialization and, when appropriate, competition, sometimes at very high levels

Adapted from reference 15.

programs do not provide sufficient opportunities for children to attain adequate amounts of physical activity.
— Physical health concerns: Children with special health care needs and those with obesity not only face additional physical challenges with exercise but may also feel self-conscious or embarrassed when participating in activities with their peers.
— Competing priorities and interests: As children get older, physical activity levels drop precipitously. Adolescents are least likely to be presented with physical education or physical activity opportunities as part of their everyday routines.
- **Help support long-term adherence.** The first 6 months of a behavior change are the most tenuous, but once a child or an adolescent consistently engages in a new behavior for 6 months, it is likely to be maintained. Children and adolescents who are active in childhood, especially in adolescence, are more likely to be active as adults, although less than 20% of physically active youth become active adults.[17] Participation in organized sports, high perceived sports competence, active parents (especially fathers), and high overall fitness and physical activity levels are a few factors in childhood and adolescence that studies have shown to be associated with lifelong physical activity.[17,18]

In Sum

- Children and adolescents involved in intensive sports training may benefit from strategic fueling and implementation of key sports nutrition principles.
- Highly active children and adolescents require increased caloric intake to fuel strenuous exercise regimens and optimize growth and development. Athletes who chronically consume insufficient calories to meet exercise needs are at risk for RED-S, a medical condition observed in physically active individuals that includes any one of the following signs: low energy availability with or without disordered eating, menstrual dysfunction in females, and low bone mineral density. Early identification and intervention can help prevent progression of the triad into clinical eating disorders, amenorrhea, and osteoporosis.
- Carbohydrates play many important roles in sports performance, including serving as the body's preferred energy source over a wide range of exercise intensities, using both aerobic and anaerobic energy systems; maintaining concentration and reducing fatigue and perception of effort during strenuous exercise; and sparing dietary protein and amino acids so they may be used for muscle building rather than as an energy source.
- Athletes should consume carbohydrates 1 to 4 hours before strenuous activity to optimize energy availability. Carbohydrate intake is unnecessary during activity lasting less than 60 minutes. However, during a prolonged exercise bout of longer than 60 minutes, consuming 10 to 15 g of carbohydrate every 15 to 20 minutes can improve athletic performance. Athletes should eat or drink some form of carbohydrate within 30 minutes of completing an intensive exercise session or competition, to replace glycogen stores.
- Athletes should consume 15 to 25 g of high-quality protein within 2 hours of a high-intensity muscle-conditioning program to optimize muscle protein synthesis.

- Adequate hydration before, during, and after exercise can help support optimal athletic performance and prevent risk of dehydration. Athletes should drink 5 to 10 mL/kg of body weight in the 2 to 4 hours before exercise and 1.7 to 3.4 c (0.4–0.8 L) of fluids per hour of exercise. Following exercise, athletes should consume 0.25–1.50 L/kg of body weight lost during exercise, if pre- and post-exercise weights are known. Water is the preferred hydration source for physical activity lasting less than 60 minutes.
- Iron, vitamin D, calcium, and antioxidants are the micronutrients at greatest risk of inadequacy for some athletes.
- Nutrient needs are best met through consumption of whole food sources whenever possible. In all cases, supplements are rarely advisable for children and adolescents, if ever, with some exceptions in the case of nutrient deficiencies.
- Although some children and adolescents are highly active and engage in sports at a high level that requires extra nutrition support to optimize their performance, most engage in insufficient levels of physical activity. Pediatricians play an important role in assessing a child's or adolescent's physical activity and providing guidance and support to help patients progress toward or meet physical activity recommendations.

References

1. Parnell JA, Wiens KP, Erdman KA. Dietary intakes and supplement use in pre-adolescent and adolescent Canadian athletes. *Nutrients.* 2016;8(9):526 PMID: 27571101 doi: 10.3390/nu8090526
2. De Souza MJ, Nattiv A, Joy E, et al; Expert Panel. 2014 Female Athlete Triad Coalition consensus statement on treatment and return to play of the female athlete triad. *Br J Sports Med.* 2014;48(4):289–309 PMID: 24463911 doi: 10.1136/bjsports-2013-093218
3. Mountjoy M, Sundgot-Borgen J, Burke L, et al. The IOC consensus statement: beyond the female athlete triad–relative energy deficiency in sport (RED-S). *Br J Sports Med.* 2014;48(7):491–497 PMID: 24620037 doi: 10.1136/bjsports-2014-093502
4. Nattiv A, De Souza MJ, Koltun KJ, et al. The male athlete triad—a consensus statement from the female and male athlete triad coalition, I: definition and scientific basis. *Clin J Sport Med.* 2021;31(4):335–348 PMID: 34091537 doi: 10.1097/JSM.0000000000000946
5. Weiss Kelly AK, Hecht S, Brenner JS, et al; American Academy of Pediatrics Council on Sports Medicine and Fitness. The female athlete triad. *Pediatrics.* 2016;138(2):e20160922 PMID: 27432852 doi: 10.1542/peds.2016-0922
6. Thomas DT, Erdman KA, Burke LM. Position of the Academy of Nutrition and Dietetics, Dietitians of Canada, and the American College of Sports Medicine: nutrition and athletic performance. *J Acad Nutr Diet.* 2016;116(3):501–528 PMID: 26920240 doi: 10.1016/j.jand.2015.12.006
7. Schneider MB, Benjamin HJ; American Academy of Pediatrics Committee on Nutrition and Council on Sports Medicine and Fitness. Sports drinks and energy drinks for children and adolescents: are they appropriate? *Pediatrics.* 2011;127(6):1182–1189 PMID: 21624882 doi: 10.1542/peds.2011-0965
8. LaBotz M, Griesemer BA, Brenner JS, et al; American Academy of Pediatrics Council on Sports Medicine and Fitness. Use of performance-enhancing substances. *Pediatrics.* 2016;138(1):e20161300 PMID: 27354458 doi: 10.1542/peds.2016-1300

9. The American Academy of Pediatrics and Kognito launch simulation to train pediatricians on addressing teen use of appearance and performance enhancing substances. News release. Kognito; January 11, 2017. Accessed October 27, 2022. http://go.kognito.com/rs/143-HCJ-270/images/Hel_PressRelease_011117_AppearancePerformanceEnhancingSubstances.pdf

10. Dietary Supplement Health and Education Act, 103rd Cong (1994). Pub L No. 103–417. Accessed October 27, 2022. https://www.congress.gov/bill/103rd-congress/senate-bill/784/text

11. Merlo CL, Jones SE, Michael SL, et al. Dietary and physical activity behaviors among high school students—youth risk behavior survey, United States, 2019. *MMWR Suppl.* 2020;69(1):64–76 PMID: 32817612 doi: 10.15585/mmwr.su6901a8

12. United States Department of Health and Human Services. *Physical Activity Guidelines for Americans.* 2nd ed. US Dept of Health and Human Services; 2018. Accessed October 27, 2022. https://health.gov/paguidelines/second-edition/pdf/Physical_Activity_Guidelines_2nd_edition.pdf

13. Stricker PR, Faigenbaum AD, McCambridge TM, et al; American Academy of Pediatrics Council on Sports Medicine and Fitness. Resistance training for children and adolescents. *Pediatrics.* 2020;145(6):e20201011 PMID: 32457216 doi: 10.1542/peds.2020-1011

14. Physical Activity Guidelines Advisory Committee. *2018 Physical Activity Guidelines Scientific Advisory Committee Scientific Report.* US Dept of Health and Human Services; 2018

15. Lobelo F, Muth ND, Hanson S, et al; American Academy of Pediatrics Council on Sports Medicine and Fitness and Section on Obesity. Physical activity assessment and counseling in pediatric clinical settings. *Pediatrics.* 2020;145(3):e20193992 PMID: 32094289 doi: 10.1542/peds.2019-3992

16. Wilkie HJ, Standage M, Gillison FB, Cumming SP, Katzmarzyk PT. Correlates of intensity-specific physical activity in children aged 9–11 years: a multilevel analysis of UK data from the International Study of Childhood Obesity, Lifestyle and the Environment. *BMJ Open.* 2018;8(2):e018373 PMID: 29431128 doi: 10.1136/bmjopen-2017-018373

17. Telama R, Yang X, Viikari J, Välimäki I, Wanne O, Raitakari O. Physical activity from childhood to adulthood: a 21-year tracking study. *Am J Prev Med.* 2005;28(3):267–273 PMID: 15766614 doi: 10.1016/j.amepre.2004.12.003

18. Jose KA, Blizzard L, Dwyer T, McKercher C, Venn AJ. Childhood and adolescent predictors of leisure time physical activity during the transition from adolescence to adulthood: a population based cohort study. *Int J Behav Nutr Phys Act.* 2011;8(1):54 PMID: 21631921 doi: 10.1186/1479-5868-8-54

Mental Health, Behavioral, and Developmental Conditions

Nutritional psychiatry is an emerging field investigating the relationship between nutrition and many common psychiatric conditions. In fact, the International Society for Nutritional Psychiatry Research advocates for "recognition of diet and nutrition as central determinants of both physical and mental health" because of "emerging and compelling evidence for nutrition as a critical factor" in mental disorders.[1] Although existing data are limited, there is some evidence to support that specific nutrition recommendations may help in the treatment of many common mental health concerns that affect children and adolescents, including depression, attention-deficit/hyperactivity disorder (ADHD), autism, severe picky eating, and eating disorders.

Depression

Many observational studies have shown that when people consume a high-quality diet, it may help protect against the development of depression. A review of 12 epidemiological studies with children and adolescent participants showed that unhealthful dietary patterns were related to poorer mental health, whereas a high-quality diet was associated with better mental health, even when controlling for income, education, and other potential confounders.[2] Although there are insufficient data for clinicians to make specific food or nutrient recommendations to prevent or treat depression, evidence does support a mental health benefit to encouraging a diet rich in fruits, vegetables, and whole grains and low in sugary and processed foods.[3] Clinicians may share this information with patients and families and use coaching strategies such as those discussed in chapters 14, Theories of Behavior Change and Motivational Interviewing, and 15, SMART Goals and Action Plans, to help patients and families take steps to improve diet quality. Additionally, it is important for clinicians to note and explore with patients the impact of depression on eating habits. Some children may have loss of appetite and decrease in intake, which can lead to nutritional concerns, whereas others may exhibit signs of emotional eating, which can contribute to excess intake. Treating the depression may help improve the nutritional concerns.

Attention-Deficit/Hyperactivity Disorder

Attention-deficit/hyperactivity disorder (ADHD) is a common neurobehavioral disorder characterized by inattention and/or hyperactivity to the extent that it interferes with performance at school, relationships with peers and family, and/or participation in organized activities such as team sports. Although not a mainstay of ADHD treatment, one or more nutrition strategies are often implemented by many families of children with ADHD in an effort to reduce ADHD symptoms. This implementation usually happens without consulting with the child's pediatrician or clinical care team. A description of these strategies is shown in **Table 19-1**, along with a summary of existing evidence to support the strategy (if available).

Table 19-1. Nutritional Interventions That Parents Often Attempt in the Treatment of Attention-Deficit/Hyperactivity Disorder

Nutritional intervention	Rationale	Evidence
Omega-3 and omega-6 fatty acid supplementation	ADHD is associated with low serum levels of long-chain polyunsaturated fatty acids.	The evidence is inconclusive, but some studies support reduced ADHD symptoms.[4,5]
Additive-free and salicylate-free diet	Immune sensitivity to these ingredients (orange and red dyes, preservatives, and salicylate foods such as apples, grapes, lunch meat, sausage, and hot dogs) may trigger ADHD symptoms.	Studies in the 1970s purported reduced hyperactivity in >50% of children studied. These findings were not replicated in controlled trials, but some studies suggest there may be benefit for certain children generally, unrelated to ADHD.[4,5]
Hypoallergenic/elimination/ "few foods" diet Eliminated foods may vary, but this diet typically involves the removal of allergenic foods (eg, eggs, nuts, wheat, dairy, soy) and foods containing artificial ingredients (artificial flavors, sweeteners, and preservatives).	Certain foods may trigger ADHD symptoms in some children. The triggering foods could vary by individual. Elimination of many foods, typically allergenic foods or foods with artificial ingredients, and then gradual reintroduction of them can help identify potential triggers.	Early studies showed that symptoms improved in 80% of children with hyperactivity, and typical behavior was achieved in nearly one-third. Subsequent studies have shown benefit of an elimination diet, but it is not intended as long-term treatment because of potential risk of nutrient deficiency.[4-6]
Sugar elimination	Parents report worsening hyperactivity after children consume a high sugar or aspartame load.	Studies have not demonstrated a relationship between sucrose/aspartame and hyperactivity.[4,5]
Ketogenic diet	This high-fat, low-carbohydrate diet is associated with reduced epileptic changes on an electroencephalogram, probably related to negative sodium and potassium balance. Children with epilepsy often have ADHD, and children with ADHD often have electroencephalographic changes.	The ketogenic diet does benefit certain forms of epilepsy, but there is no specific benefit for ADHD and this diet is not recommended in the treatment of mental disorders.[7]

Table 19-1 (*continued*)

Nutritional intervention	Rationale	Evidence
Iron supplementation	Iron deficiency causes cognitive impairment, and children with ADHD tend to have lower ferritin levels.	Supplementation may benefit children with ADHD and iron deficiency.[4,5]
Zinc supplementation	Zinc deficiency causes cognitive impairment, and children with ADHD tend to have lower zinc levels.	Supplementation may benefit children with ADHD and zinc deficiency.[4,5]
Healthful dietary pattern	A healthy diet is high in fish, vegetables, fruit, legumes, and whole grains and low in refined sugar and saturated fat. A healthful dietary pattern contains high levels of omega-3 fatty acid, iron, and zinc and is low in sugar and additives, which could help improve attention and focus.	A healthy diet is associated with improved ADHD symptoms in some studies and it benefits health overall.[8]

Abbreviation: ADHD, attention-deficit/hyperactivity disorder.

Of note, studies have shown that routine moderate to vigorous physical activity improves the cognitive, behavioral, and physical symptoms associated with ADHD.[9] More research is underway to help elucidate the optimal exercise prescription for the treatment of ADHD.

Autism

Autism spectrum disorder is characterized by varying degrees of impairment in speech and social interaction, repetitive behaviors, and sensory issues. Many children with autism struggle with nutritional concerns, such as picky or selective eating preferences and excess intake of preferred foods, which are often highly processed and high in calories, saturated fats, sodium and sugar.

Additionally, many families seek out nutritional and alternative therapies for autism. According to a survey in the United Kingdom, nearly 80% of children with autism follow some variation of a restrictive diet such as the gluten-free and casein-free diet (often referred to as the *GF/CF diet*).[10] Proponents of the gluten-free and casein-free diet believe that children with autism may process proteins in foods containing gluten and casein differently than children without autism and that the brain treats the proteins like false opiate–like chemicals that lead to difficulties in speech and social interactions. This belief has not been confirmed, and studies to date have not shown a beneficial effect of the gluten-free and casein-free diet on autism symptoms.[11] Although there is no evidence to date that supports a benefit of the gluten-free and casein-free diet in the treatment or management of autism, many families choose to follow such an eating plan. In these situations, pediatricians can play a valuable role in helping parents ensure that their child is obtaining sufficient amounts of needed nutrients by suggesting alternative sources of calcium, vitamin D, fiber, and B vitamins (refer to chapters 5, Vitamins, and 6, Minerals).

Many children with autism also take some form of nutritional supplement, such as vitamins, minerals, amino acid, omega-3 fatty acids, or herbals. A systematic review of 19 randomized controlled trials showed little evidence of the benefit of omega-3 fatty acids or vitamin supplementation in improving autism-related behaviors.[12] In conflict with the systematic review, a meta-analysis of 27 double-blind, randomized clinical trials investigating the role of dietary interventions for autism spectrum disorder showed that supplementation with omega-3 fatty acids, vitamins, or other nutritional supplements was associated with small improvements in the domains of anxiety and/or affect, autistic general psychopathology, behavioral problems and impulsivity, global severity, hyperactivity and irritability, language, social-autistic behaviors, stereotypies, and restricted and repetitive behaviors.[13]

Overall, although there is no strong evidence of clinically significant benefit of dietary interventions on autism symptoms, most parents of children with autism explore potential nutritional interventions or alternative therapies in the hope that they may help their child. Parents report that they often do so without consulting their child's pediatrician because of a perceived lack of support or willingness from the pediatrician to consider potential benefits of the dietary approaches.[12] Given this, pediatricians can aim to work collaboratively with families of children who have autism to help optimize a child's nutrition.

Severe Picky Eating and Malnutrition

On the whole, parents of young children are very concerned about feeding difficulties, with more than half of mothers reporting that at least 1 child eats poorly.[14] In most cases, poor eating is caused by neophobia or mild picky eating that resolves with repeated exposures and use of the strategies noted in Chapter 13, Culinary Medicine and Strategies for Healthy Eating and Chapter 17, Nutrition in Childhood and Adolescence. Generally, typically developing children with selective eating gain weight appropriately, have a body mass index that follows a stable percentile on the growth chart, and do not have other developmental or behavioral health concerns.

Sometimes, feeding difficulties may be an early sign of or coexist with autism and other mental and behavioral health concerns or be a sign of a feeding disorder. A child or an adolescent may have a feeding disorder if they refuse to eat certain specific foods, food groups, or textures, which results in insufficient nutrition or caloric intake to support typical growth and development.[14]

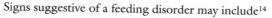

Signs suggestive of a feeding disorder may include[14]

- Prolonged mealtimes
- Food refusal lasting longer than 1 month
- Disruptive and stressful mealtimes
- Lack of appropriate independent feeding
- Nocturnal eating in a toddler
- Distraction required to increase intake
- Prolonged breastfeeding or bottle-feeding
- Failure to advance from purees to new textures

If a parent raises a concern about any of these signs, the pediatrician may investigate further, with special attention to anthropometric measures, the physical examination, and a brief dietary history to uncover any of the potential physiological or behavioral signs shown in **Table 19-2**. Note that children with autism or depression, anxiety, and other mental health challenges may have food troubles, but they always have other symptoms or behaviors that go beyond the typical and frequent occurrence of a child resisting their parents' choice of what to eat.

If a child with severe picky eating shows signs of malnutrition or growth restriction, they may need nutritional supplementation and increased caloric intake to support adequate nutrition, weight gain, and growth, in addition to identification and treatment of the underlying cause. Some strategies for increasing caloric intake are highlighted in **Box 19-1**, and featured recipes are included in Part 5, Frequently Asked Questions, Case Studies, and Recipes.

Eating Disorders

Eating disorders affect approximately 3% of children and adolescents, with a mean onset of around 12.5 years of age. Prevalence studies suggest that anywhere from 1% to 22% of females and 0.2% to 0.6% of males will have an eating disorder in their lifetime.[15,16]

Diagnostic Features of Eating Disorders

The main types of eating disorders and diagnostic features based on the *Diagnostic and Statistical Manual of Mental Disorders, Fifth Edition,* are outlined in **Box 19-2**. Binge-eating disorder is the most prevalent of the eating disorders, affecting about 1.6% of adolescents 13 to 18 years of age.[16]

Management of Eating Disorders

The appropriate evaluation and treatment of eating disorders generally includes medical monitoring, nutritional therapy, and mental health treatment. Evidence suggests that medical stabilization and nutritional rehabilitation are the most important determinants of short-term outcomes. Additionally, improved nutritional status reverses the cognitive deficits that result from malnutrition, allowing for effective mental health interventions. The goal of treatment is to restore a healthy body weight, relationship with food, and body image.[15]

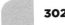

Table 19-2. Signs of Organic Disease and Behavioral Conditions Contributing to Severe Picky Eating and Recommended Next Steps

	Clinical signs	Recommended next steps
Organic disease	Dysphagia, which may manifest as refusal to eat and/or coughing and choking during eating Aspiration, which may manifest as wheezing during eating Apparent pain with feeding Vomiting and diarrhea Developmental delay Growth restriction	Basic laboratory evaluation, as appropriate. Evaluation may include complete blood cell count, comprehensive metabolic panel, erythrocyte sedimentation rate or C-reactive protein level, or urinalysis; screening for infection; and/or screening for celiac disease (immunoglobulin A and tissue transglutaminase test). Consider the following referrals: ● Oro-motor specialist, as appropriate ● Gastroenterologist, as appropriate If a patient has growth restriction, consider nutritional supplementation.
Behavioral condition	Food fixation with very selective intake and extreme limitations in what the child accepts Coercive or forceful parent feeding Abrupt cessation of feeding after a triggering event, such as refusing to eat after a choking episode Anticipatory gagging Growth restriction	Encourage responsive feeding (refer to Chapter 11, Dietary Guidelines and Principles of Healthy Eating) and strategies outlined in **Table 17-4**. Consider the following referrals: ● Feeding specialist or feeding team ● Behavioral therapist If a patient has growth restriction, consider nutritional supplementation.

CLINICAL PRACTICE TIP

Box 19-1. Strategies to Increase Caloric Intake

Adding the following healthful, high-calorie items to foods can help children or adolescents who are experiencing growth restriction or malnutrition related to insufficient caloric intake. Parents may consider including the following foods in smoothies, adding them to other foods, combining them, or encouraging children to eat them alone:

Food	Calories (Cal)
Instant breakfast powder (1 packet)	130
Infant cereal (for infants) (1 tbsp)	9
Whole milk (1 c)	276
Powdered milk (1 tbsp)	25
Evaporated milk (1 tbsp)	20
Vegetable oils (1 tbsp)	110
Avocado (½ of medium)	160
Cheese (1 oz)	100
Full-fat yogurt, plain (6–fl oz container)	100
Granola (¼ c)	140
Dried fruit (¼ c)	80
Peanut butter (1 tbsp)	95
Hummus (1 tbsp)	25
Nuts and seeds (ground for younger children to prevent choking) (¼ c)	200
Specialized drinks, such as PediaSure (8 fl oz), Boost Kid Essentials (8 fl oz), or Orgain Kids Nutritional Shake (8.25 fl oz)	240 360 180

SI conversion factor: To convert fl oz to mL, multiply by 30.

Medical Stabilization

Each of the eating disorders is associated with risk of medical instability and negative health outcomes. When evaluating patients with known or suspected eating disorders, the pediatrician's first step is to assess whether the patient's condition is medically stable. If a patient's condition is medically unstable, referral for a higher level of care is necessary. Medical risks associated with each of the eating disorders are listed in

Box 19-2. Diagnostic Features of Eating Disorders Commonly Found in Children and Adolescents

Anorexia nervosa

- Restricted caloric intake relative to energy requirements, leading to significantly low body weight for age, sex, projected growth, and physical health
- Intense fear of gaining weight or engagement in behaviors that consistently interfere with weight gain, despite being at a significantly low weight
- Altered perception of body weight or body shape, self-perception/sense of self-worth excessively influenced by body weight or body shape, or a persistent lack of acknowledgment of the seriousness of the low body weight

Subtypes

- Restricting type: Weight loss is achieved primarily through dieting, fasting, and/or excessive exercise, with no episodes of binge eating or purging repeated in the previous 3 mo.
- Binge-eating/purging type: Episodes of binge eating or purging (self-induced vomiting or misuse of laxatives, diuretics, or enemas) have repeated in the previous 3 mo.

Bulimia nervosa

- Episodes of binge eating followed by compensatory behaviors have repeated.
- Binge eating is characterized by both the following features:
  — Episodes involve eating an amount of food within a distinct time frame (eg, 2 h) that is significantly larger than most individuals would eat during a similar time frame under similar circumstances.
  — Episodes are marked by the feeling that one cannot limit or control the overeating.
- Inappropriate compensatory behaviors are repeatedly used to prevent weight gain, such as self-induced vomiting (purging); misuse of laxatives, diuretics, or other medications; fasting; or excessive exercise.
- The binge-eating and compensatory behaviors occur at least once a week for 3 mo, on average.
- Self-perception/self-worth is excessively influenced by body weight and body shape.
- The binge-eating and compensatory behaviors do not occur only during episodes of anorexia nervosa.

Box 19-2 (*continued*)

Binge-eating disorder

- Episodes of binge eating repeat, with episodes occurring at least once a week for 3 mo.
- Binge eating is characterized by both the following features:
  — Episodes involve eating an amount of food within a distinct time frame (eg, 2 h) that is significantly larger than most individuals would eat during a similar time frame under similar circumstances.
  — Episodes are marked by the feeling that one cannot limit or control the overeating.
- The binge-eating episodes include ≥ 3 of the following features:
  — Eating much more quickly than typical
  — Eating until uncomfortably full
  — Eating large amounts of food when not hungry
  — Eating alone because of embarrassment about the amount eaten
  — Feeling of guilt, disgust, depression, or anguish following the episode
- The binge eating is not associated with the use of inappropriate compensatory behavior, as in the case of bulimia nervosa, and it does not occur only in the context of bulimia nervosa or anorexia nervosa.

Avoidant/restrictive food intake disorder

- A disrupted eating pattern (eg, seeming lack of interest in eating or food, avoidance based on the sensory qualities of food, concern about unpleasant consequences of eating), as evidenced by a persistent failure to meet appropriate nutritional and/or energy needs that is associated with ≥1 of the following features:
  — Significant weight loss or, in children, failure to achieve expected growth and/or weight gain
  — Marked nutritional deficiency
  — Reliance on enteral feeding or oral nutritional supplements
  — Significant interference with psychosocial functioning
- The disrupted eating pattern cannot be better explained by lack of available food or by an associated culturally sanctioned practice.
- The disrupted eating pattern cannot be attributed to a coexisting medical condition or better explained by another mental illness or disorder.

Continued

Box 19-2 (*continued*)

Avoidant/restrictive food intake disorder (*continued*)

- If the disrupted eating pattern occurs in the context of another condition or disorder, the severity of the disrupted eating pattern exceeds that which is routinely associated with the condition or disorder.

Pica

- Episodes involve eating nonnutritive, nonfood substances over at least 1 mo. The behavior must not be appropriate for developmental stage and must not be socially typical or culturally acceptable behavior.
- The type of ingested items may vary but often include earth/clay (geophagy), raw starches (amylophagia), ice (pagophagia), charcoal, ash, paper, chalk, cloth, baby powder, coffee grounds, and eggshells.

Rumination disorder

- Regurgitation of food is repeated for at least 1 mo. Regurgitated food may be re-chewed, re-swallowed, or spit out.
- The repeated regurgitation is not caused by a medical condition (eg, gastrointestinal condition) and does not occur exclusively in the course of anorexia nervosa, bulimia nervosa, binge-eating disorder, or avoidant/restrictive food intake disorder.

Examples of other specified feeding or eating disorders

- Atypical anorexia nervosa: All criteria for anorexia nervosa are met, but body weight is within or above the reference range despite significant weight loss.
- Bulimia nervosa of low frequency and/or limited duration: All criteria for bulimia nervosa are met, but binge eating and related compensatory behaviors occur less than once a week and/or for <3 mo, on average.
- Binge-eating disorder of low frequency and/or limited duration: All criteria for binge-eating disorder are met, but binge eating occurs less than once a week and/or for <3 mo, on average.
- Purging disorder: Recurrent purging behavior, such as self-induced vomiting and/or the misuse of laxatives, diuretics, or other medications, occurs in the absence of binge eating with the intent to alter body weight or body shape.
- Night-eating syndrome: Occurs when a patient repeatedly awakens in the night to eat or consumes excessive amounts of food late in the night. To have this condition, the patient must

Box 19-2 (*continued*)

remember the nighttime eating and must feel guilt or distress or interference in typical functioning because of it. It cannot be explained by changes to a person's sleep-wake cycle or cultural practices or social norms. The disordered pattern of eating cannot be better accounted for by binge-eating disorder, another psychiatric disorder, substance use disorder or dependence, a general medical disorder, or an effect of medication.

Examples of other clinically significant feeding or eating problems that do not otherwise meet criteria for any other disorder or condition

- Orthorexia nervosa: Characterized by an obsession or preoccupation with healthy eating, distress and anxiety with lapses in adherence to self-imposed nutritional rules, and psychosocial impairments in relevant areas of life, malnutrition, and weight loss. This condition is not specifically mentioned in the *Diagnostic and Statistical Manual of Mental Disorders, Fifth Edition,* and is the subject of many scientific studies and debates about how to best diagnose, describe, and treat it.[17]

Derived from reference 15.

Table 19-3. Of particular note, patients with prolonged starvation, such as those with anorexia nervosa, are at risk for potentially fatal metabolic changes and electrolyte shifts that can occur when food and calories are reintroduced too quickly. This is referred to as *refeeding syndrome*. When refeeding syndrome occurs, it generally occurs within the first week of hospitalization in patients receiving parenteral or enteral feedings. Any patient being treated for anorexia in an inpatient setting requires monitoring of sodium, potassium, magnesium, phosphorus, and glucose levels. The hallmark sign of refeeding syndrome is hypophosphatemia. Phosphorus supplementation helps prevent refeeding syndrome.

Nutritional Rehabilitation

The primary aim of nutritional rehabilitation is to help a patient return to a safe weight and have a healthy relationship with food and body image. A patient's ideal body weight is individualized with the goal to restore premorbid height, weight, and body mass index percentile. For female patients with anorexia nervosa, resuming menstruation is one indicator of having achieved a healthier weight. Key considerations that pediatricians may share with parents to support nutritional rehabilitation are highlighted in

Table 19-3. Medical Risks Associated With Eating Disorders

Type of eating disorder	Medical risk
Restrictive (anorexia nervosa and ARFID)[a]	Electrolyte abnormalities and dehydration
	Bradycardia and dysrhythmias
	Delayed gastric emptying and constipation
	Pancreatitis
	Amenorrhea and decreased bone mass density
	Growth restriction
	Anemia and elevated ferritin level
	Depression, anxiety, and suicide
	Refeeding syndrome
Bulimia nervosa	Electrolyte abnormalities
	Gastroesophageal reflux and esophagitis
	Mallory-Weiss tears or esophageal or gastric rupture
	Acid erosion of the teeth
	Dental caries
	Xerostomia (dry mouth)
	Parotid swelling
	Laxative dependence
	Depression, anxiety, and suicide
Binge-eating disorder	Obesity and associated health conditions
	Depression, anxiety, and suicide
Pica	Generally short-term, benign, and self-resolving in children. Can become more problematic in children and adolescents with intellectual disabilities and may persist for years.
	Clay pica can cause elevated lead levels.
	Ice pica can contribute to iron deficiency.
Rumination disorder	In rare cases, esophageal damage from reflux

Abbreviation: ARFID, avoidant/restrictive food intake disorder.

[a] Anorexia nervosa and ARFID are unique restrictive eating disorders with varying manifestations and complications. Children and adolescents with ARFID tend to be younger, to have earlier age of onset, and to have a higher median percentile body mass index than children and adolescents with anorexia nervosa. Many patients with ARFID have had underweight for a prolonged period and do not tend to have the same degree of hypotension and bradycardia as patients with anorexia nervosa who are actively losing weight. Children and adolescents who are admitted with ARFID tend to have a longer hospital stay and increased reliance on enteral feeding.[18]

Table 19-4. Ideally, pediatricians will implement nutritional rehabilitation with the support of a registered dietitian who has specialized training and experience working with children and adolescents with eating disorders. Parents and other caregivers can locate dietitians with specialized training in eating disorders at EatRight (www.eatright.org/find-a-nutrition-expert) by selecting their zip code and selecting Eating Disorders as the specialty.

Table 19-4. Goals of Nutritional Therapy for Eating Disorder Rehabilitation

Food or nutrient intervention by patient/ family and clinician	Eating disorder		
	Anorexia nervosa or avoidant/ restrictive food intake disorder	Bulimia or purging disorder	Binge-eating disorder or night-eating syndrome
Meals (per day)	3	3	3
Snacks (per day)	3+ as needed to provide adequate calories	0–3 to maintain stable glucose levels, depending on the time between meals	0–3 to maintain stable glucose levels, depending on the time between meals
Meal or snack timing	Evenly spaced Times determined in advance Consistent	Timing can be based on family and patient preference and school/work schedule. Times determined in advance Consistent	Timing can be based on family and patient preference and school/work schedule. Times determined in advance Consistent
Meal or snack spacing	As needed for adequate intake	Avoid >4–5 h between meals and snacks.	Avoid >4–5 h between meals and snacks.
Meal or snack size and volume	Small portions at first, advanced to. meet energy needs	Small portions at first, advanced to meet energy needs without purging	Modify as appropriate to meet energy needs.

Continued

Table 19-4 (continued)

Food or nutrient intervention by patient/family and clinician	Eating disorder		
	Anorexia nervosa or avoidant/restrictive food intake disorder	Bulimia or purging disorder	Binge-eating disorder or night-eating syndrome
Meal or snack content	Estimate current intake. Increase by 100–200 kcal/wk until meeting goals. Use patient preferences to start, then advance to meet nutritional needs, then add variety as tolerated. Avoid foods that have triggered purging or self-harm for the patient in the past.	Include protein, carbohydrate, and fat at each meal; advance to meet macronutrient needs, then add variety as tolerated. Avoid foods that have triggered purging or self-harm for the patient in the past.	Include protein, carbohydrate, and fat at each meal; advance to meet macronutrient needs, then add variety as tolerated. Avoid foods that have triggered purging or self-harm for the patient in the past.
Meal or snack duration	Time limit of 20–40 min per meal and 10–15 min per snack	20+ min per meal recommended, with a pause partway through the meal for 3–5 min	20+ min per meal recommended, with a pause partway through the meal for 3–5 min
Meal or snack supervision	The patient • May require supervision to discourage hiding, concealing, or destroying food • May require support after eating to process feelings of distress and discourage purging or self-harm	The patient • May require supervision after eating to discourage purging or other self-harm behaviors • May require supervision when using the bathroom • May benefit from support following meals to process feelings of distress If meal preparation or cleanup triggers bingeing, tasks can be delegated to others or	The patient • May benefit from supervision or eating meals with others to encourage slow pace of eating, decrease shame-based eating behavior, and provide social interaction If meal preparation or cleanup triggers bingeing, tasks can be delegated to others or supervision provided.

Meal or snack behavior	Food rituals should be discouraged. Conversation should not focus on food.	Food rituals should be discouraged. Conversation should not focus on food. Address mindful eating and stress management before and after eating.	Food rituals should be discouraged. Conversation should not focus on food. Address mindful eating and stress management before and after eating.
Meal or snack documentation	Document intake, recorded by caregiver. Can monitor patient intake by either the percentage of meal consumed or specific foods and amounts consumed.	Document intake, bingeing, or bingeing triggers. Document compensatory behaviors.	Document intake, bingeing, or bingeing triggers. Document compensatory behaviors.
Beverage intake	If the patient has difficulty tolerating volume, limit beverages to 8 fl oz per meal or snack. Limit caffeinated and noncaloric beverages. If the patient depends on caffeine, wean caffeine intake rather than abruptly stop it.	If the patient has difficulty tolerating volume, limit beverages to 8 fl oz per meal or snack. Limit caffeinated and noncaloric beverages. Limit carbonated beverages because patients may use them to induce vomiting. If the patient depends on caffeine, wean caffeine intake rather than abruptly stop it.	If the patient has difficulty tolerating volume, limit beverages to 8 fl oz per meal or snack. Limit caffeinated and noncaloric beverages. Limit carbonated beverages because patients may use them to induce vomiting. If the patient depends on caffeine, wean caffeine intake rather than abruptly stop it.

Continued

Table 19-4 *(continued)*

Food or nutrient intervention by patient/ family and clinician	Eating disorder		
	Anorexia nervosa or avoidant/ restrictive food intake disorder	Bulimia or purging disorder	Binge-eating disorder or night-eating syndrome
Nutritional supplementation	Consider vitamin supplementation to include iron, calcium (1,000 mg for patients aged 4-8 y or 1,300 mg for patients aged 9-18 y), and vitamin D (600 IU).	Consider a multivitamin with iron.	Consider a multivitamin with iron.

Conversion factors: To convert fl oz to mL, multiply by 30; IU to mcg, by 0.025.

Adapted from reference 19. Reprinted with permission from the Academy of Nutrition and Dietetics, *Academy of Nutrition and Dietetics Pocket Guide to Eating Disorders*, Copyright 2017.

Mental Health Interventions

Patients with eating disorders should receive behavioral therapy with a mental health provider experienced in treating eating disorders. Certain therapies are more effective than others depending on the specific type of eating disorder. Family-based therapy is an intensive outpatient therapy used in the treatment of anorexia nervosa, avoidant/restrictive food intake disorder (ARFID), bulimia nervosa, and binge-eating disorder. It includes 3 phases: The first is full parental control in which the parent ensures that the patient follows the treatment plan, including supervising and monitoring all meals and snacks. The second phase allows for gradual return of control to the child or adolescent. The third phase helps the patient establish healthy independence. Cognitive behavioral therapy, in which patients learn how to recognize unhelpful or unproductive thoughts and then reframe them, is frequently used in the treatment of bulimia nervosa, anorexia nervosa, and ARFID. Mild aversion therapy consists of applying negative consequences or punishment when a child engages in the unwanted behavior, whereas positive reinforcement consists of giving praise or rewards when a child engages in the wanted behavior. Mild aversion therapy and positive reinforcement are often used in the treatment of pica. Biofeedback and diaphragmatic breathing are relaxation and mindfulness practices that may help treat rumination disorder. The therapeutic modalities most often used for each type of eating disorder are shown in **Table 19-5**. Parents and other caregivers can locate therapists with specialized training in eating disorders at Psychology Today (www.psychologytoday.com/us/therapists).

Table 19-5. Behavioral Health Therapy for Eating Disorder Rehabilitation

Eating disorder	Recommended therapy
Anorexia nervosa and avoidant/restrictive food intake disorder	Family-based therapy Cognitive behavioral therapy
Bulimia nervosa	Cognitive behavioral therapy Family-based therapy
Binge-eating disorder	Family-based therapy
Pica	Mild aversion therapy Positive reinforcement
Rumination disorder	Biofeedback Diaphragmatic breathing

The Pediatrician's Role in the Prevention of Eating Disorders

An American Academy of Pediatrics clinical report on the prevention of obesity and eating disorders encourages pediatricians to implement 6 strategies to help prevent eating disorders in children and adolescents[20]:

1. Discourage dieting, skipping meals, and using diet pills. Encourage and support sustainable healthy eating and physical activity behaviors. Focus on healthy living and healthy habits rather than weight.
2. Promote a positive body image.
3. Encourage more frequent family meals.
4. Encourage families to talk about healthy eating and physical activity to stay healthy rather than talk about weight.
5. Ask about a history of mistreatment or bullying for children and adolescents who have obesity.
6. Carefully monitor weight loss in an adolescent who has obesity and is attempting to lose weight, to ensure that medical complications of semi-starvation or indication of an eating disorder does not develop.

Children and Adolescents With Special Health Care Needs

Children and adolescents with special health care needs are more likely to experience nutritional problems because of physical disabilities that affect appetite, food intake, or ability to consume, digest, or absorb nutrients; adverse effects of long-term medication use; metabolic disturbances; psychological stressors; or environmental challenges that may affect food access and acceptance. Many of the most common nutritional concerns for children and adolescents with special health care needs according to data summarized in the *Bright Futures: Nutrition* guidebook include[21]

- Altered energy and nutrient needs
- Delayed growth
- Oro-motor dysfunction; feeding, swallowing, or digestive disorders
- Regurgitation and gastroesophageal reflux disease
- Elimination problems
- Drug/nutrient interactions
- Appetite disturbances
- Unusual food habits (eg, pica, restrictive food choices, rumination)
- Early childhood caries or gum disease

It is important that pediatricians monitor children with special health care needs closely, ensuring nutritional adequacy for appropriate growth, development, and health. Considerations for adequate caloric intake for several chronic conditions are shown in **Table 19-6**.

Referral to a registered dietitian is particularly important if a child shows signs of nutritional inadequacy that are difficult to appropriately address in the primary care setting.

Table 19-6. Energy Calculations for Children and Adolescents With Special Health Care Needs

Medical diagnosis	Energy calculation
Down syndrome[a]	For children with Down syndrome, ages 5–11 Girls: 14.3 kcal/cm (36.3 kcal/inch) Boys: 16.1 kcal/cm (40.9 kcal/inch)
Spina bifida[b-d]	For children with spina bifida > 6 years As a general recommendation, provide approximately 50% of the Dietary Reference Intake (DRI) for a child of the same age To maintain weight: 9 kcal/cm (22.9 kcal/inch) To promote weight loss: 7 kcal/cm (17.8 kcal/inch)
Prader-Willi syndrome[e]	For children and adolescents with Prader-Willi syndrome To maintain growth within a growth channel: 10–11 kcal/cm (25.4–28.0 kcal/inch) To create a slow rate of weight loss and support linear growth: 8.5 kcal/cm (21.6 kcal/inch)
Cystic fibrosis[f]	For children and adolescents with cystic fibrosis and pulmonary involvement To improve weight status, increase intake from 1.1 to 2.0 times the energy needs for healthy peers of the same age, gender, and size. Monitor for age-appropriate weight gain and adjust accordingly. Oral and enteral nutritional supplements may be required.
Pediatric HIV infection or AIDS[g,h]	For children and adolescents with HIV infection Monitor closely for growth, caloric intake, and clinical symptoms. Adjust energy requirements accordingly. For children and adolescents with mild or no symptoms related to HIV infection, adjust calories to 1.5 to 2 times the DRI if growth velocity is inappropriate for age. For children and adolescents with moderate or severe symptoms, increase calories beyond those required for children and adolescents with mild or no symptoms, particularly in response to weight loss, wasting, or fever.

Sources: [a] Culley et al, [b] Ekvall and Cerniglia, [c] Grogan and Ekvall, [d] Dustrude and Prince, [e] Pipes and Powell, [f] Stallings et al, [g] Rothpletz-Puglia, and [h] Ayoob.

Reproduced from Children and adolescents with special health care needs. In: Holt K, Wooldridge N, Story M, Sofka D, eds. *Bright Futures: Nutrition.* 3rd ed. American Academy of Pediatrics; 2011:123–129. Accessed November 23, 2022. https://downloads.aap.org/AAP/PDF/Bright%20 Futures/BFNutrition3rdEdition_issuesConcerns.pdf.

In Sum

- Many children experience mental, behavioral, and developmental health concerns, for which attention to specific nutrition strategies can help improve health outcomes and well-being.
- For example, a diet rich in fruits, vegetables, and whole grains and low in sugary and processed foods may help reduce the symptoms of depression and improve mood. This type of healthy eating pattern is also associated with improved behavior of children with ADHD.
- Although most parents of children with autism try many alternative dietary patterns, such as the gluten-free and casein-free diet, none have strong evidence to support that they lessen autism symptoms.
- Although picky eating is common during childhood, some children have severe picky eating, which can develop into a feeding disorder. Feeding disorders are generally caused by organic disease or a more serious underlying behavioral concern. If a child with severe picky eating shows signs of malnutrition or growth restriction, they may need nutritional supplementation and increased caloric intake to support adequate nutrition, weight gain, and growth, in addition to identification and treatment of the underlying cause.
- Approximately 3% of children and adolescents have an eating disorder, such as anorexia nervosa, bulimia nervosa, binge-eating disorder, ARFID, pica, or rumination disorder. The appropriate evaluation and treatment of eating disorders generally include medical monitoring, nutritional therapy, and mental health treatment. The goal of treatment is to restore a healthy body weight, relationship with food, and body image.[15]
- Children with special health care needs are more likely to experience nutritional inadequacy. It is important that pediatricians monitor patients carefully to ensure nutritional adequacy for appropriate growth, development, and health.

References

1. Sarris J, Logan AC, Akbaraly TN, et al; International Society for Nutritional Psychiatry Research. Nutritional medicine as mainstream in psychiatry. *Lancet Psychiatry.* 2015; 2(3):271–274 PMID: 26359904 doi: 10.1016/S2215-0366(14)00051-0

2. O'Neil A, Quirk SE, Housden S, et al. Relationship between diet and mental health in children and adolescents: a systematic review. *Am J Public Health.* 2014;104(10):e31–e42 PMID: 25208008 doi: 10.2105/AJPH.2014.302110

3. Khalid S, Williams CM, Reynolds SA. Is there an association between diet and depression in children and adolescents? a systematic review. *Br J Nutr.* 2016;116(12):2097–2108 PMID: 28093091 doi: 10.1017/S0007114516004359

4. Millichap JG, Yee MM. The diet factor in attention-deficit/hyperactivity disorder. *Pediatrics.* 2012;129(2):330–337 PMID: 22232312 doi: 10.1542/peds.2011-2199

5. Heilskov Rytter MJ, Andersen LBB, Houmann T, et al. Diet in the treatment of ADHD in children—a systematic review of the literature. *Nord J Psychiatry.* 2015;69(1):1–18 PMID: 24934907 doi: 10.3109/08039488.2014.921933

6. Pelsser L, Frankena K, Toorman J, Rodrigues Pereira R. Retrospective Outcome Monitoring of ADHD and Nutrition (ROMAN): the effectiveness of the few-foods diet in general practice. *Front Psychiatry.* 2020;11:96 PMID: 32226397 doi: 10.3389/fpsyt.2020.00096

7. Bostock EC, Kirkby KC, Taylor BV. The current status of the ketogenic diet in psychiatry. *Front Psychiatry.* 2017;8:43 PMID: 28373848 doi: 10.3389/fpsyt.2017.00043

8. Del-Ponte B, Quinte GC, Cruz S, Grellert M, Santos IS. Dietary patterns and attention deficit/hyperactivity disorder (ADHD): a systematic review and meta-analysis. *J Affect Disord.* 2019;252:160–173 PMID: 30986731 doi: 10.1016/j.jad.2019.04.061

9. Ng QX, Ho CYX, Chan HW, Yong BZJ, Yeo WS. Managing childhood and adolescent attention-deficit/hyperactivity disorder (ADHD) with exercise: a systematic review. *Complement Ther Med.* 2017;34:123–128 PMID: 28917364 doi: 10.1016/j.ctim.2017.08.018

10. Lange KW, Hauser J, Reissmann A. Gluten-free and casein-free diets in the therapy of autism. *Curr Opin Clin Nutr Metab Care.* 2015;18(6):572–575 PMID: 26418822 doi: 10.1097/MCO.0000000000000228

11. Keller A, Rimestad ML, Friis Rohde J, et al. The effect of a combined gluten- and casein-free diet on children and adolescents with autism spectrum disorders: a systematic review and meta-analysis. *Nutrients.* 2021;13(2):470 PMID: 33573238 doi: 10.3390/nu13020470

12. Sathe N, Andrews JC, McPheeters ML, Warren ZE. Nutritional and dietary interventions for autism spectrum disorder: a systematic review. *Pediatrics.* 2017;139(6):e20170346 PMID: 28562286 doi: 10.1542/peds.2017-0346

13. Fraguas D, Díaz-Caneja CM, Pina-Camacho L, et al. Dietary interventions for autism spectrum disorder: a meta-analysis. *Pediatrics.* 2019;144(5):e20183218 PMID: 31586029 doi: 10.1542/peds.2018-3218

14. Kerzner B, Milano K, MacLean WC Jr, Berall G, Stuart S, Chatoor I. A practical approach to classifying and managing feeding difficulties. *Pediatrics.* 2015;135(2):344–353 PMID: 25560449 doi: 10.1542/peds.2014-1630

15. Hornberger LL, Lane MA. American Academy of Pediatrics Committee on Adolescence. Identification and management of eating disorders in children and adolescents. *Pediatrics.* 2021;147(1):e2020040279 PMID: 33386343 doi: 10.1542/peds.2020-040279

16. Swanson SA, Crow SJ, Le Grange D, Swendsen J, Merikangas KR. Prevalence and correlates of eating disorders in adolescents: results from the national comorbidity survey replication adolescent supplement. *Arch Gen Psychiatry.* 2011;68(7):714–723 PMID: 21383252 doi: 10.1001/archgenpsychiatry.2011.22

17. Cena H, Barthels F, Cuzzolaro M, et al. Definition and diagnostic criteria for orthorexia nervosa: a narrative review of the literature. *Eat Weight Disord.* 2019;24(2):209–246 PMID: 30414078 doi: 10.1007/s40519-018-0606-y

18. Brigham KS, Manzo LD, Eddy KT, Thomas JJ. Evaluation and treatment of avoidant/restrictive food intake disorder (ARFID) in adolescents. *Curr Pediatr Rep.* 2018;6(2):107–113 PMID: 31134139 doi: 10.1007/s40124-018-0162-y

19. Setnick J. *Academy of Nutrition and Dietetics Pocket Guide to Eating Disorders.* 2nd ed. Academy of Nutrition and Dietetics; 2017

20. Golden NH, Schneider M, Wood C, et al; American Academy of Pediatrics Committee on Nutrition, Committee on Adolescence, and Section on Obesity. Preventing obesity and eating disorders in adolescents. *Pediatrics.* 2016;138(3):e20161649 PMID: 27550979 doi: 10.1542/peds.2016-1649

21. Hagan JF Jr, Shaw JS, Duncan PM, eds. *Bright Futures: Guidelines for Health Supervision of Infants, Children, and Adolescents.* 4th ed. American Academy of Pediatrics; 2017 doi: 10.1542/9781610020237

Obesity and Related Health Conditions

Childhood obesity is one of the most common pediatric chronic diseases, affecting 19% of children, adolescents, and young adults aged 2 to 19 years, including 13% of 2- to 5-year-olds, 20% of 6- to 11-year-olds, and 21% of 12 to 19-year-olds.[1] Obesity increases the risk of numerous health conditions, including hypercholesterolemia, hypertension, nonalcoholic fatty liver disease (NAFLD), prediabetes, and type 2 diabetes. Although each of these conditions can occur in the absence of obesity, they often coexist with obesity. In most cases, the treatment of obesity and related health conditions includes similar nutritional interventions. These nutrition best practices are highlighted in this chapter.

Obesity and Severe Obesity

Childhood obesity is defined as body mass index (BMI) at or above the 95th percentile for age and sex in children and adolescents. Body mass index is correlated with direct measures of body fat and is relatively easy to assess, even though it is a measure of excess weight rather than excess fat mass.[2] For children and adolescents with obesity, BMI is usually a good surrogate of excess body fat, although it has limited utility in the assessment of body fatness for athletes with high performance and those with a muscular habitus. For children and adolescents who have overweight (a BMI-for-age between the 85th and 94th percentiles), elevated BMI can result from increased levels of either fat or fat-free mass.[3]

Childhood obesity is further categorized into 3 classes of severity, with the risk of related health conditions increased with worsened obesity. Classes 2 and 3 obesity are commonly referred to as *severe obesity* (**Table 20-1**). Severe obesity affects 6% of all children, adolescents, and young adults aged 2 to 19 years. This number has increased 600% since the early 1970s, when just 1% of children had severe obesity.[1]

Table 20-1. Classification of Childhood Obesity

Classification	Criteria[a]
Class 1	BMI ≥ 95th percentile and < 120% of 95th percentile
Class 2	BMI ≥ 120%–140% of 95th percentile or BMI ≥ 35
Class 3	BMI ≥ 140% of 95th percentile or BMI ≥ 40

Abbreviation: BMI, body mass index.

[a] Extended BMI growth charts are available in most electronic health record systems, and these charts can be used to determine percentage of the 95th percentile.

Childhood obesity often begins at a young age and persists through adolescence and adulthood. Modeling studies predict that more than half of children will have obesity by age 35 years, with half the prevalence occurring during childhood.[4] Most children who have obesity at age 3 years also have obesity as adolescents, with the most excessive weight gain occurring between 2 and 6 years of age.[5] Likewise, only 2% of adolescents with obesity achieve a typical BMI in adulthood, whereas more than 50% of adolescents with typical BMI experience overweight or obesity by adulthood.[6] By tracking growth charts closely, recognizing risk factors early, and tailoring anticipatory guidance, pediatricians play an important role in the prevention and early identification of obesity. Of note, although childhood obesity affects children and adolescents from communities across the United States and the world, children of color, especially non-Hispanic Black girls, Mexican American boys, and American Indian and Alaska Natives; children and adolescents in rural environments; and those in families with lower income and in families with lower educational levels are disproportionately affected.[7–10] The association between ethnicity, race, and obesity most likely reflects differences in epigenetic, social, and environmental factors, such as the social determinants of health. Body mass index rates increased sharply during the COVID-19 pandemic, especially among young school-aged children and children with overweight and obesity at the onset of the pandemic.[11]

Risk Factors

Childhood obesity is caused by a complex interplay between genetic factors, environmental factors, and metabolic changes that occur in response to excess caloric intake and energy storage in relation to caloric expenditure. Studies suggest there is a 40% to 70% genetic contribution to obesity risk.[12–14] Genetic and prenatal factors affect birth weight, and many additional factors affect postnatal growth and weight gain, as discussed in Chapter 8, Anthropometric Measures. Weight gain in children of typical growth and development tends to occur in a predictable pattern, tracking across a stable percentile line over time.

Caloric overconsumption and energy storage in infancy and early childhood change a child's weight trajectory and increase the likelihood of obesity developing later in life.[5] Many individual- and family-level factors, such as those described in **Table 20-2**, influence overconsumption in infancy, childhood, and adolescence. However, overconsumption should also be considered in the context of social determinants of health and environmental exposures (refer to Chapter 10, Dietary History, Social History, and Food Insecurity Screening). Many of the factors that influence energy balance and overconsumption, such as food insecurity, food deserts (geographic areas with limited access to healthful foods), sugary drink marketing to children, high-density housing not conducive to regular activity, limited physical education and recess in schools, limited access to sports or exercise equipment and facilities, and unsafe neighborhoods, are outside a child's or family's immediate control.

Complications and Related Health Conditions

Adverse health consequences resulting from obesity can begin at a young age. A study of 2- to 18-year-olds with severe obesity in the Netherlands showed that two-thirds of the children, including some of the toddlers, already had at least 1 of the

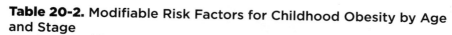

Table 20-2. Modifiable Risk Factors for Childhood Obesity by Age and Stage

Age	Risk factors	Opportunities for pediatrician intervention
All or most stages	Restrictive feeding High intake of sugary drinks Frequent consumption of fast food Eating in absence of hunger Food rewards Television/devices in bedroom Poor sleep Lack of physical activity Maternal depression Maternal obesity Psychological stress	Encourage positive food and activity modeling at home. Offer ideas for easy-to-implement healthy eating and physical activities. Teach and encourage responsive feeding. Encourage use of nonfood rewards. Advise removal of screens from bedrooms and avoidance of screen use within 1 h of bedtime. Ask about sleep duration and quality, and encourage development of regular sleep routines. Screen for maternal depression, increased family stress, and social determinants of health, and help connect the family to resources. Conduct age-appropriate screening for adverse childhood experiences, depression, and anxiety.
Prenatal period	Maternal excess weight gain and gestational diabetes Maternal smoking	Encourage healthful maternal nutrition and physical activity and avoidance of tobacco products for the benefit of both mother and baby. Help connect mothers who smoke to smoking cessation resources.
Infancy	Rapid weight gain Decreased frequency and duration of breastfeeding Use of large bottle size (≥6 fl oz) in early infancy[15] Less sleep Introduction of solid foods at <4 mo old Inappropriate bottle use and delayed transition from bottle to cup Antibiotic exposure	Recognize rapid weight gain, and share concern of increased risk of later obesity. Support breastfeeding. If a family is bottle-feeding, teach cue-based feeding. For bottle-fed infants, recommend a small bottle (<6 fl oz) in early infancy. Provide guidance to help establish sleep routines starting in infancy. Recommend introducing solid foods around 6 mo of age and no earlier than 4 mo. Recommend weaning bottle-feeding at 12 mo. Avoid antibiotics whenever possible.

Continued

Table 20-2 (*continued*)

Age	Risk factors	Opportunities for pediatrician intervention
Toddlerhood and pre-school age	Early or pronounced adiposity rebound (Refer to Chapter 8, Anthropometric Measures, for more information on adiposity rebound.) Increase in BMI *z* score of ≥0.2 in preschool years, irrespective of BMI percentile. Most electronic health records include *z* scores alongside the BMI percentile.	Review growth chart; recognize and sensitively share concern of increased risk of later obesity.
School age	Frequent snacking Skipped meals Large portions Limited or no family meals	Recommend scheduling mealtimes and snack times and sitting at a table without distractions. Ask about a patient's sense of fullness when eating. Teach and remind patients and families to use the body's cues of hunger and fullness. Encourage caregivers to allow children to choose their portion size, because adults tend to serve larger portions than children need. Recommend that families use small plates. Advise having family meals as often as possible.
Adolescence	Weight gain–promoting medication use, especially of psychiatric medications Frequent snacking Skipped meals Limited or no family meals Large portions	Identify weight gain–promoting medications, and use alternatives when possible (**Table 20-3**). Recommend scheduling mealtimes and snack times and sitting at a table without distractions. Advise having family meals at least 3 times per week. Teach adolescents to recognize non-physiological triggers to eat and how to use internal cues of hunger and fullness to guide intake, when possible.

SI conversion factor: To convert fl oz to mL, multiply by 30.

Derived from references 5, 16, and 17.

Table 20-3. Medications That Cause Weight Gain, and Potential Alternatives

Drug class/type	Common name	Alternative drugs
Insulin	Insulin lispro Insulin aspart	Metformin Glucagon-like peptide-1 receptor agonists Sodium-glucose cotransporter-2 inhibitors
Tricyclic antidepressants	Amitriptyline Mirtazapine	Bupropion Trazodone
Selective serotonin reuptake inhibitors	Paroxetine Citalopram	Sertraline Fluoxetine
Antipsychotics	Risperidone Olanzapine Quetiapine	Aripiprazole
Anti-seizure	Valproic acid	Topiramate Zonisamide Lamotrigine
Oral corticosteroids (with long-term use)	Prednisone/prednisolone Dexamethasone	Nonsteroidal anti-inflammatory drugs, when appropriate
Inhaled corticosteroids	Budesonide Fluticasone	
Contraception	Medroxyprogesterone acetate, intramuscular	Long-acting reversible contraceptive
Antihypertensives	Atenolol Metoprolol Propranolol	Timolol Enalapril Losartan Furosemide

Derived from reference 18 and Kyle T, Kuehl B. *Prescription Medications & Weight Gain: What You Need to Know.* Obesity Action Coalition. Accessed October 31, 2022. https://www.obesityaction.org/wp-content/uploads/prescription_medications.pdf.

following cardiovascular risk factors: elevated blood pressure, dyslipidemia, hyperglycemia, and type 2 diabetes.[19] US data from the National Health and Nutrition Examination Survey indicate that about half of teens with overweight and two-thirds of teens with obesity have at least 1 risk factor for cardiovascular disease (CVD).[20] Other complications of childhood obesity include fatty liver disease, asthma, obstructive sleep apnea, gallstones, slipped capital femoral epiphysis, Blount disease, bone fractures, polycystic ovary syndrome, infertility in girls,[21] depression and anxiety, low self-esteem, body dissatisfaction, disordered eating, unhealthy weight-control practices, counterproductive dietary restraint, and emotional distress.[22] Studies suggest that weight-based stigmatization and teasing, along with preoccupation with weight and size, may serve as the major mediators in the development of the mental health complications of obesity[23] (**Box 20-1**).

IN GREATER DEPTH

Box 20-1. Weight Bias and Stigmatization

Children with obesity experience weight bias and stigmatization from family members, peers, teachers, and pediatricians and other health care professionals.[24] Many patients and families with obesity report that they feel disrespected, perceive that they will not be taken seriously, believe that all their medical problems will be attributed to their weight, and report that they feel reluctant to address their weight with health care professionals. Many patients and families have avoided or delayed health supervision care because of factors related to their weight, including fear of disrespectful treatment and negative attitudes, embarrassment about being weighed, weight loss advice that is unsolicited, and medical equipment that is too small to accommodate their body size.[25] Children and adolescents who experience weight bias are more likely to experience negative physical and mental health effects, ranging from disordered eating and decreased physical activity to increased cardiovascular disease risk factors, depression, and anxiety, as shown in the following box[25]:

Mental health	Social health	Health behaviors
Depressive symptoms	Bullying and teasing at school	Increased food intake
Anxiety	Social isolation	Lower physical activity levels
Lower self-esteem	Decreased attention and compassion in health care settings	
Perceived stress		Higher exercise avoidance
Substance use		Unhealthy diet consumption
Binge eating		
Emotional overeating		Increased sedentary behavior
Disordered eating		

Derived from reference 25.

IN GREATER DEPTH

Box 20-1 (*continued*)

How pediatricians can counter weight bias

The American Academy of Pediatrics policy statement on the stigma experienced by children and adolescents with obesity advises pediatricians to take the following steps to counter weight bias[26]:

1. Model supportive and unbiased treatment of children, adolescents, and families with obesity. Acknowledge the complex cause of obesity.
2. Use non-stigmatizing language. Use words such as *weight* and *body mass index* instead of *obese, extremely obese, fat,* or *weight problem.* Use people-first language (*child with obesity* rather than *obese child*). Emphasize health rather than weight.
3. Use terms such as *unhealthy weight* and *very unhealthy weight* in the electronic health record and patient-facing resources rather than *obesity* and *morbid obesity.*
4. Use motivational interviewing and behavioral coaching skills to support patients and families in making healthful changes.
5. Create a safe, welcoming, and non-stigmatizing clinical space that accommodates patients of diverse body sizes.
6. Assess for behavioral health complications of weight bias, such as weight-based bullying and mental health conditions.

The American Academy of Pediatrics also recommends 4 advocacy goals for pediatricians to help reduce weight bias in multiple settings.

1. Work with schools to ensure that anti-bullying policies include protections for children who experience weight-based bullying.
2. Advocate for responsible and respectful portrayal of individuals with obesity in the media.
3. Advocate for medical schools and pediatric training programs to address weight bias.
4. Work with parents to recognize and reduce weight stigma experienced at home.

Childhood Obesity Treatment

The 2023 American Academy of Pediatrics (AAP) "Clinical Practice Guideline for the Evaluation and Treatment of Children and Adolescents With Obesity" outlines the optimal management of pediatric obesity, summarized in an algorithm for screening, diagnosis, evaluation, and treatment (**Figure 20-1**). This approach includes clinicians measuring BMI, assessing behaviors, appropriately screening laboratory values, and initiating treatment immediately upon diagnosis. The algorithm notes key action statements from the clinical practice guideline (referred to as *KAS* in the figure), and the full guideline can be accessed online (https://doi.org/10.1542/peds.2022-060640).

Intervention Goals

Treatment of childhood obesity focuses on health and behavior change goals in nutrition, physical activity, sleep, screen use, and stress management. Although the AAP offers guidance for appropriate weight loss based on a child's age (**Table 20-4**), the primary aim of childhood obesity interventions should be to optimize health, rather than focus on weight loss.[17] Attention to energy balance through healthful nutrition and activity habits that result in appropriate caloric intake and increased energy expenditure helps prevent obesity and may be effective in helping a young child with obesity attain and maintain a healthy weight or an older child or adolescent prevent further weight gain. However, as children get older or obesity severity increases, focusing on weight and achievement of a healthy BMI percentile through behavior changes becomes more complicated because of metabolic changes that occur with weight loss.

Fat is a highly active endocrine organ that, together with hormones from the brain and stomach, influences hunger and satiety and plays a key role in adaptive thermogenesis (also referred to as *metabolic adaptation* or *enhanced metabolic efficiency*). When a person is in negative energy balance because of "eating less" or "moving more," weight loss results in increased drive to eat and reduced energy expenditure, preventing further weight loss and usually resulting in regained weight as the body aims to maintain a set point weight. Although weight loss still occurs with dietary and activity changes, weight loss is rarely maintained beyond 1 year because of adaptive thermogenesis. It is unclear when the set point weight is determined or "programmed," but infancy and early childhood (ages 2–6 years) are likely to be critical periods.[5] It is also unclear whether there are critical periods, such as adolescence, pregnancy, or middle age, when the set point weight can be reset.[28] However, most studies suggest that once established, the set point weight is unlikely to be decreased with dietary or behavioral interventions.

Certain medications and bariatric surgery are important parts of treatment for children and adolescents with severe obesity or related health conditions. In fact, there is evidence that bariatric surgery may lower a person's set point weight, thus increasing the likelihood of long-term weight loss maintenance.[28] This section focuses on the nutritional and lifestyle intervention factors, although primary care clinicians are encouraged to increase awareness and patient access to all potential treatment options to help optimize medical and health outcomes.

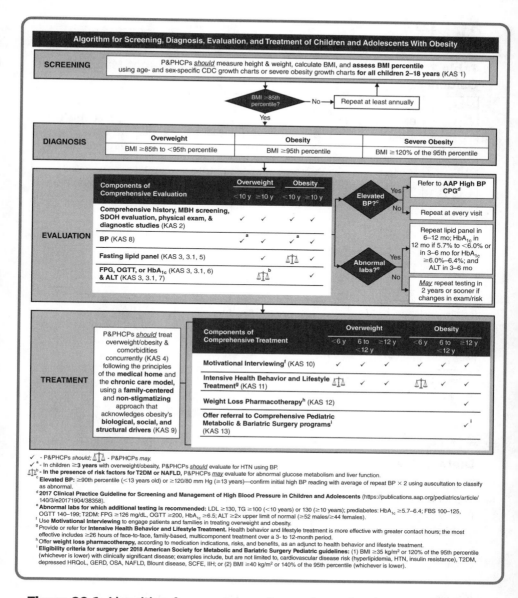

Figure 20-1. Algorithm for screening, diagnosis, evaluation, and treatment of children and adolescents with obesity.

Abbreviations: AAP, American Academy of Pediatrics; ALT, alanine transaminase; BMI, body mass index; BP, blood pressure; CDC, Centers for Disease Control and Prevention; CPG, clinical practice guideline; exam, examination; FBS, fasting blood sugar [glucose]; FPG, fasting plasma glucose; GERD, gastroesophageal reflux disease; HbA$_{1c}$, glycosylated hemoglobin; HRQoL, health-related quality of life; HTN, hypertension; IIH, idiopathic intracranial HTN; KAS, [CPG] key action statement; labs, laboratory results; LDL, low-density lipoprotein; MBH, mental and behavioral health; OGTT, 2-hour plasma glucose after 75-g oral glucose tolerance test; OSA, obstructive sleep apnea; P&PHCPs, pediatricians and other pediatric health care providers; SDOH, social determinants of health; T2DM, type 2 diabetes mellitus; NAFLD, nonalcoholic fatty liver disease; SCFE, slipped capital femoral epiphysis; TG, triglyceride.

Adapted from reference 27.

Table 20-4. American Academy of Pediatrics Weight Management Guidance

Age (y)	BMI 85th–94th percentile, no risks	BMI 85th–94th percentile, risks	BMI 95th–98th percentile	BMI ≥ 99th percentile (or ≥ 120% of the 95th percentile)
2–5	Maintain weight velocity.	Decrease weight velocity or maintain weight.	Maintain weight.	Gradually lose weight up to 1 lb/mo if BMI is very high (> 21 or 22).
6–11	Maintain weight velocity.	Decrease weight velocity or maintain weight.	Maintain weight or gradually lose weight (1 lb/mo).	Weight loss not to exceed an average of 2 lb/wk[a]
12–18	Maintain weight velocity. After linear growth is complete, maintain weight.	Decrease weight velocity or maintain weight.	Weight loss not to exceed an average of 2 lb/wk[a]	Weight loss not to exceed an average of 2 lb/wk[a]

Abbreviation: BMI, body mass index.

SI conversion factor: To convert lb to kg, multiply by 0.45.

[a] If greater loss is noted, clinicians should monitor for excessive weight loss.

Adapted from reference 17.

Dietary Changes

The AAP recommends the Cardiovascular Health Integrated Lifestyle Diet (CHILD-1) as the first stage for children who have obesity and any other CVD risk or family history of early cardiac disease or diabetes or who have smoke exposure in the home[29] (**Table 20-5**).

When talking with patients and families about nutrition strategies to support a healthy weight, a balanced meal plan including the major food groups (eg, the MyPlate plan at www.myplate.gov) in the appropriate portions, with water and milk as the main beverages, and minimal eating between scheduled mealtimes and snack times is consistent with the CHILD-1 eating plan and is likely to lead to the best overall outcomes. A focus on behavioral strategies to help support and maintain dietary changes is likely to provide the most impact. Several potential strategies are highlighted in **Table 20-6**, with several of these strategies detailed further in chapters 14, Theories of Behavior Change and Motivational Interviewing, and 15, SMART Goals and Action Plans.

The AAP advises against recommending diets as a weight loss strategy for children and adolescents. Diets are not only unlikely to be effective in promoting sustained weight loss but can also trigger disordered eating, low confidence, and an unhealthy relationship with food.[33] However, many patients may try one or more popular diets. Many

Table 20-5. The Cardiovascular Health Integrated Lifestyle Diet

	Age				
	0–6 mo	**6–12 mo**	**12–24 mo**	**2–10 y**	**11–21 y**
Fluids	Exclusive breastfeeding	Continued breastfeeding or formula, water	Whole or low-fat milk, water[a]	Low-fat or fat-free milk, water	Fat-free milk, water
Fats		25%–30% of calories from fat, 20% of which are derived from monounsaturated and polyunsaturated fats and 8%–10% of which are derived from saturated fat Avoidance of trans fat Cholesterol level < 300 mg/d			
Fiber				Age + 5 g/d	14 g per 1,000 kcal
Supportive measures			Clinicians can work with families to ● Encourage breakfast every day. ● Encourage family meals. ● Limit fast-food meals. ● Avoid or limit sugary drinks. ● Consider the Dietary Approaches to Stop Hypertension or Mediterranean-style eating plan. ● Limit sodium intake.		

[a] Or continued breastfeeding as long as mutually desired by the mother and infant, per American Academy of Pediatrics policy.

Adapted from reference 29.

studies with adult participants have looked at these diets, and variations of them, comparing weight loss and cardiovascular risk factors. The preponderance of scientific evidence supports a clear conclusion: most diets initially result in modest weight loss and improved cardiovascular risk factors, with most or all of the weight regained and risk factors returned to baseline by 12 months.[34] Because many adolescents experiment with popular diets, it is important for pediatricians to be well-informed of the most popular diets and to direct patients toward healthy, balanced eating patterns (**Table 20-7** and **Box 20-2**). Additionally, pediatricians should ask adolescent patients what they have learned about nutrition, diets, and weight loss methods and where they have learned the information. In many cases, adolescent patients may be learning this information from social media sites, which often perpetuate nutrition misinformation, dieting and food restriction, and excessive exercise. In fact, studies show a clear association between social media use and disordered eating in adolescents.[35]

In contrast to guidance to avoid encouraging or recommending weight loss diets for children and adolescents, guidance to encourage or recommend adoption of certain

Table 20-6. Behavioral Strategies to Optimize Nutrition in the Treatment of Childhood Obesity

Strategy	Highlights
Self-monitoring	Awareness is the first step of any behavior change. Tracked nutrition intake and physical activity (eg, with food and exercise logs) can help change behaviors and increase the likelihood of body mass index stabilization; however, clinicians and parents should monitor for signs of disordered eating or excessive focus on dietary tracking.
Stimulus control	Stimulus control occurs when one avoids tempting situations or triggers for an unhealthy behavior and seeks out triggers for healthy behaviors. For example, a family might remove junk food from the pantry and stock up on fruits and vegetables, spend less time with friends and neighbors with unhelpful eating and exercise habits and attitudes, make an effort to spend more time with active and healthy individuals, and eat small well-planned meals throughout the day to help prevent excessive eating or an unplanned stop at a vending machine or fast-food restaurant. To reduce psychological cues to eat (eg, boredom, habit, stress, emotional distress), families might eat only at the kitchen or dining room table.
Behavioral substitution	Behavioral substitution consists of a person identifying behaviors or habits that negatively affect health and then replacing those behaviors with more helpful positive behaviors. For example, a teen who tends to snack mindlessly while playing video games might replace video games by playing outside with friends.
Mindfulness training	When clinicians help patients be more mindful and aware of the body's cues of hunger and fullness and pay more attention to the taste and texture of food, oftentimes by slowing down when eating, patients can reestablish internal cues of hunger and fullness to guide intake and allow more overall enjoyment of eating. A review of mindfulness-based interventions showed that these methods can be effective at helping reduce binge eating and emotional eating,[30] although they may not influence energy intake or dietary quality.[31]
Accountability	Programs that have built-in accountability, to either an outside person (eg, parent, pediatrician, health coach) or oneself or others, are more likely to lead to lasting success. For example, having "homework" after appointments, such as keeping a food log; completing electronic check-ins; and verbally stating a specific goal help improve accountability.

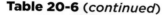

Table 20-6 (*continued*)

Strategy	Highlights
SMART (specific, measurable, attainable, relevant, and time-bound) goal setting	SMART nutrition and physical activity goals help patients move from an idea of a desired outcome to a specific plan for a healthier lifestyle. A family can increase success by posting visible reminders of the goal (refer to Chapter 15, SMART Goals and Action Plans, for more on SMART goals).
Social support	Social support improves the likelihood of making and sustaining dietary changes. Family-level dietary changes are more likely to lead to improved nutrition and outcomes for a child or an adolescent. Health-promoting social activities and family mealtimes can help families make and sustain healthful changes.
Relapse prevention	Lapses are an expected part of behavior change. By helping patients prepare for lapses, clinicians can increase the likelihood of maintaining a behavior change (refer to Chapter 15, SMART Goals and Action Plans, for more on relapse prevention).

eating plans, such as the Mediterranean-style or Dietary Approaches to Stop Hypertension (DASH) eating plan, can highly benefit the overall health and well-being of children, adolescents, and their families. These eating plans are discussed in Chapter 12, Healthy Eating Plans, and later in this chapter in the context of their role in the treatment of obesity-related health conditions.

Cardiovascular Disease Risk

Childhood obesity is strongly associated with increased cardiovascular disease (CVD) risk. Cardiovascular disease begins in childhood, with studies showing that elevated BMI at age 4 years is associated with high carotid intima-media thickness in men at 60 to 64 years of age.[36] Other risk factors for CVD include hypertension, hypercholesterolemia, hyperglycemia, excess caloric intake, and low-quality diet; low-level physical activity; and smoking. Interventions focused on reducing and optimally managing risk factors in the pediatric primary care setting can provide lifelong positive impact in the prevention of CVD, the leading cause of morbidity and mortality in adults in the United States across most race and ethnic groups, resulting mostly from suboptimal preventive measures and suboptimal control of risk factors.[7] A flow diagram of the development of CVD and possible prevention by a healthy diet is shown in **Figure 20-2**.

Pediatricians have an opportunity to intervene at each stage of the primordial, primary, and secondary prevention of CVD.

For primordial prevention, key nutrition goals include reducing excess caloric intake; increasing consumption of fruits and vegetables, whole grains, nuts, legumes, seafood,

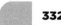

Table 20-7. Popular Diets

Diet	Details	Clinical considerations
Low carbohydrate		
Keto	<50 g/d of carbohydrate, typically around 20 g/d to promote ketosis, and use of fat as energy High fat No grains, sugar, fruit, or starchy vegetables	Early weight loss Proven for childhood epilepsy High satiety May be difficult to sustain May be deficient in some nutrients, especially fiber and fruits High in saturated fat
Paleo	Modeled on the way the hunters and gatherers ate Emphasizes meat, fish, poultry, fruits, and vegetables No refined sugar, dairy, legumes, or grains	Discourages heavily processed and refined foods Restrictive, which may lead to nutrient insufficiencies Not well studied May be expensive
Atkins	Induction phase with very low carbohydrate intake (20 g) and then gradual increase	Early weight loss Well studied High satiety May be difficult to sustain May be deficient in some nutrients, especially fiber and fruits High in saturated fat
Balanced macronutrients		
Vegan	No meat, fish, poultry, eggs, or dairy Rich in high-fiber foods	Similar to vegetarian diet, provides health and environmental benefits Very restrictive Risk of nutrient insufficiencies, especially iron and vitamin B_{12} Associated with development of eating disorders
Low glycemic index	Encourages a diet rich in "good" (low glycemic index) carbohydrates Emphasizes whole foods and minimizes processed foods	Difficult to know glycemic index of all foods Studies demonstrating mixed results

Table 20-7 (*continued*)

Diet	Details	Clinical considerations
Prepared and packaged foods and shakes		
Medifast	Five 100-Cal meal-replacement shakes and Medifast products per day plus 1 meat-and-vegetables entrée per day Very low calories (800–1,000 Cal/d)	Quick weight loss Nutritionally balanced Because of very low calorie levels, requires medical supervision May be cost prohibitive for many patients
Nutrisystem	Patients and families purchase prepackaged meals online and shop for vegetables and fruits to supplement these meals. Calorie goals: 1,200–1,550 Cal	Adherence made easier initially by prepacked foods Behavioral support in online group environment May be cost prohibitive for many patients
Other		
Intermittent fasting or time-restricted eating	Based on cycling between fasting and eating. Length of each cycle varies, with patients and families sometimes limiting number of hours per day of eating (typically a 16-h fast) and other times rotating fasting days with non-fasting days over a week (typically fasting 24 h, 2 times per week). Typically, there are no "rules" during eating time.	Weight loss achieved by decreased caloric intake
Detox, cleanse, "clean eating"	Claim for quick weight loss and "cleansing the body of toxins"	Not scientifically based Not nutritionally balanced
Gluten-free	Eliminates all foods that contain gluten (wheat, grain, and barley)	Treats celiac disease and may help treat gluten sensitivity Not in itself associated with weight loss Poorly studied for those without celiac disease Could interfere with workup and diagnosis of celiac disease

Derived from U.S. News & World Report. Best diets 2022. Accessed October 31, 2022. https://health.usnews.com/best-diet.

CLINICAL PRACTICE TIP

Box 20-2. U.S. News & World Report Best Diets

Families who have questions about diets can be directed to the annual U.S. News & World Report ranking of "best diets" for a credible, comprehensive review of >30 of the most popular diets and eating plans. Each year, a panel of medical and nutrition experts reviews detailed assessments of dozens of the most popular diets. Then they rate each diet on categories including weight loss, sustainability, safety, and nutritional value. Pediatricians can encourage parents and adolescents to note that the Mediterranean-style and Dietary Approaches to Stop Hypertension eating plans consistently rank at the top of the list, as No. 1 and 2, and the fad diets consistently rank at the bottom of the list.

---

and water; and decreasing consumption of processed meats, refined grains, sugar-sweetened beverages, added sugar, trans fat, sodium, and saturated fat. This is consistent with the dietary guidelines and MyPlate recommendations (refer to chapters 11, Dietary Guidelines and Principles of Healthy Eating, and 12, Healthy Eating Plans) and the CHILD-1 eating plan detailed in **Table 20-5**. Pediatricians can provide nutritional counseling accounting for drivers of poor diet quality, which include lack of knowledge, lack of food availability, price of healthful food, scarcity of time, social and cultural norms, marketing and branding, and food taste or flavor. These considerations and how to approach coaching families through dietary changes are detailed in Part 3, Nutritional Counseling.

The primary and secondary prevention of CVD includes dietary and lifestyle changes to help optimally manage elevated blood pressure, cholesterol level, and glucose level.

Hypercholesterolemia and Dyslipidemia

Lipoprotein disorders in childhood are strongly associated with obesity and future risk of CVD. The most common dyslipidemia in childhood consists of moderate to severe increase in triglyceride levels, reduction in high-density–lipoprotein cholesterol (HDL-C) level, and normal or mild elevation of low-density–lipoprotein cholesterol (LDL-C) level. Non–HDL-C level, calculated by subtracting HDL-C from total cholesterol, leaving only the "bad" types of cholesterol, can be measured without fasting and is a significant predictor of atherosclerosis. **Table 20-8** provides reference values for low, acceptable, borderline-high, and high lipid and lipoprotein values for children and adolescents. Strong evidence supports that early identification and control of dyslipidemias in childhood and adolescence decreases CVD in adulthood.[29] The AAP recommends universal non-fasting cholesterol screening at least once for children

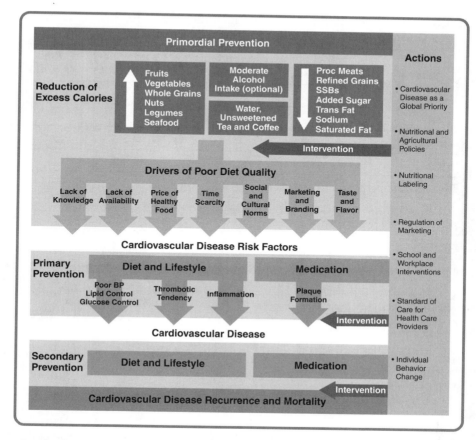

Figure 20-2. Flow diagram of the development of cardiovascular disease (CVD) and possible prevention by a healthy diet. Avoiding excess calories is an integral part of halting the development of CVD risk factors (ie, primordial prevention). Unfavorable eating patterns are driven by a variety of biological, social, economic, and psychological factors, and a robust intervention from all levels of society may steer populations toward a healthier diet and prevent disease progression. Diet and other lifestyle changes remain crucial steps in primary and secondary prevention of CVD, although the relative importance of medication and clinical procedures increases over time with disease progression.

Abbreviations: BP, blood pressure; proc, processed; SSB, sugar-sweetened beverage.
Reproduced with permission from reference 23.

Table 20-8. Low, Acceptable, Borderline-High, and High Plasma Lipid Concentrations in Children and Adolescents

Category	Low (mg/dL)[a]	Acceptable (mg/dL)	Borderline-high (mg/dL)	High (mg/dL)[a]
Total cholesterol	—	<170	170–199	≥200
LDL-C[b]	—	<110	110–129	≥130
Non–HDL-C[c]	—	<120	120–144	≥145
HDL-C	<40	>45	40–45	—
Triglycerides[b]				
0–9 y	—	<75	75–99	≥100
10–19 y	—	<90	90–129	≥130

Abbreviations: HDL-C, high-density–lipoprotein cholesterol; LDL-C, low-density–lipoprotein cholesterol.

SI conversion factor: To convert mg/dL to mmol/L, multiply by 0.0259 (cholesterol) or 0.0113 (triglycerides).

[a] Low cut points for HDL-C represent approximately the 10th percentile. The cut points for high represent approximately the 95th percentile; for borderline-high, the 75th percentile.

[b] Disregard LDL-C and triglyceride levels in a non-fasting sample. Normal and elevated levels vary by age (0–9 y vs 10–19 y).

[c] Non-fasting lipid panel, rely on non–HDL-C for interpretation. If non–HDL-C ≥145 mg/dL ± HDL-C <40 mg/dL, perform a fasting lipid panel twice, with 2 wk–3 mo between samples, and average the results.

Adapted from reference 29.

aged 9 to 11 years and in adolescents and young adults aged 17 to 21 years. Universal lipid screening is not recommended for adolescents aged 12 to 16 years because of the variability in cholesterol levels during puberty, which results in decreased sensitivity and specificity for predicting adult LDL-C levels and high rates of false-negative results in this age-group.[29,37] However, the AAP recommends that pediatricians screen for lipid disorders in children 10 years and older with obesity and of adolescents with overweight or obesity. They may also consider screening of children aged 2 to 9 years who have obesity. Although a fasting lipid panel is advised for accurate LDL-C and triglyceride values, pediatricians may obtain a non-fasting level and base recommendations on the non–HDL-C level. If levels are within reference range, a lipid panel should be repeated in 2 years. If they are abnormal, pediatricians should repeat testing every 6 to 12 months in conjunction with lifestyle treatment.[27]

Children and adolescents who have elevated LDL-C level, non–HDL-C level, or triglyceride levels benefit from progression of a CHILD-1 eating plan to the CHILD-2 eating plan, which further reduces saturated fat to 7% or less of total calories and cholesterol to 200 mg/d (**Table 20-9**). If the average LDL-C value from 2 fasting lipid panels performed 2 weeks and 3 months apart remains 190 mg/dL or greater (≥4.921 mmol/L) after a 6-month trial of CHILD-2 in children and adolescents 10 years and older, medication therapy may be considered. Low-density–lipoprotein

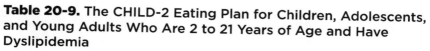

Table 20-9. The CHILD-2 Eating Plan for Children, Adolescents, and Young Adults Who Are 2 to 21 Years of Age and Have Dyslipidemia

	Elevated LDL-C level	Elevated triglyceride levels or non–HDL-C level
Referral	Registered dietitian for medical nutritional therapy	
Dietary fat composition	25%–30% calories from fat ≤7% from saturated fat 10% from monounsaturated fat <200 mg/d of cholesterol Avoidance of trans fat	
Carbohydrates		Decrease in sugar intake Replacement of simple carbohydrates with complex carbohydrates Avoidance of sugary drinks
Supportive actions	Plant sterols and stanols up to 2 g/d can be used to replace usual fat sources. They are most commonly used in pediatrics for familial hypercholesterolemia. They work by binding to cholesterol receptors and preventing cholesterol from being absorbed into the bloodstream. They decreased total cholesterol by 4%–11% and LDL-C by 7%–15% in adult studies. There are no known harmful effects. The water-soluble fiber psyllium can be used at a dose of 6 g/d for children aged 2–12 y and 12 g/d for adolescents and young adults aged >12 y.	Increase in dietary fish or initiation of supplementation to increase omega-3 fatty acids. Fish oils in adults can lower triglyceride levels by 30%–40% and raise HDL-C levels by 6%–17%. There have been no randomized controlled trials of fish oil in children, but there are no known safety concerns. Pediatricians may consider supplementation if a patient has persistent fasting triglyceride levels of ≥200–499 mg/dL or non–HDL-C levels of >145 mg/dL.

Abbreviations: HDL-C, high-density–lipoprotein cholesterol; LDL-C, low-density–lipoprotein cholesterol.

SI conversion factor: To convert mg/dL to mmol/L, multiply by 0.0259 (cholesterol) or 0.0113 (triglycerides).

Adapted from reference 29.

cholesterol cutoffs for starting medication therapy may be lower for children and adolescents with risk factors such as family history of premature CVD in first-degree relatives or high-level risk factors such as severe obesity, hypertension, and type 2 diabetes.[29]

Part 5, Frequently Asked Questions, Case Studies, and Recipes, includes recipes high in plant stanols and sterols and omega-3 fatty acids to help promote improved cholesterol levels.

Similar eating plans have shown benefit in improving lipid profile in adult populations, including the Therapeutic Lifestyle Change eating plan, which was specifically developed to improve cholesterol level; the Ornish and Mediterranean-style eating plans; and the DASH eating plan (**Table 20-10**). Although they have not been as well studied in children and adolescents, they are likely to similarly benefit the pediatric population. All these eating plans are high in vegetables, fruits, and whole grains; are moderate in protein-rich foods; are limited in added sugars; and emphasize oils over solid fats. The plans are generally lower in sodium, saturated fat, and caloric density than the typical American diet and higher in fiber and potassium. They tend to contain high amounts of cardioprotective nutrients.

Table 20-10. Cardioprotective Eating Plans

Eating plan	Details	Clinical considerations
Dietary Approaches to Stop Hypertension	High in fruits and vegetables, low-fat milk products, whole grains, fish, poultry, nuts, and lean red meats Limited intake of sugar, sweets, and sodium	Lowers systolic blood pressure by approximately 5–6 mm Hg and diastolic blood pressure by 3 mm Hg Lowers total cholesterol and LDL-C
Mediterranean-style	All variations high in fruits and vegetables, whole grains, beans, nuts, and seeds and olive oil Fish and seafood at least 2–3 times per week Moderate intake of poultry, eggs, and dairy Minimal intake of sweets and red meat Detailed more in Chapter 12, Healthy Eating Plans	Recommended in the *Dietary Guidelines for Americans* Improves cardiovascular disease markers such as weight, blood pressure, fasting glucose level, total cholesterol level, and C-reactive protein level and is associated with reduced incidence of stroke and myocardial infarction in adults
Ornish	Foods rated as most (1) to least (5) healthful, with emphasis on fruits and vegetables and whole grains Emphasizes exercise	Strong evidence for cardiovascular benefits

Table 20-10 (continued)

Eating plan	Details	Clinical considerations
Therapeutic Lifestyle Change	Developed by the National Heart, Lung, and Blood Institute specifically to help people improve cholesterol level[38] by 1. Decreasing saturated fat to <7% of calories (8%–10% reduction in LDL-C) 2. Decreasing cholesterol to <200 mg/d (3%–5% reduction in LDL-C) 3. Losing 10 lb (for adults), if the person has overweight (5%–8% reduction in LDL-C) 4. Adding 5–10 g/d of soluble fiber 5. Adding 2 g/d of plant stanols and sterols (5%–15% reduction in LDL-C)	Following these 5 recommendations leads to a 20%–30% reduction in LDL-C, on par with the lipid profile lowering noted with many cholesterol-lowering medications.

Abbreviation: LDL-C, low-density–lipoprotein cholesterol.
SI conversion factor: To convert lb to kg, multiply by 0.45.

High-Density–Lipoprotein Cholesterol

Optimal high-density–lipoprotein cholesterol (HDL-C) levels provide cardioprotective benefits, offsetting other CVD risk factors such as obesity. Few foods substantially improve HDL-C levels, although high levels of physical activity can raise HDL-C levels. Diets rich in polyunsaturated fats improve HDL-C's anti-inflammatory properties, with particular benefit from omega-3 fatty acids, which also increase overall concentration of HDL-C, especially when used to replace dietary carbohydrate.[39]

Hypertension

Hypertension is diagnosed in children and adolescents if blood pressure is at or above the 95th percentile for sex, age, and height, and/or is 130/80 mm Hg or greater for adolescents, at 3 different visits. Obesity is a significant risk factor for hypertension, especially in children with BMI at or above the 99th percentile. The AAP recommends that pediatricians monitor blood pressure at every visit for children with overweight or obesity. Obesity and hypertension are often accompanied by other cardiometabolic risk factors, such as dyslipidemia, fatty liver disease, and type 2 diabetes. The goal of treatment of pediatric hypertension is to attain a blood pressure that is less than the 90th percentile for sex, age, and height or is less than 130/80 mm Hg, whichever is lower. Most children and adolescents can achieve this goal through nutritional changes proven to treat hypertension.

The DASH Eating Plan and Nutrients That Affect Blood Pressure

The Dietary Approaches to Stop Hypertension (DASH) eating plan is a proven treatment of hypertension and should be recommended for children and adolescents who have hypertension. The main reason it is so effective is its strict limits on sodium intake. Refer to Chapter 12, Healthy Eating Plans, for a detailed description of the DASH eating plan along with strategies to support families in making dietary changes that are consistent with the plan. In addition to sodium, several other nutrients and their effects on blood pressure have been studied with mixed results. In most cases, the strength of evidence is too weak to make any definitive conclusions or recommendations. **Table 20-11**

Table 20-11. Foods and Nutrients Proposed to Affect Blood Pressure, and Related Strength of Evidence

Food/nutrient	Effect on blood pressure	Strength of evidence[a]
Sodium	↑	Strong
Omega-3 fatty acids	None	Fair
Dietary protein	Unclear	Weak
Soluble fiber	Unclear	Weak
Potassium	↓	Fair
Vitamin C	Unclear	Weak
Vitamin D	Inconclusive	Weak
Vitamin E	Unclear	Weak
Magnesium	Unclear	Weak
Calcium	↓	Fair
Fruits and vegetables	When at least 5–10 servings per day, ↓	Strong
Soy foods	Unclear	Weak
Garlic	Inconclusive	Weak
Cocoa and chocolate	Inconclusive	Weak
Caffeine	Immediate intake ↑ Long-term intake unclear	Weak

↑ indicates increases; ↓, decreases.

[a] The strength of evidence is based on the Academy of Nutrition and Dietetics "Evidence-Based Nutrition Practice Guidelines" recommendation ratings. A detailed rubric outlining criteria for ratings is available at www.andeal.org/recommendation-ratings.

Derived from Academy of Nutrition Dietetics Evidence Analysis Library. Hypertension guideline, 2008 and 2015. Accessed October 31, 2022 (registration required). https://www.andeal.org/topic.cfm?menu=5285&pcat=5140&cat=5679.

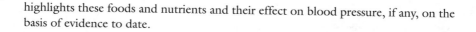

highlights these foods and nutrients and their effect on blood pressure, if any, on the basis of evidence to date.

Prediabetes and Type 2 Diabetes

Prediabetes and type 2 diabetes are increasingly common in children and adolescents because the rates and severity of childhood obesity have increased over time. The American Diabetes Association defines *prediabetes* as a hemoglobin A_{1c} level that falls between 5.7% and 6.4% (0.057 and 0.064), a fasting glucose level that falls between 100 and 125 mg/dL (5.55 and 6.94 mmol/L), or a 2-hour oral glucose tolerance test result that falls between 140 and 199 mg/dL (7.77 and 11.04 mmol/L). *Type 2 diabetes* is defined as a hemoglobin A_{1c} level of 6.5% or greater (≥ 0.065), a fasting glucose level of 126 mg/dL or greater (≥ 6.99 mmol/L), or a 2-hour oral glucose tolerance test result of 200 mg/dL or greater (≥ 11.10 mmol/L).[40] Children and adolescents with type 2 diabetes generally have a BMI at or above the 85th percentile for age and sex; a strong family history of type 2 diabetes; substantial residual insulin secretory capacity at diagnosis, reflected by typical or elevated insulin and C-peptide concentrations; insidious onset of disease; and insulin resistance, including clinical evidence of PCOS or acanthosis nigricans. Children and adolescents with type 2 diabetes have increased risk of hypertension, dyslipidemia, and NAFLD. Although a small proportion of children and adolescents have type 2 diabetes, many more have its precursor, prediabetes.

The AAP recommends that pediatricians screen children and adolescents 10 years and older who have obesity for abnormal glucose metabolism with fasting plasma glucose level, 2-hour plasma glucose level after a glucose tolerance test, or hemoglobin A_{1c} (HbA_{1c}) level. Pediatricians may also consider screening children 10 years and older who have overweight and risk factors for type 2 diabetes or NAFLD. Of note, HbA_{1c} levels can be 0.1% to 0.2% higher in children or adolescents with iron deficiency anemia. Hemoglobin A_{1c} is the preferred test for monitoring prediabetes. For children with a hemoglobin A_{1c} level of 5.7% to less than 6% and one or more risk factors for progression, the AAP recommends repeating the testing in 12 months. Otherwise, testing can be repeated in 2 years or sooner if new risk factors occur. If the HbA_{1c} level is greater than or equal to 6% to 6.4%, testing should be repeated in 3 to 6 months.

Risk factors for progression of prediabetes include severe obesity, weight gain, signs of insulin resistance such as acanthosis nigricans, and use of obesogenic psychotropic medication. Some children from racial and ethnic groups who have higher risk resulting from a combination of genetic predisposition and social determinants of health may also have increased risk of progression.[27]

For many children and adolescents, the progression of prediabetes to type 2 diabetes can be slowed or reversed with the following lifestyle changes[41]:

- Weight loss of 5% to 7% through eating regular meals and snacks; decreasing portion sizes; choosing calorie-free drinks and plain milk; increasing consumption of fruits and vegetables; consuming 3 servings of dairy per day; limiting intake of high-fat foods; limiting the frequency and size of snacks; and reducing calories from fast food.

- Physical activity of 1 hour per day, ideally of moderate to vigorous intensity. Exercise performed in shorter bouts of 10- to 15-minute increments provides equivalent benefit as continuous exercise.
- Healthy behavior changes, which include avoiding eating while watching television or using computers or smartphones; using smaller plates; and leaving small amounts of food on the plate.

The DASH, Mediterranean-style, Therapeutic Lifestyle Change, vegetarian, low glycemic, and other healthy, balanced eating plans can all improve insulin sensitivity and blood glucose level in children with prediabetes while improving cardiovascular risk profile. These lifestyle changes, together with metformin, are first-line treatment of type 2 diabetes.

Nonalcoholic Fatty Liver Disease

Approximately 38% of children with obesity have signs of nonalcoholic fatty liver disease (NAFLD), typically manifesting as an alanine aminotransferase (ALT) level that is greater than 2 times the high typical value. Children and adolescents of older age; of higher weight; of male assignment at birth; who have a sibling with NAFLD; who have prediabetes, obstructive sleep apnea, or dyslipidemia; and of Hispanic or Asian ancestry are at increased risk of developing NAFLD. Nonalcoholic fatty liver disease is a manifestation of hepatic insulin resistance, which results in hepatic inflammation that can progress to fibrosis and cirrhosis. Children and adolescents with NAFLD are at elevated risk of developing type 2 diabetes.

Weight loss is the only proven treatment of NAFLD. A sustained decrease in ALT level from baseline is a good surrogate measure of effectiveness of treatment. Additionally, interventions that decrease adiposity also improve dyslipidemia, insulin resistance, high blood pressure, and central adiposity, all of which are associated with NAFLD, type 2 diabetes, and CVD risk. All children with signs of NAFLD should be offered lifestyle behavioral intervention to help improve their diet and increase physical activity if their BMI is greater than 85%.

For adolescents, the most effective treatment includes a 5% to 10% weight loss, whereas for younger children, the goal is generally to maintain weight. Focused dietary counseling should include recommendations to avoid sugary drinks, eat a healthy and balanced diet, engage in moderate to high intensity exercise daily, and aim for less than 2 hours per day of screen time. No medications have been proven to benefit most patients with NAFLD.[42]

The AAP recommends that pediatricians check ALT levels for children 10 years and older who have overweight with risk factors for NAFLD or obesity. Higher ALT levels correlate with more advanced liver disease with steatosis and fibrosis. Pediatricians should exclude other causes of elevated ALT levels if the level is persistently at twice the upper limit of reference (ALT $\geq$ 52 IU/L for males and ALT $\geq$ 44 IU/L for females for $\geq$ 3 months or if ALT > 80 IU/L while concurrently treating the child for overweight or obesity. Other causes of elevated ALT levels include conditions such as hepatitis, autoimmune disease, or genetic disease (eg, Wilson disease, lipodystrophies,

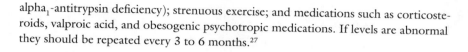

alpha$_1$-antitrypsin deficiency); strenuous exercise; and medications such as corticosteroids, valproic acid, and obesogenic psychotropic medications. If levels are abnormal they should be repeated every 3 to 6 months.[27]

Polycystic Ovary Syndrome

Polycystic ovary syndrome (PCOS) is associated with obesity and excess adiposity. Polycystic ovary syndrome in adolescence includes irregular menstrual cycles (<21 or >45 days in the 1–3 years post-menarche and <21 days or >35 days or <8 cycles per year for >3 years post-menarche, or >90 days for any one cycle) and hyperandrogenism (as assessed by calculated free testosterone level, free androgen index or bioavailable testosterone level, and clinical signs of severe acne and hirsutism). Polycystic ovary syndrome is a strong risk factor for the development of type 2 diabetes. There is a high association of PCOS with depression, anxiety, and disordered eating in women, with a likely increased prevalence among adolescents as well. In adolescents, features of PCOS that do not meet criteria for diagnosis are a risk factor for developing PCOS, and the adolescent may be monitored for the development of PCOS over time.[43]

Treatment of PCOS generally includes

- Lifestyle interventions, including attention to improved nutrition and adoption or continuance of a healthy eating plan; physical activity, including at least 60 minutes of moderate to vigorous intensity per day and at least 3 days of bone- and muscle-strengthening exercises per week; behavioral strategies, such as SMART (specific, measurable, attainable, relevant, and time-bound) goal setting, self-monitoring, and stimulus control (refer to **Table 20-6**); and minimized sedentary and screen time.
- Pharmacological treatment with a combined oral contraceptive pill and/or metformin. Treatment with a combined oral contraceptive pill alone should be considered in adolescents with a clear diagnosis of PCOS and those at risk for developing PCOS. Metformin may be considered in combination with this pill in adolescents with PCOS and obesity when lifestyle changes do not achieve desired goals and in patients with diabetes risk factors.[43]

In Sum

- Obesity increases risk of multiple cardiovascular and other related health conditions, including hypertension, hypercholesterolemia, prediabetes and type 2 diabetes, fatty liver disease, and PCOS.
- Treatment of childhood obesity and related health conditions focuses on health and behavior change goals in nutrition, physical activity, sleep, screen use, and stress management. The primary aim of childhood obesity interventions should be to optimize health, rather than focus on weight loss.[17] As changes are made that optimize health, oftentimes BMI reduction occurs as well. Certain anti-obesity medications and bariatric surgery are important parts of treatment for children with severe obesity or related conditions.
- Children and adolescents with obesity experience weight bias and stigma in multiple settings, including at home, at school, and in health care settings. Pediatricians

should actively strive to counter weight bias. They should always use people-first language (ie, *child with obesity* rather than *obese child*). When communicating with patients and families, they should use language such as *weight* and *body mass index,* rather than *obese, extremely obese, fat,* or *weight problem.* Pediatricians should also use motivational interviewing and behavioral coaching skills to support patients and families in making healthful changes; create a safe, welcoming, and non-stigmatizing clinical space that accommodates patients of diverse body sizes; and assess for behavioral health complications of weight bias, such as weight-based bullying and mental health conditions.

- The AAP recommends the CHILD-1 as the first stage for children and adolescents who have obesity and any other CVD risk or family history of early cardiac disease or diabetes or who have smoke exposure in their home. Children and adolescents who have elevated LDL-C level, non–HDL-C level, or triglyceride levels benefit from progression of a CHILD-1 eating plan to the CHILD-2 eating plan, which further reduces saturated fat to 7% or less of total calories and cholesterol to 200 mg/d.
- The DASH eating plan is a proven treatment of hypertension and should be recommended for children and adolescents who have hypertension.
- Healthy eating patterns, weight loss, and physical activity can help slow or reverse prediabetes and the progression to type 2 diabetes.
- Healthful nutrition and ample amounts of physical activity are the first-line treatments for prediabetes and NAFLD.
- Treatment of PCOS includes intensive lifestyle intervention plus medication management with oral contraceptives and/or metformin, when appropriate.

References

1. Fryar CC, Carroll MD, Afful J. Prevalence of overweight, obesity, and severe obesity among children and adolescents aged 2–19 years: United States, 1963–1965 through 2017–2018. *NCHS Health E-Stats.* 2020
2. Freedman DS, Sherry B. The validity of BMI as an indicator of body fatness and risk among children. *Pediatrics.* 2009;124(suppl 1):S23–S34 PMID: 19720664 doi: 10.1542/peds.2008-3586E
3. Centers for Disease Control and Prevention. Body mass index: considerations for practitioners. Accessed October 31, 2022. https://www.cdc.gov/obesity/downloads/bmiforpactitioners.pdf
4. Ward ZJ, Long MW, Resch SC, Giles CM, Cradock AL, Gortmaker SL. Simulation of growth trajectories of childhood obesity into adulthood. *N Engl J Med.* 2017;377(22):2145–2153 PMID: 29171811 doi: 10.1056/NEJMoa1703860
5. Geserick M, Vogel M, Gausche R, et al. Acceleration of BMI in early childhood and risk of sustained obesity. *N Engl J Med.* 2018;379(14):1303–1312 PMID: 30281992 doi: 10.1056/NEJMoa1803527
6. Ng CD, Cunningham SA. In, out, and fluctuating: obesity from adolescence to adulthood. *Ann Epidemiol.* 2020;41:14–20 PMID: 31901410 doi: 10.1016/j.annepidem.2019.12.003
7. Arnett DK, Khera A, Blumenthal RS. 2019 ACC/AHA guideline on the primary prevention of cardiovascular disease: part 1, lifestyle and behavioral factors. *JAMA Cardiol.* 2019;4(10):1043–1044 PMID: 31365022 doi: 10.1001/jamacardio.2019.2604

8. Ogden CL, Carroll MD, Fakhouri TH, et al. Prevalence of obesity among youths by household income and education level of head of household—United States 2011–2014. *MMWR Morb Mortal Wkly Rep.* 2018;67(6):186–189 PMID: 29447142 doi: 10.15585/mmwr.mm6706a3

9. Johnson JA III, Johnson AM. Urban-rural differences in childhood and adolescent obesity in the United States: a systematic review and meta-analysis. *Child Obes.* 2015;11(3):233–241 PMID: 25928227 doi: 10.1089/chi.2014.0085

10. Bell S, Deen JF, Fuentes M, et al; American Academy of Pediatrics Committee on Native American Child Health. Caring for American Indian and Alaska Native children and adolescents. *Pediatrics.* 2021;147(4):e2021050498 PMID: 33753539 doi: 10.1542/peds.2021-050498

11. Lange SJ, Kompaniyets L, Freedman DS, et al. Longitudinal trends in body mass index before and during the COVID-19 pandemic among persons aged 2–19 years—United States, 2018–2020. *MMWR Morb Mortal Wkly Rep.* 2021;70(37):1278–1283 PMID: 34529635 doi: 10.15585/mmwr.mm7037a3

12. Maes HH, Neale MC, Eaves LJ. Genetic and environmental factors in relative body weight and human adiposity. *Behav Genet.* 1997;27(4):325–351 PMID: 9519560 doi: 10.1023/A:1025635913927

13. Stunkard AJ, Foch TT, Hrubec Z. A twin study of human obesity. *JAMA.* 1986;256(1):51–54 PMID: 3712713 doi: 10.1001/jama.1986.03380010055024

14. Elks CE, den Hoed M, Zhao JH, et al. Variability in the heritability of body mass index: a systematic review and meta-regression. *Front Endocrinol (Lausanne).* 2012;3:29 PMID: 22645519 doi: 10.3389/fendo.2012.00029

15. Wood CT, Skinner AC, Yin HS, et al. Bottle size and weight gain in formula-fed infants. *Pediatrics.* 2016;138(1):e20154538 PMID: 27273748 doi: 10.1542/peds.2015-4538

16. Taveras EM, Gillman MW, Kleinman K, Rich-Edwards JW, Rifas-Shiman SL. Racial/ethnic differences in early-life risk factors for childhood obesity. *Pediatrics.* 2010;125(4):686–695 PMID: 20194284 doi: 10.1542/peds.2009-2100

17. Barlow SE; Expert Committee. Expert committee recommendations regarding the prevention, assessment, and treatment of child and adolescent overweight and obesity: summary report. *Pediatrics.* 2007;120(suppl 4):S164–S192 PMID: 18055651 doi: 10.1542/peds.2007-2329C

18. Wharton S, Raiber L, Serodio KJ, Lee J, Christensen RA. Medications that cause weight gain and alternatives in Canada: a narrative review. *Diabetes Metab Syndr Obes.* 2018;11:427–438 PMID: 30174450 doi: 10.2147/DMSO.S171365

19. van Emmerik NM, Renders CM, van de Veer M, et al. High cardiovascular risk in severely obese young children and adolescents. *Arch Dis Child.* 2012;97(9):818–821 PMID: 22826539 doi: 10.1136/archdischild-2012-301877

20. May AL, Kuklina EV, Yoon PW. Prevalence of cardiovascular disease risk factors among US adolescents, 1999–2008. *Pediatrics.* 2012;129(6):1035–1041 PMID: 22614778 doi: 10.1542/peds.2011-1082

21. Halfon N, Larson K, Slusser W. Associations between obesity and comorbid mental health, developmental, and physical health conditions in a nationally representative sample of US children aged 10 to 17. *Acad Pediatr.* 2013;13(1):6–13 PMID: 23200634 doi: 10.1016/j.acap.2012.10.007

22. Russell-Mayhew S, McVey G, Bardick A, Ireland A. Mental health, wellness, and childhood overweight/obesity. *J Obes.* 2012;2012:281801 PMID: 22778915 doi: 10.1155/2012/281801

23. Yu E, Malik VS, Hu FB. Cardiovascular disease prevention by diet modification: JACC health promotion series. *J Am Coll Cardiol.* 2018;72(8):914–926 PMID: 30115231 doi: 10.1016/j.jacc.2018.02.085

24. Puhl RM, Heuer CA. The stigma of obesity: a review and update. *Obesity (Silver Spring).* 2009;17(5):941–964 PMID: 19165161 doi: 10.1038/oby.2008.636

25. Rubino F, Puhl RM, Cummings DE, et al. Joint international consensus statement for ending stigma of obesity. *Nat Med.* 2020;26(4):485–497 PMID: 32127716 doi: 10.1038/s41591-020-0803-x

26. Pont SJ, Puhl R, Cook SR, Slusser W; American Academy of Pediatrics Section on Obesity, Obesity Society. Stigma experienced by children and adolescents with obesity. *Pediatrics.* 2017;140(6):e20173034 PMID: 29158228 doi: 10.1542/peds.2017-3034

27. Hampl SE, Hassink SG, Skinner AC, et al. Clinical practice guideline for the evaluation and treatment of children and adolescents with obesity. *Pediatrics.* 2023;151(2):e2022060640 doi: 10.1542/peds.2022-060640

28. Schwartz MW, Seeley RJ, Zeltser LM, et al. Obesity pathogenesis: an Endocrine Society scientific statement. *Endocr Rev.* 2017;38(4):267–296 PMID: 28898979 doi: 10.1210/er.2017-00111

29. Expert Panel on Integrated Guidelines for Cardiovascular Health and Risk Reduction in Children and Adolescents: summary report. *Pediatrics.* 2011;128(suppl 5):S213–S256 PMID: 22084329 doi: 10.1542/peds.2009-2107C

30. O'Reilly GA, Cook L, Spruijt-Metz D, Black DS. Mindfulness-based interventions for obesity-related eating behaviours: a literature review. *Obes Rev.* 2014;15(6):453–461 PMID: 24636206 doi: 10.1111/obr.12156

31. Grider HS, Douglas SM, Raynor HA. The influence of mindful eating and/or intuitive eating approaches on dietary intake: a systematic review. *J Acad Nutr Diet.* 2021;121(4):709–727.e1 PMID: 33279464 doi: 10.1016/j.jand.2020.10.019

32. Muth ND. Practical applications of nutrition in weight management. In: *ACE Weight Management Specialist Program.* American Council on Exercise; 2015

33. Golden NH, Schneider M, Wood C, et al; American Academy of Pediatrics Committee on Nutrition, Committee on Adolescence, and Section on Obesity. Preventing obesity and eating disorders in adolescents. *Pediatrics.* 2016;138(3):e20161649 PMID: 27550979 doi: 10.1542/peds.2016-1649

34. Ge L, Sadeghirad B, Ball GDC, et al. Comparison of dietary macronutrient patterns of 14 popular named dietary programmes for weight and cardiovascular risk factor reduction in adults: systematic review and network meta-analysis of randomised trials. *BMJ.* 2020; 369:m696 PMID: 32238384 doi: 10.1136/bmj.m696

35. Wilksch SM, O'Shea A, Ho P, Byrne S, Wade TD. The relationship between social media use and disordered eating in young adolescents. *Int J Eat Disord.* 2020;53(1):96–106 PMID: 31797420 doi: 10.1002/eat.23198

36. Johnson HM, Douglas PS, Srinivasan SR, et al. Predictors of carotid intima-media thickness progression in young adults: the Bogalusa Heart Study. *Stroke.* 2007;38(3):900–905 PMID: 17272779 doi: 10.1161/01.STR.0000258003.31194.0a

37. Daniels SR, Greer FR; American Academy of Pediatrics Committee on Nutrition. Lipid screening and cardiovascular health in childhood. *Pediatrics.* 2008;122(1):198–208 PMID: 18596007 doi: 10.1542/peds.2008-1349

38. National Heart, Lung, and Blood Institute. *Your Guide to Lowering Your Cholesterol With the Therapeutic Lifestyle Change Diet.* National Institutes of Health; 2005. NIH publication 06–5235. Accessed October 31, 2022. https://www.nhlbi.nih.gov/files/docs/public/heart/chol_tlc.pdf

39. Siri-Tarino PW. Effects of diet on high-density lipoprotein cholesterol. *Curr Atheroscler Rep.* 2011;13(6):453–460 PMID: 21901431 doi: 10.1007/s11883-011-0207-y

40. American Diabetes Association. Diagnosis and classification of diabetes mellitus. *Diabetes Care.* 2004;27(suppl 1):s5–s10 PMID: 14693921 doi: 10.2337/diacare.27.2007.S5

41. Copeland KC, Silverstein J, Moore KR, et al; American Academy of Pediatrics. Management of newly diagnosed type 2 diabetes mellitus (T2DM) in children and adolescents. *Pediatrics.* 2013;131(2):364–382 PMID: 23359574 doi: 10.1542/peds.2012-3494

42. Vos MB, Abrams SH, Barlow SE, et al. NASPGHAN clinical practice guideline for the diagnosis and treatment of nonalcoholic fatty liver disease in children: recommendations from the Expert Committee on NAFLD (ECON) and the North American Society of Pediatric Gastroenterology, Hepatology and Nutrition (NASPGHAN). *J Pediatr Gastroenterol Nutr.* 2017;64(2):319–334 PMID: 28107283 doi: 10.1097/MPG.0000000000001482

43. Teede HJ, Misso ML, Costello MF, et al; International PCOS Network. Recommendations from the international evidence-based guideline for the assessment and management of polycystic ovary syndrome. *Fertil Steril.* 2018;110(3):364–379 PMID: 30033227 doi: 10.1016/j.fertnstert.2018.05.004

CHAPTER 21

Nutrition for Common Gastrointestinal, Autoimmune, and Inflammatory Conditions

Gastrointestinal and immune-related concerns, such as constipation and food allergies, are among the most common topics of discussion between pediatricians and parents. From questions of prevention to the need for a diagnosis and treatment plan when concerning symptoms develop, nutritional guidance is an important part of these conversations. Key nutrition principles for the most common gastrointestinal and immune-related pediatric conditions are the focus of this chapter.

Constipation

Constipation is among the most common chief concerns in primary care pediatric practice. Epidemiological studies suggest that functional constipation, as defined by the Rome IV criteria (**Box 21-1**), affects 0.7% to 29.6% of children (median: 12%).[1] Studies suggest that the median age of onset of constipation is 2.3 years. Approximately 5% of infants and 9% of toddlers have functional constipation.[2] In some cases, the transition from breastfeeding to formula feeding and the introduction of solid foods can mark the onset of constipation. Overall, nutritional factors are an important component of the effective prevention and, to a lesser degree, management of functional constipation.

Priorities in treating constipation include

1. Increase the amount of fluid in the stool.
2. Propel or stimulate the stool through the colon.
3. Add bulk to the stool, which stimulates the colon to contract and push out the stool.

Nutrition strategies that can help achieve these aims include increasing fluids, fiber, fruit, and physical activity. Supplemental prebiotics and probiotics are also often used for the management of pediatric constipation, but studies have not shown clear benefit.[3] **Table 21-1** provides an overview of nutrition strategies that can help prevent and treat functional constipation, and **Table 21-2** details the role of fibers in the prevention of functional constipation. **Table 21-3** details nutrition information about fruits that aid in the prevention of functional constipation. In most cases, pharmacological management is necessary to treat functional constipation in children and adolescents, of which polyethylene glycol 3350 is first-line treatment.[3]

Certain foods can promote constipation. Examples include processed and refined carbohydrates, which are low in fiber and fluid content. Dairy products are also low in fiber and, when consumed in large amounts, can contribute to constipation. When children are consuming a large amount of milk, this amount should be cut back to the

Box 21-1. Rome IV Criteria for the Diagnosis of Functional Constipation

Children 6 mo–4 y of age

≥ 2 of the following symptoms occurring for at least 1 mo:

- ≤ 2 defecations per week
- Excessive stool retention
- Painful or hard bowel movements
- Large-diameter stools
- Large fecal mass in the rectum

In toilet-trained children,

- At least 1 episode per week of incontinence
- History of large-diameter stools that may obstruct the toilet

Children and adolescents ≥ 4 y of age

≥ 2 of the following symptoms occurring at least 1 time per week for at least 1 mo:

- ≤ 2 defecations in the toilet per week.
- At least 1 episode of fecal incontinence per week.
- History of retentive posturing or excessive volitional stool retention.
- History of painful or hard bowel movements.
- Presence of a large fecal mass in the rectum.
- History of large-diameter stools that can obstruct the toilet.
- The symptoms cannot be explained by another medical condition.

Adapted with permission from Benninga MA, Nurko S, Faure C, Hyman PE, St. James Roberts I, Schechter NL. Childhood functional gastrointestinal disorders: neonate/toddler. *Gastroenterology*. 2016;150(6)1443–1455.e2 and Hyams JS, Di Lorenzo C, Saps M, Shulman RJ, Staiano A, van Tilburg M. Childhood functional gastrointestinal disorders: children and adolescents. *Gastroenterology*. 2016;150(6)1456–1468.e2.

amount recommended for age and not completely eliminated from the diet while treating the constipation with medications.

Irritable Bowel Syndrome

Irritable bowel syndrome (IBS) is a complex pathology and falls under the umbrella of disorders of gut-brain interaction. Irritable bowel syndrome causes recurrent abdominal pain, bloating, discomfort, and changed frequency and consistency of bowel movements. The symptoms include abdominal pain at least 4 days per month for at least 2 months with one or more of the following signs: abdominal pain related to defecation,

Table 21-1. Dietary and Lifestyle Changes to Prevent and Treat Constipation in Children and Adolescents

Dietary or lifestyle change	Prevention of constipation	Treatment of constipation
Fiber	Daily fiber intake (age in years + 5 g/d at a minimum). Fibers have a laxative effect by stimulating and irritating gut mucosa to increase secretion and peristalsis. Short-chain fatty acids, the end products of fermentation of soluble dietary fibers by the gut microbiota, increase motility-stimulating bowel movements. Soluble, nonviscous, readily fermentable fibers promote bacterial growth, adding mass to stool (**Table 21-2**).	Fiber supplements or additional dietary fiber is not an effective treatment of functional constipation if adequate dietary fiber is being consumed.
Fluids	Patients should consume at least the Dietary Reference Intake–recommended total water amount (refer to **Table A-1** in the Appendix). Studies show a correlation between low fluid intake and constipation.[4]	Fluid intake beyond the Dietary Reference Intake–recommended amount is not an effective treatment of functional constipation.
Fruit	Patients should consume the *Dietary Guidelines for Americans*–recommended fruit intake to help prevent constipation. Fruits are high in fiber and may help prevent constipation (**Table 21-3**).	Several studies have shown improved constipation symptoms in children and adolescents with high fruit intake. Multiple randomized controlled trials with adult participants have shown similar benefit.[5]
Physical activity	60 min/d of physical activity helps prevent constipation.	No randomized studies have evaluated the effect of increased physical activity on the treatment of constipation.
Prebiotics and probiotics	Prebiotics from vegetables and fruits may help prevent constipation; however, supplements and probiotics do not seem to prevent constipation.	Evidence does not support prebiotic or probiotic supplementation in the treatment of constipation.

Derived from reference 3.

Table 21-2. Fibers and Other Dietary Compounds That May Help Prevent Constipation

Structure	Dietary sources
Soluble fibers, fermentable (prebiotic)	
Oligosaccharides	Chicory root, Jerusalem artichokes (sunchokes)
Fructo-oligosaccharides	Ripe bananas, artichoke, onion, asparagus, chicory
Galacto-oligosaccharides	Beans, root vegetables, dairy
Inulin oligofructose	Wheat, onion, banana, leek, artichoke, asparagus
Wheat dextrin	Products extracted from wheat starch (eg, Benefiber)
Soluble fibers, viscous	
β-Glucan	Oats, barley, flax, berries, bananas
Gums	Guar gum (fiber from the seed of the guar plant)
Pectin	Apples, citrus fruits
Psyllium	From the herb *Plantago ovata,* Metamucil
Insoluble fiber	
Cellulose and hemicellulose	Prunes, root and leafy vegetables, nuts and legumes, whole grains, skins of produce (eg, pears, apples)
Lignin	Flaxseed, whole grains, carrots, cauliflower, broccoli, tomatoes, strawberries, peaches
Other	
Sennoside A (stimulant)	Rhubarb, senna plant (The leaves of the senna fruit are used to create senna–docusate sodium laxative.)
Sorbitol (osmotic laxative)	Stone fruits (plums, prunes, peaches, nectarines, apricots, cherries, and dates) and pome fruit (apples and pears)
Ficain (enzyme)	Figs
Actinidin (enzyme)	Kiwifruit

changed frequency of stool, and/or changed form (appearance) of stool. In children and adolescents who have constipation caused by IBS, the pain does not resolve with resolution of the constipation. If the pain does resolve with resolution of the constipation, the patient has functional constipation, not IBS. Children and adolescents with suspected IBS should be fully medically evaluated and not be diagnosed with IBS unless the symptoms cannot be explained by another medical condition after appropriate evaluation.[6]

Table 21-3. Fiber, Sugar, and Caloric Content in Fruits

Fruit source	Serving size	Estimated fiber components					Sugar (starch) (100-g)	Energy density (kcal/g)	Energy (kcal) (100-g)
		Total (100-g)	Insoluble (100-g)	Soluble (100-g)	Pectin (100-g)				
Fresh fruit									
Apples	1 (182 g)	2.4	1.7	0.5	0.8	10	0.5	52
Avocados	⅓ (50 g)	6.8	4.4	2.4	2.4	<1.0	1.6	160
Bananas	1 (118 g)	2.6	1.8	0.8	0.6	12 (5)	0.9	89
Blackberries	1 cup (144 g)	5.3	4.7	0.6	1.4	4.9	0.4	43
Blueberries	1 cup (148 g)	2.8	2.4	0.3	0.8	10	0.6	57
Cherries	1 cup (138 g)	2.2	1.6	0.6	0.7	13	0.6	63
Figs	1 (100 g)	3.0	2.4	0.6	1.0	16	0.7	74
Grapefruits	1 cup (154 g)	1.6	1.1	0.5	0.6	7.0	0.4	42
Guavas	1 cup (165 g)	5.4	4.2	1.8	1.5	9.0	0.7	68
Kiwis	2 (138 g)	3.0	2.2	0.9	0.7	9.0	0.6	61
Mangoes	1 cup (165 g)	1.6	1.0	0.6	0.5	14	0.6	60
Oranges	1 (131 g)	2.4	1.4	1.0	0.8	9.1	0.5	47
Papayas	1 cup (145 g)	1.7	1.4	0.3	0.5	7.6	0.4	43
Pears	1 (166 g)	3.1	2.2	0.9	1.0	10	0.6	60

Continued

Table 21-3 (*continued*)

Fruit source	Serving size	Estimated fiber components							
		Total (100-g)	Insoluble (100-g)	Soluble (100-g)	Pectin (100-g)	Sugar (starch) (100-g)	Energy density (kcal/g)	Energy (kcal) (100-g)
Fresh fruit (*continued*)								
Plantains	½ (134 g)	2.2	1.5	0.7	0.4	2.2 (30)	1.5	149
Pomegranate arils	1 cup (122 g)	5.7	4.1	1.6	2.0	12	0.8	81
Raspberries	1 cup (123 g)	6.5	5.3	1.2	1.6	4.4	0.5	52
Strawberries	1 cup (152 g)	2.0	1.5	0.5	0.7	4.7	0.3	33
Apricots	2 (70 g)	2.0	1.0	1.0	0.7	9.1	0.5	49
Cantaloupes	1 cup (177 g)	0.9	0.6	0.3	0.3	7.9	0.3	34
Green grapes	1 cup (92 g)	0.9	0.6	0.3	0.2	17	0.7	69
Peaches	1 (150 g)	1.5	0.9	0.6	0.5	9.0	0.4	39
Pineapples	1 cup (165 g)	1.4	1.1	0.3	0.5	10	0.5	50
Plums	2 (132 g)	1.4	0.9	0.5	0.4	11	0.5	45
Watermelons	1 wedge (286 g)	0.4	0.3	0.1	0.1	6.3	0.3	29

Dried fruit

Apricots	6 (40 g)	10	7.5	2.5	3.0	37	2.6	258
Cranberries	¼ cup (40 g)	7.5	5.0	2.5	2.5	72	3.3	325
Dates, pitted	5–6 (40 g)	7.5	6.0	1.5	2.5	72	3.0	300
Dried figs	⅓ cup (40 g)	12	8.8	37	4.3	50	2.8	275
Prunes	7 (40 g)	7.5	5.0	2.5	2.5	37	2.5	250
Raisins	¼ cup (40 g)	5.0	3.7	1.2	1.7	73	3.0	300

Reproduced with permission from reference 5.

A diet low in fermentable oligosaccharides, disaccharides, monosaccharides, and polyols (FODMAP) may help relieve symptoms. FODMAPs are short-chain, poorly absorbed, highly fermentable carbohydrates found in wheat, onions, some fruits and vegetables, sorbitol, and some dairy products. FODMAPs increase colonic water secretion, which may contribute to diarrhea. Additionally, the high rate of fermentation by the gut microbiota leads to increased production of short-chain fatty acids and gas, which may contribute to a patient's experience of abdominal pain, bloating, and flatulence. The low FODMAP diet is generally implemented in 3 phases, starting with restriction, followed by reintroduction and personalization for long-term management. A FODMAP-gentle eating plan focuses on avoidance of the foods most highly concentrated in FODMAPs. This approach is advised for children and adolescents to help prevent over-restriction and nutritional inadequacy while providing clinical benefit from reducing FODMAP intake (**Table 21-4**).[7] A low FODMAP diet is very restrictive and should not be suggested to children with poor nutritional status or risk factors for restrictive eating. Also, such a diet should be implemented only with guidance from a registered dietitian.

Gastroesophageal Reflux

Gastroesophageal reflux is defined as the passage of stomach contents into the esophagus with or without regurgitation and vomiting. Gastroesophageal reflux disease (GERD) results when reflux leads to troubling symptoms that affect daily functioning and/or leads to complications.[8] Nutritional changes are an important component of therapy for infants, children, and adolescents with signs and symptoms of GERD (**Box 21-2**).

Inflammatory Bowel Disease

Inflammatory bowel disease (IBD) exists on a spectrum and includes Crohn disease and ulcerative colitis, both of which are relapsing and remitting chronic inflammatory diseases that are usually first diagnosed in adolescence or young adulthood, although they can occur at any stage in life. The first signs of IBD usually include abdominal

Table 21-4. FODMAP Gentle Eating Plan

Food group	Food to restrict	FODMAP of concern
Grains	Wheat, rye	Fructosans (oligosaccharide)
Vegetables	Onion, leek	Fructosans (oligosaccharide)
	Cauliflower, mushrooms	Polyols
Fruits	Apple, pear, dried fruit, stone fruit, watermelon	Fructose (monosaccharide)
Dairy	Milk and yogurt	Lactose (disaccharide)
Protein	Legumes	Galacto-oligosaccharides

Abbreviation: FODMAP, fermentable oligosaccharide, disaccharide, monosaccharide, and polyol.
Adapted with permission from reference 7.

Box 21-2. Nutritional Treatment of Gastroesophageal Reflux Disease

Infants	Children and adolescents
Thickened feedings	A Mediterranean-style eating plan may be beneficial.[9]
Reduced feeding volume	Weight loss if obesity is present
More frequent feedings	Avoidance of late-night eating
Cow milk may be a trigger for gastroesophageal reflux disease in some infants, but this is not an allergy. Trial elimination of cow milk protein for 2 wk. During this trial, formula-fed infants may benefit from transitioning to an extensively hydrolyzed milk formula or amino acid–based formula. If symptoms improve, they should be followed closely, with reintroduction of cow milk protein and monitoring for recurrence. If symptoms do not improve during the trial, cow milk protein should be resumed.	Avoidance of food and beverages that trigger gastroesophageal reflux disease symptoms. These foods and beverages may vary, but common triggers include spicy food, chocolate, citrus fruits, tomatoes, caffeinated drinks, and peppermint.
Breastfed infants may benefit from maternal elimination of all dairy, including casein and whey.[8] Trial for 2 wk. If symptoms improve, they should be followed closely, with reintroduction of maternal dairy and monitoring for recurrence. If symptoms do not improve during the trial, maternal dairy intake should be resumed.	
The infant should be kept upright following feedings.	
Prebiotics and probiotics have not been adequately studied to provide a recommendation.	

pain, diarrhea, bloody stool, and weight loss; however, about 20% of the time, IBD first manifests with non-classic symptoms, such as poor growth or anemia. The cause of IBD is not fully understood, but some combination of genetic, environmental, and microbial factors converge, creating a dysregulated immune response to the gut microbiota. Risk factors for IBD include birth by cesarean delivery, lack of exposure to human (breast) milk, high intake of dietary fat, low intake of dietary fiber, and early exposure to antibiotics.[10]

Nutritional factors play an important role in the management of IBD. During exacerbation or a disease flare, low fiber intake may be necessary. Exclusive enteral feeding with liquid formula for 8 to 12 weeks is as effective as corticosteroids in inducing remission in children with Crohn disease.[10] During remission, nutritional management for both ulcerative colitis and Crohn disease is focused on preventing severe nutritional deficiency, insufficient caloric intake, increased nutrient losses from the gut, and drug-nutrient interactions. Encouraging a high-calorie diet with a particular emphasis on iron (ie, lean beef, beans), calcium (dairy products), vitamin D (fortified dairy products or supplementation), folate (ie, dark leafy greens, fortified grains, strawberries), vitamin B_{12} (lean beef and other meat products), and zinc (ie, seafood, spinach) intake is important in the nutritional management for children and adolescents with IBD.[11]

Celiac Disease and Gluten Sensitivity
Celiac disease is an autoimmune disease triggered by the ingestion of gluten in genetically predisposed individuals. About 40% of the population carries the genotype HLA-DQ2 or HLA-DQ8, which is required for the development of celiac disease, but just 2% to 3% of carriers, or about 1% of the total population, experience celiac disease, which can first develop at any age. Children who have celiac disease are at risk for other autoimmune diseases, such as type 1 diabetes and thyroid disease (eg, autoimmune thyroiditis, Hashimoto thyroiditis).

Gluten is present in all food products made from wheat, barley, rye, and oats contaminated with gluten (**Box 21-3**). Gluten is a protein compound made up of gliadin and glutenin proteins joined with starch. Intestinal enzymes are able to only partially digest gluten. The partially digested gluten produces a mix of peptides that can trigger an immune response, causing blunting of the small intestinal villi and negatively affecting nutrient absorption. When the gut is unable to absorb nutrients, vitamin deficiency, anemia, weight loss, and diarrhea occur. Other symptoms include abdominal pain and distention. Celiac disease can be diagnosed through serum screening with tissue transglutaminase and total immunoglobulin A and through biopsy of the small intestine. The only definitive treatment of the disease is strict avoidance of gluten-containing foods.[12]

Non-celiac Gluten Sensitivity
Non-celiac gluten sensitivity manifests with symptoms such as tiredness, abdominal pain, diarrhea, or constipation after consumption of gluten-containing grains. The

Box 21-3. Gluten-Containing and Gluten-free Grains

Gluten-containing grains	Gluten-free grains
Wheat	Rice
Barley	Corn
Rye	Soy
Contaminated oats	Tapioca
	Quinoa
	Millet
	Buckwheat
	Flax
	Nut flours
	Uncontaminated oats

symptoms improve when gluten is removed from the diet and recur when gluten is reintroduced. It is unclear what causes these symptoms or the body's actual response to the gluten. Although there is limited research explaining the role of gluten in causing gastrointestinal symptoms, preliminary evidence suggests that although some people without celiac disease may experience gluten sensitivity, the number of people who have a physiological reaction to gluten is probably much smaller than the number of people who perceive benefit from a gluten-free diet. Because gluten is only partially digested and because gluten-containing grains such as wheat are also a source of FODMAPs, there may be some overlap between non-celiac gluten sensitivity and IBS. Children and adolescents with presumed non-celiac gluten sensitivity may benefit from following a gluten-free and fructosan-free diet for 6 weeks and then undergoing retesting of gluten tolerance.[13]

Gluten-free Nutrition Considerations

Many foods contain gluten, so without appropriate dietary planning, complete elimination of gluten from the diet can lead to nutritional deficiency of B vitamins, calcium, vitamin D, iron, zinc, magnesium, and/or fiber. Most standard grains, such as bread, cereal, and pasta, contain wheat, rye, or barley and thus include gluten. Additionally, more than 25% of children with celiac disease exhibit high rates of nutrient deficiencies at diagnosis, including iron (28%), folate (14%), vitamin B_{12} (1%), and vitamin D (27%).[12]

Although a poorly planned gluten-free diet can lead to micronutrient deficiencies, with appropriate planning, a child or an adolescent can safely follow a gluten-free diet without risk to nutritional adequacy. Although gluten is present in many foods, an increasing number of gluten-free products are on the market and are clearly labeled "gluten-free." Bread, pasta, cereal, and various other products that typically contain gluten have been reformulated into gluten-free products, although these products tend to cost more than their gluten-containing counterparts.

Of note, although a gluten-free diet is essential for a patient with celiac disease and may help reduce symptoms in a patient with non-celiac gluten sensitivity, a gluten-free diet is neither recommended nor effective as a method to lose weight or improve health. A gluten-free diet is restrictive and can lead to serious vitamin deficiencies. It may also contribute to disordered eating behaviors.

Food Allergies

Up to 8% of children in the United States have food allergies. The 9 most common food allergens, which account for more than 90% of all allergic reactions, are milk, eggs, peanuts, tree nuts (eg, almonds, cashews, walnuts), shellfish, fish, soy, wheat, and sesame.[14,15] More detailed information about the most common food allergens is high-lighted in **Table 21-5**. The US Food and Drug Administration requires that all food products containing any of the most common food allergens as an ingredient list the specific allergen on the product label.

Food allergies can be categorized according to the kind of immunoglobulin E (IgE) reaction: IgE-mediated, non–IgE-mediated, or mixed.

IgE-Mediated Reactions

IgE-mediated reactions are type 1 hypersensitivity reactions. For IgE-mediated food allergies, symptom onset after sensitization is typically immediate (minutes to <2 hours) because of the IgE-mediated release of antibodies that results in mast cell degranulation and release of histamine and inflammatory mediators, causing local and/or systemic inflammation. Symptoms may include hives, angioedema, cough, wheezing, congestion, vomiting, abdominal pain, hypotension, or anaphylaxis.

Risk Factors and Prevention of IgE-Mediated Food Allergies

Infants with severe eczema have the highest risk of developing an IgE-mediated food allergy. Risk is also increased in infants with mild to moderate eczema, other known food allergies, and genetic predisposition, including allergic disease in a first-degree relative. In some cases, infants with no known risk factors experience food allergies. As described in Chapter 16, Nutrition in Infancy, the Learning Early About Peanut clinical trial showed that offering infants with egg allergy and/or severe atopic dermatitis at least 6 g of peanut protein over 3 or more meals per week decreased the risk of peanut allergy. Only 3% of babies who had risk factors for peanut allergy and regularly consumed peanut developed allergy by age 5 years, compared to 17% of babies who avoided peanut.[23] Following **Table 21-5** is advice from the American Academy of Pediatrics to help in the primary prevention of atopic diseases.

Table 21-5. Facts About the Most Common Food Allergens in Children

Allergen	Prevalence (approximate)	Clinical considerations
Egg	1.3% in children <5 y of age; 0.9% in all children[16]	<ul><li>Most children and adolescents who are allergic to concentrated egg can tolerate baked egg in a muffin or waffle.</li><li>Egg allergy is associated with increased rates of asthma, eczema, and allergic rhinitis.</li><li>Many children with egg allergy are also allergic to other foods, most commonly, milk and peanut.</li><li>Egg is the most common trigger for anaphylaxis in infants.</li><li>About half of children outgrow egg allergy by 6 y of age.[17]</li></ul>
Milk	1.9%	<ul><li>Milk frequently triggers immunoglobulin E reactions, mediated and non-mediated.</li><li>In infants, human (breast) milk is the preferred nutrition source. When breastfeeding is not possible, extensively hydrolyzed casein formula is recommended for mild to moderate cow milk allergy. In the case of severe cow milk allergy, including when there has been anaphylaxis, failure to thrive, or poor response to extensively hydrolyzed casein formula, amino acid formulas are recommended.[18]</li><li>Most children and adolescents who are allergic to milk are able to tolerate baked milk.</li><li>Most children outgrow milk allergy by early adolescence.</li></ul>
Peanut	2.2%	<ul><li>Peanut is the most common food allergen.</li><li>Peanut allergy is associated with egg allergy and severe atopic dermatitis.</li><li>Peanut allergy poses increased risk for severe allergic reaction.</li><li>Peanut allergy is usually not outgrown.</li></ul>
Tree nut (almond, Brazil nut, cashew, hazelnut, pecan, pistachio, or walnut)	1.2%	<ul><li>Rates of almond, cashew, walnut, pecan, and hazelnut allergies are similar (about 0.6%).</li><li>Cashew and pistachio are closely related to each other, and pecan and walnut are closely related to each other.</li><li>Tree nuts pose increased risk for severe allergic reaction.</li><li>Approximately 10%–15% of children and adolescents with tree nut allergies outgrow them over time.</li></ul>

Continued

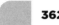

Table 21-5 (*continued*)

Allergen	Prevalence (approximate)	Clinical considerations
Soy	0.3%	Nearly half of children outgrow soy allergy by 6 y of age.
Wheat	0.2%–1.0%	Mean age of resolution of wheat allergy is 6.5 y.
Fish and shellfish	0.6% for finfish and 1.3% for shellfish[19]	<ul><li>Shrimp, crab, and lobster are the most common shellfish allergies.</li><li>Shellfish pose increased risk for severe allergic reaction.</li><li>Any food in a restaurant that serves shellfish may contain shellfish because of cross contact.</li><li>Very few children and adolescents outgrow fish or shellfish allergy.</li></ul>
Sesame	0.1%–0.2%[15]	<ul><li>Sesame is the most common seed to cause hypersensitivity reaction.</li><li>Serological and clinical cross-reactivity with peanut and tree nuts is common.</li><li>As of January 1, 2023, sesame is required to be included as an allergen on food labels.</li><li>20%–30% of children outgrow sesame allergy.[15]</li></ul>

Derived from references 14 and 19–22.

Do recommend

- Exclusive breastfeeding for at least 3 to 4 months, to reduce the risk of eczema, and breastfeeding (even if not exclusively) for longer, to protect against wheezing and asthma
- Introduction of complementary foods between 4 and 6 months of age, including allergenic foods such as peanuts, eggs, and fish

Do not recommend

- Avoidance diets during pregnancy and lactation
- Partially or extensively hydrolyzed formula in an attempt to prevent atopic disease[24]

Oral Allergy Syndrome

Oral allergy syndrome (pollen food allergy syndrome) occurs in some children and adolescents who have allergic rhinitis caused by cross-reacting allergens found in pollens and in raw fruits, vegetables, or tree nuts. Swelling of the lips, tongue, and throat; watery, itchy eyes; runny nose; sneezing; and itchy ears occur immediately following ingestion of the protein. Symptoms are usually confined to the mouth and face because the triggering protein passes quickly through the digestive process once the food is swallowed. Although oral allergy symptoms do not usually progress, systemic reactions can and do occur. The triggering protein is heat labile, so cooking or processing of the fruits and vegetables easily breaks down the proteins in them that cause oral allergy syndrome; thus, the allergic reaction does not occur with intake of cooked, baked, or processed fruits and vegetables.

Children and adolescents with birch pollen allergy are more likely to have a reaction to raw almond, carrot, celery, cherry, hazelnut, kiwifruit, peach, pear, and plum. Children and adolescents with grass pollen allergy are more likely to have a reaction to celery, melons, oranges, peaches, and tomato. Those with ragweed pollen allergy are more likely to have a reaction to banana, cucumbers, melons, sunflower seeds, and zucchini. Children with pollen allergy are not advised to avoid these fruits and vegetables. Rather, they should avoid consumption of only the raw forms of the foods that cause symptoms. Oral allergy syndrome is rare in children younger than 3 years, because in children of this age, allergic rhinitis often has not yet developed.[25]

Non–IgE-Mediated Reactions

Non–IgE-mediated reactions are cell-mediated reactions with a delayed onset of symptoms of 2 or more hours following exposure. They are characterized by subacute or chronic gut inflammation. The most common non–IgE-mediated conditions that pediatricians will encounter and that are described in detail in this section include food protein–induced enterocolitis syndrome (FPIES), food protein–induced allergic proctocolitis (FPIAP), food protein–induced enteropathy (FPE), and the eosinophilic gastrointestinal disorders such as eosinophilic esophagitis (EoE).[26] Other non–IgE-mediated reactions include food protein–induced GERD and constipation (described in the Gastroesophageal Reflux and Constipation sections earlier in this chapter) and the extremely rare Heiner syndrome (cow milk–induced pulmonary disease).

Food Protein–Induced Enterocolitis Syndrome

Food protein–induced enterocolitis syndrome (FPIES) is a non–IgE-mediated food allergy characterized by vomiting and diarrhea following acute or repeated consumption of a specific food. The most common triggers are cow milk, soy, rice, barley, oats, chicken, turkey, and fish. FPIES is classified as acute or chronic. Acute FPIES manifests with repetitive, profuse, and protracted vomiting 1 to 4 hours after ingestion of the triggering food. Vomiting is generally followed by watery diarrhea. Symptoms can progress to cause dehydration, pallor, lethargy, and hypovolemic shock. They generally resolve within 24 hours as long as the offending food is not reintroduced. Chronic FPIES manifests as intermittent but progressive vomiting and watery diarrhea, which can lead to weight loss, failure to thrive, dehydration, and lethargy. It typically results from repeated ingestion of the offending food, which is usually cow milk or soy-based formula. Diagnosis is clinical on the basis of history and response to elimination of the triggering food. Characteristics of acute and chronic FPIES are shown in **Table 21-6**.[27]

Because of the delayed manifestation of symptoms, because of the nonspecific laboratory findings, and because blood and skin-prick test results for allergies are typically negative, FPIES is difficult to diagnose. Clinicians often mistake FPIES for recurrent episodes of severe gastroenteritis or suspected sepsis. FPIES typically first develops in infancy after the introduction of milk- or soy-based formula, although it can also first occur around 4 to 6 months of age, when an infant starts to eat rice, oats, and barley. FPIES is rare among exclusively breastfed infants.

Table 21-6. Features of Acute and Chronic FPIES

	Acute FPIES	Chronic FPIES
Age of onset	2–7 mo	
Symptom onset	Follows intermittent food exposures and includes vomiting (within 1–4 h), diarrhea (within 24 h), lethargy, and pallor	Follows daily food ingestion and includes vomiting (within hours), diarrhea (within 24 h, usually 5–10 h after ingestion, and may be chronic), poor weight gain, and malnutrition
Clinical features	Vomiting, pallor, lethargy without skin or respiratory symptoms May also include watery or bloody diarrhea, hypotension, abdominal distention, or hypothermia	Intermittent but progressive vomiting and diarrhea, dehydration, metabolic acidosis, poor weight gain, and malnutrition
Laboratory findings	Leukocytosis, neutrophilia, thrombocytosis, metabolic acidosis, methemoglobinemia	
Medical treatment	Mild symptoms • Oral rehydration • Ondansetron (for ages ≥6 mo) • Close monitoring at home for 4–6 h from onset of symptoms Moderate or severe symptoms (>3 episodes of vomiting or lethargy) • Emergency care and/or hospitalization may be required. • Aggressive fluid resuscitation • Single dose of intravenous methylprednisolone • Ondansetron • Close attention to electrolyte abnormalities (eg, acidemia) • Correction of methemoglobinemia • Intensive cardiorespiratory support if hypovolemic shock	Supportive care based on clinical signs and symptoms

Table 21-6 (*continued*)

	Acute FPIES	**Chronic FPIES**
Medical nutritional therapy	Elimination of triggering food Use of extensively hydrolyzed or amino acid–based formula or breastfeeding Guided introduction of low-risk solid foods, progressing to moderate and higher-risk solid foods with close supervision (**Table 21-7**)	
Symptom resolution	Resolves within 24 h after food elimination	Resolves within 3–10 d of food elimination and switch to hypoallergenic formula
Average age of resolution based on triggering food	Soy: 12 mo (range: 6 mo to >22 y) Grains: 35 mo Milk: 3 y Other solid foods: 42 mo	

Abbreviation: FPIES, food protein–induced enterocolitis syndrome.

Adapted with permission from reference 27: *ImmunoTargets Ther.* 2021;10:431–446. Originally published by and used with permission from Dove Medical Press Ltd.

Untreated FPIES can result in growth failure, dehydration, lethargy, hypothermia, and hypotension. Treatment is symptomatic care as detailed in **Table 21-6** and avoidance of the triggering food. Infants who are formula fed and have FPIES should be transitioned to hypoallergenic formula, and infants who are consuming solid foods should have guided introduction of low-risk solid foods, progressing to moderate-risk and more high-risk solid foods under close supervision (**Table 21-7**).[27] Clinicians should ensure close follow-up of patients with FPIES, ideally with support of an allergist and a registered dietitian to ensure adequate growth and nutritional status and a gradual reintroduction of potential triggering foods over time as the patient develops tolerance.[28,29] FPIES is generally outgrown by 1 to 5 years of age. Allergists will typically conduct an oral food challenge around 12 to 18 months after the most recent reaction to assess whether a child has outgrown FPIES.[30]

Food Protein–Induced Allergic Proctocolitis

Food protein–induced allergic proctocolitis (FPIAP) is a common cause of bloody stools in an otherwise well-appearing infant. It usually appears in the first few weeks to months after birth, most often in exclusively breastfed infants. Cow milk and soy protein are the most common triggers, although sometimes, egg, corn, or wheat can trigger FPIAP. Bloody stools generally resolve within 72 to 96 hours from maternal elimination of the triggering food. Pediatricians may advise a breastfeeding mother to eliminate dairy and soy from her diet. If the infant's bloody stools subsequently resolve, cow milk or soy was the most likely trigger. If the bloody stools do not resolve, the mother may next trial egg elimination—and so on. Food protein–induced allergic proctocolitis usually resolves by 1 to 2 years of age, if not sooner.[29]

Table 21-7. Empirical Guidelines for Selecting Weaning Foods in Infants With FPIES

Food group	Low-risk foods	Moderate-risk foods	High-risk foods
Vegetables	Broccoli Cauliflower Parsnip Turnip Pumpkin	Squash Carrot White potato Green bean (legume)	Sweet potato Green pea (legume)
Fruits	Blueberries Strawberries Plum Watermelon Peach Avocado	Apple Pear Orange	Banana
Grains	Fortified quinoa cereal Millet	Grits and corn cereal Wheat Barley cereal	Infant rice cereal Infant oat cereal Soy
Protein	Lamb Tree nuts and seed butters	Peanut and other legumes (other than green pea) Beef	Poultry Egg Fish
Dairy			Milk

Abbreviation: FPIES, food protein–induced enterocolitis syndrome.

Adapted with permission from reference 30.

Food Protein–Induced Enteropathy

Food protein–induced enteropathy (FPE) is an uncommon condition that typically manifests with symptoms of chronic diarrhea, steatorrhea, and failure to thrive in a formula-fed infant once the infant transitions to cow milk, although FPE can also be triggered by soy, wheat, and egg. Symptoms resolve with the elimination of cow milk or other triggering food. Like FPIAP, FPE generally resolves between 1 and 2 years of age.[29]

Eosinophilic Esophagitis

Eosinophilic esophagitis (EoE) occurs when eosinophils infiltrate the esophagus and release cytokines, which inflame the esophagus. Most of the time, EoE results from a delayed immune-mediated reaction to dairy, egg, soy, or wheat intake in a child or adolescent who has atopy, although other foods and environmental allergens can also trigger EoE. Unlike symptoms of IgE-mediated food allergies, symptoms of EoE do not occur immediately following ingestion of the causative antigen. Instead, they can develop over days after exposure.

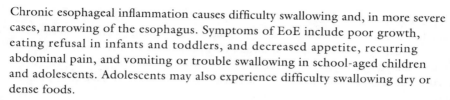

Chronic esophageal inflammation causes difficulty swallowing and, in more severe cases, narrowing of the esophagus. Symptoms of EoE include poor growth, eating refusal in infants and toddlers, and decreased appetite, recurring abdominal pain, and vomiting or trouble swallowing in school-aged children and adolescents. Adolescents may also experience difficulty swallowing dry or dense foods.

Gastroenterologists diagnose EoE by esophageal biopsy during endoscopy. Eosinophils are not typically present in the esophagus. The presence of greater than 15 eosinophils per high-power field on biopsy indicates EoE if the clinical manifestation is consistent with the condition and once other causes of eosinophilic presence in the esophagus are ruled out. Once the diagnosis is made and the causative food-based antigen is eliminated, symptoms typically improve within a few weeks. Eosinophilic esophagitis is a manageable lifelong diagnosis.

In many cases, children and adolescents with EoE are advised to follow an elimination diet in which they eliminate either 1 (milk), 2 (milk and wheat), 4 (milk, wheat, egg, and soy), or 6 (milk, egg, soy, wheat, peanuts/tree nuts, and fish/shellfish) of the major food allergens until symptoms resolve (approximately 6–8 weeks) and then gradually add the foods back to their diets, one at a time, with follow-up endoscopies to identify the causative food. The preferential order and number of specific antigens to avoid and the order of reintroduction are an area of active investigation.[31] Food allergy testing is unhelpful in identifying the causative agents of EoE. Children and adolescents who follow an elimination diet should be referred to a registered dietitian who is experienced in food allergies and EoE to help ensure adequate caloric and nutrient intake.[26] Initial treatment of EoE is typically dietary changes or pharmacological therapy, which may include swallowed topical corticosteroids (eg, fluticasone, budesonide), proton pump inhibitors, and/or the monoclonal antibody dupilumab, which was approved by the US Food and Drug Administration in 2022 as the first treatment approved specifically for EoE.

Food Intolerance

Food intolerance is not a food allergy. Rather, food intolerance often results from a deficiency in an enzyme that is needed to break down a food. For example, lactose intolerance results from a deficiency in the enzyme lactase, which is necessary to digest the sugar. Undigested lactose can cause gastrointestinal symptoms such as abdominal pain, bloating, and diarrhea. Another fairly common food intolerance is fructose intolerance, or fructose malabsorption. This results from an ineffective carrier protein that impedes the absorption of fructose in the small intestine. Children and adolescents with fructose malabsorption experience gastrointestinal symptoms such as bloating, abdominal pain, vomiting, and flatulence after eating fructose-containing foods. Foods high in fructose include many fruits, some vegetables, and processed foods containing high-fructose corn syrup. Lactose intolerance and fructose intolerance are detailed more in Chapter 2, Carbohydrates. Unlike with food allergy, the immune system plays no role in the dysfunction of food intolerance, and symptoms are not life threatening.

Type 1 Diabetes

Type 1 diabetes is an autoimmune disorder that is characterized by insulin deficiency and chronic hyperglycemia. Therapy includes daily exogenous, subcutaneous long-acting insulin injections and short-acting insulin boluses to correct glucose spikes and to cover for carbohydrate intake. The management of type 1 diabetes includes medical nutritional therapy, exercise, and medication.

The goals of medical nutritional therapy are to regulate glucose level, blood pressure, and lipid levels and to maintain a healthy weight and growth.[22] Most children with type 1 diabetes follow an individualized insulin to carbohydrate ratio in which preprandial insulin dosing is matched to carbohydrate intake. The insulin to carbohydrate ratio is individualized on the basis of the child's age, sex, pubertal status, diagnosis duration, and physical activity level. Children and families learn to quantify carbohydrate intake on the basis of carbohydrate gram increments, 10- to 12-g carbohydrate portions, and/or 15-g carbohydrate exchanges. For instance, a serving of most grains, starchy vegetables, beans, and fruits is about 15 g of carbohydrate, 8 fl oz (237 mL) of milk is 12 g, and a serving of non-starchy vegetables is about 5 g. Generally, an insulin bolus of 1 U per 12 to 15 g of carbohydrates consumed is given 15 to 20 minutes before eating.

Nutrition education and nutritional management for a child with type 1 diabetes are part of the multidisciplinary comprehensive care provided by diabetes specialty clinics, which include the support of a highly trained and experienced registered dietitian and certified diabetes educators. Overall recommended macronutrient distribution, micronutrient needs, and physical activity recommendations to promote optimal health are the same for children with type 1 diabetes as for other children. Dietary management for children and adolescents with type 1 diabetes should be individualized, considering family habits, food preferences, religious or cultural needs, schedules, physical activity, and family health literacy and self-management skills.[32] Pediatricians should be aware that adolescent girls with type 1 diabetes exhibit higher rates of disordered eating patterns (eg, fasting, binge eating, and purging) than their peers without type 1 diabetes. In an adolescent, disordered eating is a risk factor for poor diabetes management. Key nutrition, physical activity, and self-management principles for pediatricians to consider when helping children with type 1 diabetes optimize blood glucose control, reduce health risks, and improve overall quality of life are highlighted in **Table 21-8**.

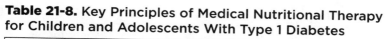

Table 21-8. Key Principles of Medical Nutritional Therapy for Children and Adolescents With Type 1 Diabetes

Lifestyle factor	Key principles	Recommendations for the primary care pediatrician
Nutritional therapy	• Individualized medical nutritional therapy • Monitoring of carbohydrate intake to achieve optimal glycemic control • Comprehensive nutrition education at diagnosis followed by annual updates with an experienced registered dietitian • Healthy, balanced lifelong eating patterns incorporating social, cultural, and psychological well-being • Healthy habits including regular physical activity, healthy weight, and healthy relationship with food • Routine of 3 meals per day and 2–3 healthy snacks (avoidance of grazing) • Meeting of nutritional macronutrient and micronutrient needs • Reduction of risk of microvascular and macrovascular complications	• Encourage families to make and keep appointments with registered dietitian and multidisciplinary diabetes team. • Encourage family-level changes to prevent isolation or resentment on the part of the child or adolescent if they have to make changes the rest of the family is not making; encourage incorporation of the child's or adolescent's favorite foods. • Encourage families to engage children in food choices and preparation and in age-appropriate nutrition education and understanding of diabetes. • Help families prepare for adolescent behaviors that can disrupt meal patterns and glucose control, such as staying out late or sleeping in. • Recognize that energy intake, nutritional demands, and insulin needs increase during puberty. Monitor behaviors for disordered eating and excessive weight gain. • Counsel against alcohol use.
Physical activity and exercise	• Meeting of physical activity recommendations of 60 min/d of moderate to vigorous activity daily and at least 3 d/wk of muscle- and bone-strengthening exercise (same as for children who do not have diabetes) • Frequent monitoring of glucose level before, during, and after exercise and adjustments to insulin and carbohydrate intake as indicated	Ensure that patients and families have a plan for diabetes management related to physical activity and sports participation.

Continued

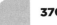

Table 21-8 (*continued*)

Lifestyle factor	Key principles	Recommendations for the primary care pediatrician
Behavioral self-management	• Age- and developmentally appropriate division of care between parent, child, and other caregivers • Recognition and support to help with social adjustment, diabetes-related distress, family stresses, school factors, and disordered eating patterns that often accompany type 1 diabetes diagnosis	• Assess psychosocial and family stresses that could affect diabetes management, and refer families and patients to a mental health professional when indicated. • Recognize signs of disordered or disrupted eating, such as unexplained weight loss or unexplained hyperglycemia. Refer to Chapter 19, Mental Health, Behavioral, and Developmental Conditions, for further discussion of the management of eating disorders.

Derived from reference 32.

In Sum

- Nutritional guidance plays an important role in the prevention and treatment of many gastrointestinal and immune-related health conditions.
- High fluids, fiber, and fruit intake and engagement in recommended levels of physical activity can help prevent functional constipation, whereas dairy products and processed and refined carbohydrates can increase risk of constipation. Although prebiotic or probiotic supplements are often used in an attempt to prevent and/or treat constipation, there is no evidence that they provide benefit in constipation prevention or treatment.
- A diet low in FODMAPs may help relieve IBS symptoms, but such a diet is very restrictive and should not be pursued without the guidance of a registered dietitian. A FODMAP-gentle eating plan, in which specific high-FODMAP foods are avoided, is advised for children and adolescents to help prevent over-restriction and nutritional inadequacy while providing clinical benefit from reducing FODMAP intake. On this plan, wheat, rye, onion, leeks, cauliflower, mushrooms, apples, pear, dried fruit, stone fruits, watermelon, milk, yogurt, and legumes are usually avoided.
- Infants with GERD are likely to experience improved symptoms with thickened feedings, reduced feeding volume, more frequent feedings, upright positioning following feedings, and temporarily eliminated cow milk protein through use of an extensively hydrolyzed or amino acid–based formula for formula-fed infants and through maternal dietary elimination of dairy products for breastfed infants. Children and adolescents with GERD may experience improved symptoms by

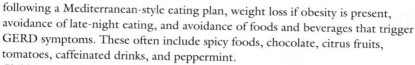

following a Mediterranean-style eating plan, weight loss if obesity is present, avoidance of late-night eating, and avoidance of foods and beverages that trigger GERD symptoms. These often include spicy foods, chocolate, citrus fruits, tomatoes, caffeinated drinks, and peppermint.

- Children and adolescents with IBD may benefit from a low-fiber diet during disease flares. During remission, a high-calorie diet high in iron, calcium, vitamin D, folate, vitamin B_{12}, and zinc can help support typical growth and nutritional adequacy.

- Children with celiac disease must avoid all gluten-containing food products. Gluten is present in all food products made from wheat, barley, rye, and oats contaminated with gluten.

- The 9 most common food allergens, which account for more than 90% of all allergic reactions, are milk, eggs, peanuts, tree nuts (eg, almonds, cashews, walnuts), shellfish, fish, soy, wheat, and sesame. Many food allergies are outgrown over time, but the likelihood of outgrowing peanut allergy and shellfish and fish allergies in childhood or adolescence is low.

- Oral allergy syndrome (pollen food allergy syndrome) generally results from cross-reacting allergens found in pollens and raw fruits, vegetables, or some tree nuts. Cooking or processing of the fruits and vegetables easily breaks down the proteins in them that cause oral allergy syndrome; thus, the allergic reaction does not occur with intake of cooked, baked, or processed fruits and vegetables.

- FPIES, FPIAP, and FPE are delayed non–IgE-mediated food allergies. Treatment is avoidance of the inciting foods, which are most often cow milk and soy. FPIES is outgrown by 1 to 5 years of age, whereas FPIAP and FPE are outgrown by 1 to 2 years of age.

- Eosinophilic esophagitis is most often triggered by a delayed immune-mediated reaction to dairy, egg, soy, or wheat intake in a child or adolescent who has atopy. Symptoms of EoE include poor growth, decreased appetite, recurring abdominal pain, and vomiting or trouble swallowing. Treatment includes dietary elimination of 1 (milk), 2 (milk and wheat), 4 (milk, wheat, egg, and soy), or 6 (milk, egg, soy, wheat, peanuts/tree nuts, and fish/shellfish) of the major food allergens until symptoms resolve and then gradual addition of the foods back to the diet, one at a time, with follow-up endoscopies to identify the causative food. Pharmacological therapy may include swallowed topical corticosteroids (eg, fluticasone, budesonide), proton pump inhibitors, and/or the monoclonal antibody dupilumab. Generally, initial therapy for EoE is dietary or pharmacological; typically, both are not needed. Eosinophilic esophagitis is a manageable lifelong condition.

- Food intolerance results from a deficiency in an enzyme that is needed to break down a food. Food intolerance often develops with gastrointestinal symptoms such as bloating, abdominal pain, vomiting, and flatulence after specific foods are eaten.

- The goals of medical nutritional therapy in the management of type 1 diabetes are to regulate glucose level, blood pressure, and lipid levels and maintain a healthy weight and growth. Overall recommended macronutrient distribution, micronutrient needs, and physical activity recommendations to promote optimal health are the same for children with type 1 diabetes as for other children.

References

1. Mugie SM, Benninga MA, Di Lorenzo C. Epidemiology of constipation in children and adults: a systematic review. *Best Pract Res Clin Gastroenterol.* 2011;25(1):3–18 PMID: 21382575 doi: 10.1016/j.bpg.2010.12.010

2. Malowitz S, Green M, Karpinski A, Rosenberg A, Hyman PE. Age of onset of functional constipation. *J Pediatr Gastroenterol Nutr.* 2016;62(4):600–602 PMID: 26488119 doi: 10.1097/MPG.0000000000001011

3. Tabbers MM, DiLorenzo C, Berger MY, et al; European Society for Pediatric Gastroenterology, Hepatology, and Nutrition; North American Society for Pediatric Gastroenterology. Evaluation and treatment of functional constipation in infants and children: evidence-based recommendations from ESPGHAN and NASPGHAN. *J Pediatr Gastroenterol Nutr.* 2014;58(2):258–274 PMID: 24345831 doi: 10.1097/MPG.0000000000000266

4. Boilesen SN, Tahan S, Dias FC, Melli LCFL, de Morais MB. Water and fluid intake in the prevention and treatment of functional constipation in children and adolescents: is there evidence? *J Pediatr (Rio J).* 2017;93(4):320–327 PMID: 28450053 doi: 10.1016/j.jped.2017.01.005

5. Dreher ML. Whole fruits and fruit fiber emerging health effects. *Nutrients.* 2018;10(12):1833 PMID: 30487459 doi: 10.3390/nu10121833

6. Hyams JS, Di Lorenzo C, Saps M, Shulman RJ, Staiano A, van Tilburg M. Childhood functional gastrointestinal disorders: child/adolescent. *Gastroenterology.* 2016;150(6):1456–1468.e2

7. Halmos EP, Gibson PR. Controversies and reality of the FODMAP diet for patients with irritable bowel syndrome. *J Gastroenterol Hepatol.* 2019;34(7):1134–1142 PMID: 30945376 doi: 10.1111/jgh.14650

8. Rosen R, Vandenplas Y, Singendonk M, et al. Pediatric gastroesophageal reflux clinical practice guidelines: joint recommendations of the North American Society for Pediatric Gastroenterology, Hepatology, and Nutrition and the European Society for Pediatric Gastroenterology, Hepatology, and Nutrition. *J Pediatr Gastroenterol Nutr.* 2018;66(3):516–554 PMID: 29470322 doi: 10.1097/MPG.0000000000001889

9. Maret-Ouda J, Markar SR, Lagergren J. Gastroesophageal reflux disease: a review. *JAMA.* 2020;324(24):2536–2547 PMID: 33351048 doi: 10.1001/jama.2020.21360

10. Rosen MJ, Dhawan A, Saeed SA. Inflammatory bowel disease in children and adolescents. *JAMA Pediatr.* 2015;169(11):1053–1060 PMID: 26414706 doi: 10.1001/jamapediatrics.2015.1982

11. Owczarek D, Rodacki T, Domagała-Rodacka R, Cibor D, Mach T. Diet and nutritional factors in inflammatory bowel diseases. *World J Gastroenterol.* 2016;22(3):895–905 PMID: 26811635 doi: 10.3748/wjg.v22.i3.895

12. Leonard MM, Sapone A, Catassi C, Fasano A. Celiac disease and nonceliac gluten sensitivity: a review. *JAMA.* 2017;318(7):647–656 PMID: 28810029 doi: 10.1001/jama.2017.9730

13. Khan A, Suarez MG, Murray JA. Nonceliac gluten and wheat sensitivity. *Clin Gastroenterol Hepatol.* 2020;18(9):1913–1922.e1 PMID: 30978535 doi: 10.1016/j.cgh.2019.04.009

14. Gupta RS, Warren CM, Smith BM, et al. The public health impact of parent-reported childhood food allergies in the United States. *Pediatrics.* 2018;142(6):e20181235 PMID: 30455345 doi: 10.1542/peds.2018-1235

15. Sokol K, Rasooly M, Dempsey C, et al. Prevalence and diagnosis of sesame allergy in children with IgE-mediated food allergy. *Pediatr Allergy Immunol.* 2020;31(2):214–218 PMID: 31657083 doi: 10.1111/pai.13143

16. Samady W, Warren C, Wang J, Das R, Gupta RS. Egg allergy in US children. *J Allergy Clin Immunol Pract.* 2020;8(9):3066–3073.e6 PMID: 32376485 doi: 10.1016/j.jaip.2020.04.058

17. Sicherer SH, Wood RA, Vickery BP, et al. The natural history of egg allergy in an observational cohort. *J Allergy Clin Immunol.* 2014;133(2):492–499.e8 PMID: 24636473 doi: 10.1016/j.jaci.2013.12.1041

18. Vandenplas Y, Brough HA, Fiocchi A, et al. Current guidelines and future strategies for the management of cow's milk allergy. *J Asthma Allergy.* 2021;14:1243–1256 PMID: 34712052 doi: 10.2147/JAA.S276992

19. Moonesinghe H, Mackenzie H, Venter C, et al. Prevalence of fish and shellfish allergy: a systematic review. *Ann Allergy Asthma Immunol.* 2016;117(3):264–272.e4 PMID: 27613460 doi: 10.1016/j.anai.2016.07.015

20. Savage J, Johns CB. Food allergy: epidemiology and natural history. *Immunol Allergy Clin North Am.* 2015;35(1):45–59 PMID: 25459576 doi: 10.1016/j.iac.2014.09.004

21. McWilliam VL, Perrett KP, Dang T, Peters RL. Prevalence and natural history of tree nut allergy. *Ann Allergy Asthma Immunol.* 2020;124(5):466–472 PMID: 32044450 doi: 10.1016/j.anai.2020.01.024

22. Konek S, Becker P. *Samour & King's Pediatric Nutrition in Clinical Care.* 5th ed. Jones & Bartlett; 2020

23. Du Toit G, Roberts G, Sayre PH, et al; LEAP Study Team. Randomized trial of peanut consumption in infants at risk for peanut allergy. *N Engl J Med.* 2015;372(9):803–813 PMID: 25705822 doi: 10.1056/NEJMoa1414850

24. Greer FR, Sicherer SH, Burks AW, et al; American Academy of Pediatrics Committee on Nutrition and Section on Allergy and Immunology. The effects of early nutritional interventions on the development of atopic disease in infants and children: the role of maternal dietary restriction, breastfeeding, hydrolyzed formulas, and timing of introduction of allergenic complementary foods. *Pediatrics.* 2019;143(4):e20190281 PMID: 30886111 doi: 10.1542/peds.2019-0281

25. American College of Allergy, Asthma & Immunology. Pollen food allergy syndrome. Reviewed March 21, 2019. Accessed October 31, 2021.https://acaai.org/allergies/allergic-conditions/food/pollen-food-allergy-syndrome

26. American Academy of Allergy, Asthma & Immunology. Eosinophilic esophagitis. Revised May 23, 2022. Accessed October 31, 2022. https://www.aaaai.org/Conditions-Treatments/relatedconditions/eosinophilic-esophagitis

27. Zhang S, Sicherer S, Berin MC, Agyemang A. Pathophysiology of non-IgE-mediated food allergy. *ImmunoTargets Ther.* 2021;10:431–446 PMID: 35004389 doi: 10.2147/ITT.S284821

28. American College of Allergy, Asthma & Immunology. Food protein-induced enterocolitis syndrome (FPIES). Reviewed March 21, 2019. Accessed October 31, 2022. https://acaai.org/allergies/allergic-conditions/food/food-protein-induced-enterocolitis-syndrome-fpies

29. Labrosse R, Graham F, Caubet JC. Non-IgE-mediated gastrointestinal food allergies in children: an update. *Nutrients.* 2020;12(7):2086 PMID: 32674427 doi: 10.3390/nu12072086

30. Nowak-Węgrzyn A, Chehade M, Groetch ME, et al. International consensus guidelines for the diagnosis and management of food protein-induced enterocolitis syndrome: executive summary—Workgroup Report of the Adverse Reactions to Foods Committee, American Academy of Allergy, Asthma & Immunology. *J Allergy Clin Immunol.* 2017;139(4):1111–1126.e4 PMID: 28167094 doi: 10.1016/j.jaci.2016.12.966

31. Gonsalves NP, Aceves SS. Diagnosis and treatment of eosinophilic esophagitis. *J Allergy Clin Immunol.* 2020;145(1):1–7 PMID: 31910983 doi: 10.1016/j.jaci.2019.11.011

32. Chiang JL, Maahs DM, Garvey KC, et al. Type 1 diabetes in children and adolescents: a position statement by the American Diabetes Association. *Diabetes Care.* 2018;41(9):2026–2044 PMID: 30093549 doi: 10.2337/dci18-0023

Frequently Asked Questions, Case Studies, and Recipes

Part 5, Frequently Asked Questions, Case Studies, and Recipes, offers real-world applications of the nutrition information and strategies detailed throughout this book, including many of the most frequently asked nutrition questions in pediatric practice and several case studies of common nutrition-related pediatric concerns. This part culminates in a thorough sampling of recipes that can be used and shared with parents to help turn much of the guidance and advice offered throughout this book into positive behavior changes, including a transformation of what children and their families choose to eat.

Frequently Asked Questions

Caregivers and patients frequently rely on primary care pediatricians to answer their nutrition questions. Based on an informal survey of pediatricians and the authors' own experiences as primary care pediatricians, several of the most common nutrition questions that parents and patients ask and recommended answers are included here, divided by child age and stage of development.

Infancy and Early Childhood

1. How long should preterm newborns and infants continue 22 kcal/fl oz of fortified breast milk or formula? Likewise, how long should they continue an iron supplement?

Pediatricians should encourage feeding of fortified human (breast) milk (preferred) or preterm formula (22–24 kcal/fl oz) until 4 months of corrected age. However, pediatricians should monitor the infant's growth chart and may choose to recommend discontinuation of fortified breast milk and/or formula earlier or later, depending on the infant's growth trajectory. Most preterm newborns and infants who breastfeed or those whose diet consists of regular newborn formula benefit from iron supplementation of 2 to 3 mg/kg/d until 6 to 12 months of (uncorrected) age. Infants who have very low birth weight or significant anemia of prematurity may need supplementation up to 6 to 8 mg/kg/d. Infants who consume preterm formula do not usually need empirical iron supplementation but should undergo a complete blood cell count and iron studies at 12 months after birth or sooner if there is low intake of iron-rich foods. Pediatricians may choose to monitor an infant's iron status by following their ferritin level. If an infant's ferritin level is less than 35 ng/mL (35 mcg/L), iron supplementation should be increased. If an infant's ferritin level is greater than 300 ng/mL (300 mcg/L), supplementation should be stopped. A ferritin level from 35 to 300 ng/mL (35–300 mcg/L) is acceptable.

2. When should parents introduce water? How should they introduce it and how much should they offer?

Water should be introduced in an open cup when an infant is about 6 months of age. Water needs at this age are minimal; however, introducing water in this way helps infants improve fine motor skills and helps them develop a preference for water, which will make it more likely that they will choose it as a preferred drink in childhood and adolescence.

3. What should pediatricians advise parents regarding European formulas, organic formulas, and specialty formulas?

The American Academy of Pediatrics (AAP) recommends exclusive breastfeeding until 6 months of age and "supports continued breastfeeding, along with appropriate complementary foods introduced at about 6 months, as long as mutually desired by mother and child for 2 years or beyond."[1] For infants who are not breastfed or who receive supplemental formula, parents have many formulas from which to choose. Parents are advised to choose US Food and Drug Administration–registered formulas. All formulas available for purchase at US stores are US Food and Drug Administration–registered formulas.

Many online parenting groups assert the benefits of European formulas because some are made with milk from goats or pasture-free cows, the hypoallergenic forms use lactose sugars rather than corn syrup, and most contain higher levels of docosahexaenoic acid than US formulas. In hopes of providing their infants the "best" nutrition, parents spend large amounts of money importing these formulas, but the safety cannot be ensured. Additionally, many labels are not in English, which can lead to formula mixing errors. The nutritional value of European formulas is mostly equivalent to that of US formulas.

There is no evidence that organic formulas are nutritionally superior to conventional formulas or that additions such as prebiotics and probiotics add health benefit for healthy, full-term infants.

There are some times when infants may benefit from specialty formula use. For example, formula-fed babies who have cow milk protein allergy are likely to also have soy allergy and may do better with extensive milk protein hydrolysates. A small minority of infants with severe cow milk protein allergy may require elemental (amino acid) formula. Additionally, infants with clinically significant reflux and growth restriction may benefit from thickened formulas. Refer to Chapter 16, Nutrition in Infancy, for a more extensive discussion of formula options and considerations.

4. Should pediatricians recommend baby-led weaning?

Baby-led weaning refers to an initiation of complementary feeding in which infants are provided textured whole foods rather than purees. The infant drives the feeding amount and the parent encourages self-feeding of all foods, thus eliminating purees because infants do not have the coordination to spoon-feed themselves. Overall, studies have shown that there is insufficient evidence currently available to draw conclusions about baby-led weaning. Parents may choose to follow baby-led weaning or to follow a more traditional advancement of foods—from purees to more textured table foods over time, on the basis of developmental readiness. As a general rule, infants exposed to a variety of both textures (including purees) and tastes from foods, as well as in breast milk and amniotic fluid in utero, are more likely to continue to accept and prefer those tastes and textures once they become toddlers. As with the traditional methods of introducing complementary foods, the infant still initially obtains most nutrition intake from breast milk or formula. The AAP recommends exclusive breastfeeding for about 6 months after birth and "supports continued breastfeeding, along with appropriate complementary foods introduced at about 6 months, as long as mutually desired by mother and child for 2 years or beyond."[1] Refer to Chapter 16, Nutrition in Infancy, for further discussion of baby-led weaning.

5. Are vegetable pouches, plant-based milks, and toddler formula healthy for children?

Although vegetable pouches are a convenience and contain mostly pureed fruits and vegetables, pediatricians are advised to encourage parents to continue offering vegetables with other meals and snacks, helping children become familiar with and learn to like the taste and texture of vegetables in their natural forms. Overconsumption of pouches can lead to excess caloric intake and may impede oro-motor development. Pouches often also have preservatives and added coloring and flavoring that are unnecessary and may be best avoided. Offering fresh, home-prepared whole foods for snacks is preferable.

Although popular with many parents, plant-based "milks" have not been studied sufficiently to promote their use. Many are lower in protein, calcium, and vitamin D than their animal-based equivalents, except for soy milk and pea protein, which are nutritionally equivalent to cow or fortified goat milk. Milk (cow or soy without added sugars) and water are the preferred drinks at this age and throughout childhood. Unfortified goat milk is deficient in vitamin B_6 and folate and is not recommended.

Although heavily marketed to parents of toddlers, especially those who exhibit picky eating or have low weight, toddler/follow-on formulas are rarely recommended for children who are otherwise healthy and growing well. These products are sometimes used in specialty clinics in the treatment of avoidant/restrictive food intake disorder or rumination disorder or in other clinical situations when a child is otherwise unable to obtain adequate nutrition intake for typical growth and development. Refer to Chapter 17, Nutrition in Childhood and Adolescence, for more information.

6. What should pediatricians recommend to help parents of children who exhibit picky eating, children who eat only 1 or 2 foods, or a toddler who refuses milk? How can parents encourage their children to eat vegetables?

Young children often refuse new foods. In most cases, the most advisable first step is to encourage parents to be patient and continue to offer the rejected food or milk. Rather than consider the rejected food off-limits, parents or other caregivers can reintroduce it 3 to 14 days later. A child may be more willing to accept it. In fact, it can take 8 to 10 tries or more for a child to accept a new food. In many cases, with repeated exposures, a child eventually accepts and sometimes even prefers the previously rejected food. Parents may continue to offer rejected foods such as vegetables but not force or pressure their child to eat them. Encouragement is best provided through a gentle nudge, increased accessibility and exposure, foods made to look and taste good, and parental modeling. Refer to Chapter 17, Nutrition in Childhood and Adolescence, for further discussion of picky eating and Chapter 19, Mental Health, Behavioral, and Developmental Conditions, for discussion of severe picky eating and feeding disorders.

7. Do children need a multivitamin supplement? Do they need a vitamin D supplement? How about a docosahexaenoic acid (DHA) supplement?

When children consume a diet that resembles MyPlate and the *Dietary Guidelines for Americans*, supplementation with vitamins and minerals is generally unnecessary. However, many children may not be eating in an optimally nutritious way and may not be obtaining all the nutrients they need. When a pediatrician suspects that a child may not be consuming sufficient vitamins and minerals, advising the use of a multivitamin may be warranted. All infants breastfeeding and infants consuming less than 27 fl oz/d of formula fortified with vitamin D should take a 400-IU (10-mcg) vitamin D supplement until 12 months of age. Additionally, children and adolescents who do not consume at least 600 IU (15 mcg) of vitamin D through fortified dairy products, fish such as canned tuna or salmon, eggs, or other vitamin D–containing foods should take a 400-IU (10-mcg) vitamin D supplement. Docosahexaenoic acid is best obtained from food sources such as fatty fish (eg, salmon, tuna). Small amounts of alpha-linolenic acid from plant sources are converted to DHA. In some cases, such as when following a vegan diet or experiencing hypertriglyceridemia, children and adolescents may benefit from supplementation. The benefits of DHA for children with attention-deficit/hyperactivity disorder are inconclusive. Note that DHA comes as a fish oil supplement, which can have a fishy taste and cause halitosis.

Middle Childhood and Adolescence

8. How can parents encourage children and adolescents to eat better, including choosing healthier foods when not at home, eating breakfast each morning, and/or increasing their fruit and vegetable consumption?

Parents can help prepare their children to make healthy choices when their children are not at home by providing mostly healthful foods at home while not being too restrictive, because this often leads to increased intake of nutritionally poor foods outside the home.

Having a family routine of eating 3 balanced meals per day that are consistent with MyPlate recommendations, including breakfast, helps children and adolescents develop a healthy eating pattern and access to and familiarity with healthful foods, including fruits and vegetables, thus increasing liking for these foods and the likelihood that they will be eaten even when a parent is not overseeing the meal.

Many children and adolescents skip breakfast for various reasons, including lack of time or no feeling of hunger. Parents can help children and adolescents establish a routine of eating breakfast by helping or encouraging them to plan breakfast the night before and by having healthy options available that are easy to incorporate into busy schedules, such as pieces of fruit, or by planning to have them eat a healthy choice from the school breakfast program, if available. Notably, many "breakfast foods," such as sugary cereals, high-sugar yogurt, cereal or nutrition bars, and fruit juice, are not healthy breakfast options. Alternatives such as low-sugar cereals, plain yogurt, oatmeal, and water or plain milk are more healthful. Parents can encourage these healthier options by having them available in the home and avoiding purchasing the less desirable items.

Children and adolescents may make healthier choices when nutrition information is linked to their goals, such as improved performance in sports and increased concentration at school. Parents can play a particularly important role by modeling not only healthy eating and activity habits but also a healthy relationship with food and a healthy body image. Additionally, children enrolled in school meal programs benefit from breakfast and lunch food offerings aligned with the dietary guidelines and MyPlate recommendations for their age.

9. How can pediatricians best encourage families to eat family meals?

Pediatricians might share the following data, compiled by The Family Dinner Project (https://thefamilydinnerproject.org), to help support the recommendation to eat family meals together as often as possible:

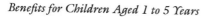

Benefits for Children Aged 1 to 5 Years

- Conversation and language stimulation supports language development and learning to read.
- Meals tend to be healthier and to support improved dietary intake and decreased risk for overweight and obesity.
- Parents who eat meals together tend to demonstrate improved marriage satisfaction, which supports a stronger family bond and connectedness.

Benefits for Children Aged 6 to 12 Years

- Children who eat family meals tend to demonstrate improved academic performance.
- Children who eat family meals eat more fruits and vegetables and consume fewer fried foods and sugary drinks.
- Children who eat family meals report improved connectedness to parents and siblings.

Benefits for Adolescents Aged 13 to 18 Years

- Adolescents who eat family meals demonstrate improved academic performance.
- Adolescents who eat family meals have lower risk of smoking, substance use, eating disorders, pregnancy, and violence.
- Adolescents who eat family meals demonstrate stronger relationships and connectedness with their parents and caregivers.
- Adolescents who eat family meals display higher self-esteem and have lower risk of depression.

Although much of the focus tends to be on family dinners, evening family meals may not always be possible for families for many reasons, such as conflicting work, school, and extracurricular schedules. The meals eaten together need not always be dinner; they could be breakfast or lunch. The benefits of family meals are realized if the family meals occur 3 or more times per week. Families might create a weekly meal plan and schedule to help facilitate family meals, might explore whether work or extracurricular schedules can be adapted to prioritize eating together, or might commit to eating together as often as possible when schedules allow.

Pediatricians and parents can learn more about the benefits of family meals and more of the suggested strategies that families can use to prioritize family meals at The Family Dinner Project (https://thefamilydinnerproject.org).

10. What are key points to ensure optimal nutrition for children and adolescents who follow a vegetarian or vegan eating plan?

A well-planned vegetarian eating plan can optimize nutrition and health benefits while promoting environmental health through use of fewer natural resources and less environmental damage. Vegetarian diets tend to be low in saturated fat and animal protein and high in fiber, folate, vitamins C and E, carotenoids, and some phytochemicals. Children and adolescents who follow a vegetarian eating plan tend to consume more fruits and vegetables and less sweets, salty snacks, and saturated fat than their nonvegetarian peers. They also tend to have lower risk for overweight and obesity.

Although in the past there was concern that following a vegetarian diet might lead to inadequate intake of certain key nutrients, this is not generally the case in well-planned vegetarian eating plans. However, several nutrients could be consumed in inadequate amounts if a vegetarian eating plan is not well designed.

- **Protein:** Children who follow a vegetarian plan tend to consume sufficient protein variety and quantity. Regular intake of legumes (eg, beans, peas, lentils, peanuts, soy) ensures adequate protein intake. Children and adolescents who follow a vegan diet may require higher protein intake than children who do not follow a vegan diet because of decreased protein quality.
- **Iron:** Iron from vegetarian sources (nonheme iron) is lower in quality than that from nonvegetarian sources because nonheme iron is not absorbed as well as heme iron. Overall, vegetarians need about 1.8 times higher iron intake than nonvegetarians. Inadequate iron intake is generally common in children and more so common in children who follow a vegetarian eating plan. Excellent vegetarian sources of iron include soy, lentils, chickpeas, black-eyed peas, beans, seeds such as sesame, and hemp. Vitamin C enhances iron absorption. Refer to chapters 5, Vitamins, and 6, Minerals, for more information.
- **Zinc:** Zinc levels may be lower in children following a vegetarian diet, although deficiency is rare. Vegetarian sources of zinc include soy, legumes, grains, cheese, seeds, and nuts. Additionally, soaking and sprouting beans, grains, nuts, and seeds and leavening bread can help the body better use zinc. Citric acid can also increase zinc absorption. Refer to Chapter 6, Minerals, for more information.
- **Vitamin B$_{12}$:** Vitamin B$_{12}$ is naturally present primarily in animal products. It is present in very small amounts in some fermented foods, nori, spirulina, *Chlorella* algae, and unfortified nutritional yeast. Although most vegetarian plans contain sufficient vitamin B$_{12}$, children and breastfeeding mothers who follow a vegan eating plan should take a vitamin B$_{12}$ supplement or eat fortified foods, such as fortified nutritional yeast.
- **Calcium:** The body's ability to use calcium from plant foods can be compromised by high content of oxalates, phytates, and fiber in foods. For instance, although spinach, beet greens, and Swiss chard contain high levels of calcium, they also contain high levels of oxalates, making them a poor calcium source. Low-oxalate greens such as kale, turnips, Chinese cabbage, and bok choy are good sources of calcium, as are fortified plant milks and soy products, white beans, almonds, tahini, figs, and oranges.
- **Vitamin D:** Few foods naturally contain vitamin D. Mushrooms treated with UV light and eggs contain some vitamin D. Cow milk, some nondairy milks, fruit juices, breakfast cereals, and margarines are often fortified with vitamin D.
- **Eicosapentaenoic acid and docosahexaenoic acid omega-3 fatty acids:** Intake of these acids is generally low in vegetarian (and absent in vegan) eating plans. A small proportion of alpha-linolenic acid (omega-3 fatty acid from plants) is converted to eicosapentaenoic acid and docosahexaenoic acid. The best sources of alpha-linolenic acid include seeds (flaxseeds, chia, *Camelina,* canola, and hempseeds), walnuts, and their oils. Refer to Chapter 4, Fats, for more information.

Starting with an idea such as "meatless Mondays" can help families sample vegetarian eating 1 day per week to determine whether it is something they would like to continue. Additionally, trying new recipes and involving children and adolescents in meal preparation and cooking can help make new foods seem more familiar and increase intake. Resources for vegetarian recipes include Part 5 of this book, Frequently Asked Questions, Case Studies, and Recipes; HealthyChildren.org, the official AAP website for parents (www.healthychildren.org/recipes); ChopChop Family (www.chopchopfamily.org); and the Bonus Bites section of Raddish (www.raddishkids.com).

11. What are healthy snack ideas to recommend to families?

In helping families choose healthy snacks, pediatricians may consider recommending that snacks include 2 food groups, with extra attention to include fruits and vegetables, whole grains, and healthful protein and dairy sources. The following list is a sampling of ideas that patients and families can be encouraged to mix and match for a balanced snack:

- **Fruit:** strawberries, bananas, blueberries, watermelon, pineapple, cantaloupe, grapes, peaches, nectarines, clementines, pears, apple slices, frozen fruit, persimmon, cherries, mango, pomegranate, honeydew, raspberries, blackberries, blueberries, or raisins
- **Vegetables:** bell pepper slices, sugar snap peas, edamame, salad/greens, baby carrots, celery sticks, cherry tomatoes, cucumber slices, jicama, snow peas, cauliflower, or broccoli
- **Proteins and dairy:** hummus, peanut or nut butter, nuts or seeds, boiled eggs, string cheese, yogurt, or cottage cheese
- **Whole grains:** plain popcorn, whole grain crackers, or whole grain bread
- **Mix-and-match ideas:** "ants on a log" (celery + peanut butter + raisins), apples and peanut butter, whole grain crackers with cottage cheese and sliced pineapples, or cucumbers with lemon and salt and sliced grapes

12. How can parents encourage children and adolescents to be more active?

The AAP recommends that children and adolescents engage in at least 60 minutes of physical activity per day; however, many children and adolescents do not meet this recommendation. Pediatricians and parents alike can support children in increasing physical activity by applying some or all of the following strategies:

- **Model being active.** Parents and pediatricians can serve as positive role models for activity. Pediatricians can share their favorite activities and strategies for finding the time and energy to meet physical activity recommendations. Parents can make a commitment to prioritize physical activity in their own lives.
- **Tailor recommendations to a child's age, stage, and ability.** Physical activity recommendations should be tailored to a child's or adolescent's development stage because activities provide varying degrees of engagement and results based on a youth's ability. Chapter 18, Sports and Athletic Performance (refer to **Table 18-4**), highlights key fitness priorities for children and adolescents by developmental stage from ages 0 to 18 years.
- **Identify and focus on a child's interests.** Enjoyment and the perception of fun are especially important for children and adolescents. Every child's preferences are different, and parents should make an effort to identify activities that their child enjoys. Children and adolescents who participate in sports, spend more time outdoors, and walk or ride their bike to and/or from school are most likely to meet physical activity guidelines.

- **Incorporate physical activity into the day.** The best chance for children and adolescents to meet physical activity guidelines is when the physical activity is built into the day. This is one reason why school is an ideal place for children and adolescents to obtain their recommended 60 minutes of activity. Parents should consider how a child or an adolescent can take steps to increase physical activity before, during, and after school.

- **Encourage screen limits.** Screen time is a key cause of reduced physical activity in children and adolescents. The AAP Family Media Plan (https://healthychildren. org/mediaplan) includes recommendations to support families in structuring and limiting screen time, such as avoiding or restricting screen time during mealtimes and within 1 hour of bedtime.

- **Pair physical activity with a focus on sleep and sleep quality.** One of the many benefits of physical activity is that it helps improve sleep quality. The 2018 Physical Activity Guidelines Advisory Committee found strong evidence that acute bouts of activity and regular physical activity improve sleep of adults, including total sleep time, sleep efficiency, time to fall asleep, sleep quality, and rapid eye movement sleep. Insufficient evidence was available to draw conclusions for children and adolescents. This is most likely owing to lack of studies rather than lack of benefit. The adult findings likely apply to children and adolescents.

13. What should pediatricians recommend to a family in which one child has overweight and another child has underweight?

Many families have children of varying body types, including one child who has overweight or obesity and another who may have slow weight gain or underweight. The general principles for healthy eating apply to both categories of children, and it is advisable that parents treat children similarly to avoid stigmatization or poor body image. In general, a balanced meal plan including the major food groups (eg, the MyPlate plan) in the appropriate portions, with water and milk as the main beverages, and minimal eating between scheduled mealtimes and snack times is likely to lead to the best overall outcomes. It is important to assess for and treat any root causes of body mass index percentiles outside the healthy body mass index range. This situation is explored in more detail in the Case Studies.

14. How can parents help children and adolescents build self-confidence and a positive body image?

Parents play an important role in helping their children and adolescents build self-confidence and a positive body image. The following suggestions are recommendations adapted from the AAP *Bright Futures: Nutrition* "Tool I: Tips for Fostering a Positive Body Image Among Children and Adolescents"[2]:

For Parents

- Model healthy eating and physical activity behaviors, and avoid extreme eating and physical activity behaviors.
- Focus on non–appearance-related traits when discussing yourself and others.
- Praise your child or adolescent for academic and other successes.
- Analyze media messages with your child or adolescent.

- Show that you love your child or adolescent regardless of what they weigh.
- If your child or adolescent has overweight, do not criticize their appearance; offer support instead.
- Share with a health care professional any concerns you may have about your child's or adolescent's eating behaviors or body image.

For Children and Adolescents

- Look in the mirror and focus on features that you perceive to be positive, not negative.
- Say something nice to your friends about how they look.
- Think about your positive traits that are unrelated to appearance.
- Look at magazines (and social media images) with a critical eye, and find out what photographers and graphic designers do to make models look the way they do.
- If you have increased weight and want to lose weight, be realistic in your expectations and aim for gradual change.
- Realize that everyone has a unique size and shape.
- If you have questions about your size or weight, ask a health care professional.

For Health Care Professionals

- Discuss changes that occur during adolescence.
- Assess weight concerns and body image. If a child or an adolescent has a distorted body image, explore causes and discuss potential consequences.
- Discuss how the media negatively affects body image.
- Discuss typical variation in body sizes and shapes among children and adolescents.
- Educate parents, physical education instructors, and coaches about realistic and healthy body weights.
- Emphasize each patient's positive characteristics and strengths.

In addition, parents and pediatricians can help support a child's or adolescent's positive body image by discouraging dieting, skipped meals, and the use of diet pills and encouraging and supporting healthy eating and physical activity behaviors.

In addition, pediatricians should focus on healthy living and healthy habits rather than weight and encourage families to talk about eating healthy and being active as a way to stay healthy rather than as a way to lose weight.

Ask about a history of mistreatment or bullying when children and adolescents have obesity. If a patient expresses that they have experienced bullying, help the patient and family develop a plan to stop the bullying and seek additional help and supports.

15. What should pediatricians say to an older child who has picky eating preferences?

In some cases, picky eating persists beyond early childhood and parents find themselves struggling with an older child's or adolescent's picky eating preferences. Following are a few strategies that pediatricians might suggest to older children and adolescents to help them become more open to trying new foods:

1. Share that it can take 8 to 10 or more tries to like a new food. The taste buds change as children and adolescents try foods, and a food or beverage that they did not like at one point can start to taste better with repeated exposures.

2. Encourage children and adolescents to try growing, choosing, and cooking their own foods. The more engaged they are, the more likely they will be to eventually try the foods.
3. Encourage children and adolescents to explore more and to learn about food, nutrition, farming, and cooking. As they do, they will naturally become more interested in trying new foods.

Although these strategies tend to be helpful, the following list includes additional tips for parents that are tailored to a child's age and developmental stage:

- **School-age:** Help children learn where their food comes from by growing a miniature garden. Plant easy-to-grow foods that your child might otherwise resist trying (eg, spinach, sweet peppers).
- **Adolescence:** Make a commitment to eat family meals together at least 2 to 3 times per week. This not only makes it more likely that a teen will eat a balanced meal but also helps strengthen family relationships and decrease the likelihood of risk-taking behaviors. Require a teen to occasionally help choose and prepare meals to support their development of cooking skills. Require that the meal contain a protein, grain, fruit, and vegetable; otherwise, avoid the urge to micromanage what your teen chooses to include in the meal.

References

1. Meek JY, Noble L; American Academy of Pediatrics Section on Breastfeeding. Breastfeeding and the use of human milk. *Pediatrics.* 2022;150(1):e2022057988 doi: 10.1542/peds.2022-057988
2. Tool I: tips for fostering a positive body image among children and adolescents. In: Holt K, Wooldridge NH, Story M, Sofka D, eds. *Bright Futures Nutrition.* 3rd ed. American Academy of Pediatrics; 2011:257–258

Case Studies

Case 1. Nutritional Needs of the Preterm Infant

J.S. is a former 32-weeks'-gestation infant who presents as a new patient for his 4-month health supervision visit. His birth history includes a 4-week neonatal intensive care unit stay caused by difficulty feeding, but ever since his discharge, he has been doing well on fortified human (breast) milk of 22 kcal/fl oz. His corrected weight is at the 50th percentile for age. Per his prior pediatrician's recommendations, his parents are giving him a vitamin D supplement of 400 IU (10 mcg) and an iron supplement of 2 mg/kg/d. What would be key nutrition recommendations at this health supervision visit?

- Advise J.S.'s parents to continue with fortified breast milk (preferred) or preterm formula (22–24 kcal/fl oz) until 4 months of corrected gestational age, or in J.S.'s case until the 6-month health supervision visit. If J.S. is directly breastfeeding, then fortifying 1 to 2 bottles of expressed breast milk to 24 Cal may be necessary until the 6-month visit.
- Recommend that J.S's parents continue iron supplementation of 2 to 3 mg/kg/d until J.S. is 12 months of age (uncorrected) if he continues to breastfeed. If J.S.'s mother stops breastfeeding and transitions to iron-fortified formula, additional iron supplementation may be unnecessary.

   You may consider monitoring J.S.'s iron status by checking his complete blood cell count and conducting an iron panel ± ferritin level. If his hemoglobin and iron levels are low or if his ferritin level is less than 35 ng/mL (35 mcg/L), iron supplementation should be increased. If his ferritin level is greater than 300 ng/mL (300 mcg/L), supplementation should be stopped. A ferritin level from 35 to 300 ng/mL (35–300 mcg/L) is acceptable.

- Advise J.S's parents to continue vitamin D supplementation until at least 12 months of age.
- Encourage J.S.'s parents to help J.S. develop a feeding routine, while practicing responsive feeding and being attuned to J.S.'s signs of hunger and satiety.
- Advise J.S.'s parents to wait until his 6-month health supervision visit to introduce complementary foods.

Case 2. A Toddler With Severe Picky Eating and Poor Weight Gain, Complicated by Anemia and Constipation

S.M. is a 22-month-old who has severe picky eating habits, preferring to drink milk (about 30 fl oz/d) and eat only chicken nuggets, cheese pizza, or noodles with butter. Assessment of S.M.'s growth chart indicates a decrease in weight-for-length from the 40th percentile at the 18-month health supervision visit to the 20th percentile at the current visit. S.M.'s hemoglobin level is 10 g/dL (100 g/L). S.M. experiences constipation, having about 2 large, hard bowel movements per week. What nutritional advice and next steps would help address nutritional concerns for S.M.?

- Given that S.M.'s severe picky eating behaviors are showing medical complications of poor weight gain, anemia, and constipation, additional resources are indicated. If services are available, a referral for occupational therapy or to a feeding team for feeding therapy will help.

- Although picky eating is typical and expected of children in S.M.'s age range, given the extent of the pickiness, to the point of affecting weight gain and causing medical complications, consideration of other potential developmental or medical concerns is warranted (refer to **Table 19-2** in Chapter 19, Mental Health, Behavioral, and Developmental Conditions).

- Parents may be unaware of recommended nutrition practices at this age, so sharing nutrition guidelines for toddlers may help. Parents may find the guidance from Healthy Eating Research for children aged 2 to 8 years to be helpful (https://healthyeatingresearch.org/tips-for-families/ages-2-8-feeding-recommendations). Reference MyPlate (https://choosemyplate.gov/myplateplan) for details of a recommended eating plan and examples of portion sizes. For S.M.'s case, nutritional needs include 1,000 kcal/d, consisting of 1 c (150 g) of fruits, 1 c (150 g) of vegetables, 3 oz (85 g) of grains, 2 oz (57 g) of protein, and 2 c (473 mL) of dairy. Encourage S.M.'s parents to aim to offer S.M. meals and snacks that resemble this plan, but acknowledge that S.M. may refuse to follow it. Encourage S.M's parents to consistently offer but not coerce or force S.M. to eat the foods. If services are available, consider referral to a registered dietitian for nutrition education and assistance with behavioral strategies to support healthier dietary intake.

- Guide S.M.'s parents through best practices for managing picky eating but recognizing that addressing picky eating is a process that requires time and patience. Provide support and close follow-up to assess progress and ensure appropriate weight gain. Best practices for parents and other caregivers for managing picky eating include
  - Offer a balanced mix of 3 meals and 2 snacks per day, including fruits, vegetables, and other healthful food options. Include at least 1 food that the child likes at each meal and snack, but do not cater to their preferences. Even if a child does not eat the offered foods, repeated exposure and familiarity increase later intake. Offer foods in small portions to limit food waste.
  - Limit food or drink to 2 hours before offering a meal or a snack to increase typical appetite and the likelihood that S.M. will be hungry at mealtimes and snack times and thus more likely to eat the offered foods.
  - Aim to increase accepted foods by *bridging* foods, from a preferred food to a new exposure. For instance, build a bridge from chicken nuggets to fish sticks or from plain cheese pizza to cauliflower-crust pizza.
  - Eat the same meals together as a family as often as possible. Model healthy, balanced eating practices.

- Given the anemia, recommend iron supplementation of 2 to 3 mg/kg/d.
- Given S.M.'s constipation and severe picky eating, consider a stool softener (titrated to 1 soft bowel movement per day) in addition to recommendations to offer water at and between meals, and limit milk to only mealtimes.
- Ensure close follow-up.

Case 3. A Family With 2 School-aged Children, 1 With Obesity and 1 With Underweight

T.Y. is an 8-year-old with a body mass index (BMI) in the 98th percentile for age and sex. J.Y. is a 10-year-old with a BMI in the 3rd percentile for age and sex. Their parents feel frustrated and confused because they had been advised by a previous pediatrician at T.Y.'s health supervision visit to stop purchasing desserts and processed foods to improve T.Y.'s weight, whereas they had been told at J.Y.'s health supervision visit to offer J.Y. ice cream and pizza to help her gain weight. What would be the most helpful nutritional advice for this family?

- Acknowledge the family's feelings of frustration and confusion. Affirm their commitment to help both their children be healthy and strive toward optimal nutrition.
- Encourage the family to focus on health more than weight, and note that eating a variety of vegetables, fruits, whole grains, and lean protein helps support good nutrition for the whole family.
  - Encourage the parents to adopt similar structure and routines for the whole family to support healthy eating and a healthy relationship with food and to prevent over-restriction and stigmatization or shame around food, which can sometimes lead children and adolescents to sneak food or binge later.
  - Encourage the parents to offer J.Y. healthy options to increase caloric intake if needed (refer to **Box 19-1** in Chapter 19, Mental Health, Behavioral, and Developmental Conditions, for examples) rather than desserts and processed foods.
- Investigate any potential medical or behavioral underlying causes of increased or decreased BMI and potential associated risk factors or related health conditions. For example, given that T.Y. has a BMI in the 98th percentile, evaluate cholesterol level, blood glucose level, and liver function to assess for related health conditions. Consider checking J.Y.'s hemoglobin level and, potentially, other nutritional laboratory test results or conducting a celiac panel if any concerns are raised on history or physical examination. Signs other than low BMI percentile or weight loss that suggest possible celiac disease may include abdominal pain after eating, gas, chronic diarrhea, foul-smelling stools, or skin or mouth lesions.
- Share a recommended eating plan for both children. According to the plan available at MyPlate (www.myplate.gov/myplate-plan), T.Y. needs about 1,400 kcal/d and J.Y. needs about 1,800 kcal/d. J.Y. might attain the additional calories by adding a small amount of healthy high-calorie/high-fat options to foods, such as extra olive oil to prepared foods.
- Encourage the family to develop a plan for incorporating desserts and preferred foods that are not as healthful (eg, having dessert days twice per week), so the

children can have these foods but in a balanced, equitable way. Avoid storing these foods in the house because this can lead to unnecessary conflicts and a perception of "unfair" feeding practices.

Case 4. An Adolescent With an Eating Disorder

A.M. presents for a 14-year adolescent health supervision visit. Her height is 5 ft 5 inches (165 cm), and her weight is 115 lb (52 kg). Her growth chart reveals a 15-lb (52-kg) weight loss since her 13-year health supervision visit, with her BMI percentile decreasing from the 75th percentile to the 47th percentile. When the growth chart is discussed during the examination, A.M. confides that she has been trying to lose weight for the past 3 months by restricting intake and exercising more and that she has a goal weight of 100 lb (45 kg). What would be the best next steps?

- Share with A.M. and her parents concern about the quick weight loss that has occurred and concern for a possible eating disorder. Assess A.M.'s readiness to change. Check A.M.'s orthostatic blood pressure, and assess for medical stability (refer to **Table 19-3** in Chapter 19, Mental Health, Behavioral, and Developmental Conditions).
- Advise a focused follow-up visit to review A.M.'s laboratory test results, obtain a more complete history, and make a referral to a therapist and registered dietitian who have expertise working with adolescents with eating disorders. Continue to medically monitor A.M. once care has been established with a therapist and registered dietitian.
- Emphasize the importance of eating in a healthful, balanced way to support optimal nutrition, health, and brain development and maturation.
- Offer the following nutritional guidance:
  — Consume 3 meals and 3 snacks per day. Aim for meals that last about 20 to 40 minutes and snacks that last 10 to 15 minutes.
  — Aim for meals and snacks to be evenly spaced at consistent times.
  — Parents or other caregivers should oversee eating and discourage hiding, concealing, or destroying food.
  — Parents or other caregivers should discourage food rituals.
  — Consider a multivitamin with iron, a 1,300-mg calcium supplement, and a 600-IU (15-mcg) vitamin D supplement.

Case 5. A School-aged Child With Celiac Disease

G.L. is an 8-year-old who was recently diagnosed with celiac disease. His family is experiencing challenges in making dietary changes to eliminate gluten from its diet. They have an appointment with a registered dietitian who specializes in celiac disease, but it is not for another month. What guidance would best help this family avoid gluten and prevent potential nutritional deficiencies resulting from a poorly planned gluten-free diet?

- Note that gluten is a component of wheat, rye, and barley. Oats do not contain gluten, but most are processed in plants that also process wheat, rye, and barley, so there is risk of contamination. This means that most breads, cereals, and pasta should be avoided, unless they are specially formulated to be gluten-free.

- Grains should not be avoided altogether because this avoidance increases risk for many micronutrient deficiencies. Rice, corn, soy, tapioca, quinoa, millet, buckwheat, flax, nut flours, and uncontaminated oats are all gluten-free grains.
- All Nutrition Facts labels must note whether products contain gluten. Many food products that normally contain gluten have "gluten-free" offerings, such as breads, cereals, and pastas, available in stores, although these gluten-free products are often much more expensive than their gluten-containing counterparts.
- All fruits and vegetables and all unprocessed protein foods, including meats, fish, eggs, and beans, are naturally gluten-free. Incorporate them into the daily eating plan, and continue to encourage G.L. to eat them.
- Choose iron-rich and vitamin-D fortified foods. Consider supplementation if hemoglobin or vitamin D laboratory tests are assessed and levels fall below the reference range.

Case 6. A Family Who Has Adopted a Vegan Diet

A family of 6 that includes 2 parents, a breastfeeding 8-month-old, a 3-year-old, a 7-year-old, and a 13-year-old has recently adopted a vegan eating plan. The parents want to follow this plan while ensuring that their children do not develop nutritional deficiencies. What nutritional advice do they need to consider?

- A well-planned vegan eating plan can be healthy and nutritionally adequate for the whole family, including any breastfeeding infant. A poorly planned vegan eating plan can be detrimental to health, so it is important to carefully plan the family's meals and snacks.
- Key nutrients to consider when following a vegan eating plan include calories, protein, iron, zinc, vitamin B$_{12}$, calcium, vitamin D, and omega-3 fatty acids. Beans, peas, lentils, peanuts, tree nuts, and soy are high-quality vegan sources of protein, iron, and zinc. Soaking beans and legumes overnight can help increase zinc absorption. Low-oxalate greens such as kale, turnips, Chinese cabbage, and bok choy are good sources of calcium, as are white beans, almonds, tahini, figs, oranges, and fortified plant milks and soy. Families should ensure varied sources of calcium intake because it can be difficult to get adequate calcium from greens alone. Mushrooms treated with UV light, eggs, and some nondairy milks, fruit juices, and breakfast cereals are fortified with vitamin D. Eicosapentaenoic acid and docosahexaenoic acid are absent in vegan eating plans, although a small proportion of alpha-linolenic acid is converted into eicosapentaenoic acid and docosahexaenoic acid. The best sources of alpha-linolenic acid include seeds (eg, flaxseeds, chia, *Camelina*, canola, hempseeds), walnuts, soybeans, and oils derived from seeds, walnuts, or soybeans (eg, flaxseed, canola, walnut, soybean).
- The parents should pay close attention to nutrition labels and their children's nutritional needs by age. Providing them a report of each child's recommended needs based on the DRI Calculator for Healthcare Professionals (www.nal.usda.gov/human-nutrition-and-food-safety/dri-calculator) and highlighting the key nutrients or summarizing key nutrient needs may help.

- Should their infant stop breastfeeding, soy infant formula is an appropriate vegan option until 12 months of age, when their infant should transition to soy or pea protein–based milk. Low-allergy formulas, including protein hydrolysate and elemental formulas, may contain some animal products. Soy tends to taste better and be more affordable than pea protein–based milk. Other plant-based "milks" are a possible substitute for soy, but they are not nutritionally equivalent.
- Anyone following a vegan eating plan should take a vitamin B_{12} supplement, especially breastfeeding mothers and their babies, because a breastfeeding newborn or infant with vitamin B_{12} deficiency is at risk for neurological damage, poor weight gain, developmental delays, and anemia. Many people who follow a vegan eating plan also benefit from vitamin D and omega-3 fatty acid supplementation.
- Laboratory evaluation is important to monitor nutritional status, in particular to track hemoglobin levels to assess iron intake and vitamin B_{12} levels to ensure adequate intake or supplementation.
- General nutrition and parent feeding principles for children and adolescents apply for the youths in this family, with substitution of nutrient-dense, plant-based products for animal products as noted previously.

Recipes

Chapter 2

Healthy Recipes to Satisfy a Child's Desire for Sweet Foods

 Frozen Yogurt Banana Pops

Serving size: 6

Ingredients:

3 bananas

1 c vanilla or strawberry yogurt

Toppings: sprinkles, mini chocolate chips, shredded coconut, chopped nuts

Special equipment: wooden craft sticks/chopsticks

Directions:

Peel bananas and cut each banana in half crosswise. Insert craft stick/chopstick into cut end of each banana half. Dip each banana half into yogurt, using a spoon to evenly coat the banana. Place the banana half onto a plate or small baking sheet lined with parchment or wax paper. Sprinkle toppings onto yogurt-covered bananas. Place them into the freezer for 2 to 3 hours.

American Academy of Pediatrics

DEDICATED TO THE HEALTH OF ALL CHILDREN®

Watermelon Lime Granita

Serving size: 4 to 6

Ingredients:

4 to 5 c seedless watermelon, cut into 1-inch chunks (½ a seedless watermelon)

2 to 3 tbsp honey or agave nectar/syrup, as needed, depending on the sweetness of the watermelon

1 lime, juiced

Special equipment: blender

Directions:

Place all ingredients into the blender and blend them. Pour mixture into a 13 × 9–inch baking dish or another deep dish of similar size. Freeze mixture for 2 hours. Remove the mixture from the freezer and, with a fork, rake the semi-frozen watermelon puree, breaking it into larger ice clumps. Place the mixture back into the freezer for another hour. Remove the mixture from the freezer and rake it again, breaking the ice clumps into smaller clumps, resembling the texture of shaved ice. Place the mixture back into the freezer for another 30 minutes, then serve.

 Chia Seed Pudding

Serving size: 4

Ingredients:

¼ c chia seeds

1½ c milk (cow milk or plant-based variety)

½ c low-fat plain yogurt

¼ tsp salt

2 tbsp maple syrup or honey

Directions:

Mix chia seeds, desired milk, yogurt, salt, and desired sweetener together in a medium bowl and place into the refrigerator overnight. The next day, top the pudding with fruit if desired and serve.

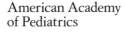
American Academy of Pediatrics

DEDICATED TO THE HEALTH OF ALL CHILDREN®

Single copies of these recipes may be made for noncommercial, educational purposes. The information contained herein should not be used as a substitute for the medical care and advice of a pediatric health care professional.

The American Academy of Pediatrics is an organization of 67,000 primary care pediatricians, pediatric medical subspecialists, and pediatric surgical specialists dedicated to the health, safety, and well-being of all infants, children, adolescents, and young adults.

American Academy of Pediatrics website—www.HealthyChildren.org   © 2023 American Academy of Pediatrics. All rights reserved.

Three-Ingredient Peanut Butter Cookies

Yield: approximately 2 dozen cookies

Ingredients:

1 c peanut butter, creamy or chunky

½ c sugar

1 egg

Directions:

Preheat oven to 350 °F. Mix all ingredients together with a large spatula. Scoop 1 tbsp of dough and roll it into a ball. Place rolled dough onto a nonstick cookie sheet. If the cookie sheet is not nonstick, line it with parchment paper or a silicone baking mat. Gently press down on dough ball with a fork. Repeat steps with remaining dough, placing each dough ball about 2 inches apart because they will spread when baking. Bake at 350 °F for 8 to 10 minutes. Let cookies cool for 5 minutes, then transfer them to a cooling rack to cool completely.

American Academy of Pediatrics

DEDICATED TO THE HEALTH OF ALL CHILDREN®

Single copies of these recipes may be made for noncommercial, educational purposes. The information contained herein should not be used as a substitute for the medical care and advice of a pediatric health care professional.

The American Academy of Pediatrics is an organization of 67,000 primary care pediatricians, pediatric medical subspecialists, and pediatric surgical specialists dedicated to the health, safety, and well-being of all infants, children, adolescents, and young adults.

American Academy of Pediatrics website—www.HealthyChildren.org   © 2023 American Academy of Pediatrics. All rights reserved.

Recipes High in Prebiotics

 Creamy Broccoli and Cheese Soup

Serving size: 4

Ingredients:

3 tbsp olive oil

1 leek, chopped into ¼-inch slices (if leek is unavailable, can substitute 1 onion, chopped)

3 garlic cloves, chopped

1 lb broccoli, top cut into florets and stalk cut into 1-inch pieces

1 (15-oz) can cannellini or great northern beans, drained

4 c water or vegetable/chicken broth

2 c frozen spinach (no need to defrost)

2 tsp salt

½ c shredded cheddar cheese, divided

Special equipment: blender

Directions:

Warm the olive oil in a large pot over medium-low heat. Place the chopped leek and garlic into the pot and stir occasionally for 2 to 3 minutes. Add the broccoli pieces to the pot and stir for another 2 to 3 minutes. Add the drained beans and the water or broth to the pot and stir. Reduce heat to low and cook mixture for 15 to 20 minutes, until broccoli is soft. Add the frozen spinach and salt and stir until the spinach is defrosted.

Add half the soup and ¼ c of the cheddar cheese to the blender and blend until smooth. Pour the blended soup into a medium-sized bowl and repeat these steps with the remaining soup and cheese. Place all the soup back into the original pot and turn the heat back to medium. Simmer for 10 minutes, then serve.

"All the Greens" Salad

Serving size: 4 to 6

Ingredients:

Salt

2 c broccoli, cut into small florets

2 c asparagus, cut into 1-inch pieces

1 c shelled edamame (if shelled edamame is not available, can substitute the same amount of frozen green peas, defrosted)

1 medium-sized cucumber, sliced into rounds and quartered (approximately 1½ c)

1 avocado, cubed

Dressing of choice (Refer to the Dressings section later in these recipes.)

Directions:

Bring a medium pot of water to a boil and add a pinch of salt. Once the water is boiling, add cut broccoli and asparagus (and edamame, if frozen) to the pot and stir. Cook for 30 seconds, then drain the vegetables and edamame in a colander. Run water over the vegetables and edamame until cool or place them into a bowl with ice water until cool, then drain them well. Mix the cooked vegetables and edamame with the cucumber and avocado. Drizzle the mixture with dressing and toss the two until well combined.

Simple Roasted Vegetables

Roasting at high heat brings out the natural sweetness in vegetables. It is important not to overcrowd the baking sheet because overcrowding can lead to uneven cooking and often steams the vegetables. These vegetables are delicious with salt and pepper but can be served with one of the dressings from the Dressings section that follows for variety.

Serving size: 4 to 6

Ingredients:

1½ lb vegetables (brussels sprouts, broccoli, asparagus, root vegetables, or cabbage; refer to the following table for preparation methods for each)

2 to 3 tbsp olive oil

1 to 2 tsp salt

1 tsp ground black pepper

Directions:

Preheat oven to 425 °F. Rub the olive oil and salt over the vegetables. Refer to the following table for cooking times.

Tip: Frozen vegetables can be roasted without the need to defrost them first. Add 2 to 3 minutes to the cooking time if using frozen vegetables.

Vegetable	Cutting preparation	Cooking time (min)
Asparagus	Cut off tough ends.	10
Broccoli or cauliflower	Cut into smaller florets.	10–12
Brussels sprouts	Cut in half (or quarters, if larger) and place cut side down on baking tray.	15–20
Cabbage	Cut in half, then cut in quarters. (There is no need to remove the core, which will keep the cabbage wedges together as they roast.) Cut each quarter in half lengthwise, for a total of 8 wedges.	15–20
Green beans	Trim ends.	10
Root vegetables (such as sweet potatoes, beets, parsnips, or carrots)	Cut vegetables into similarly sized pieces, about 1½-inch cubes.	20–25

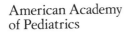

Dressings

 Tahini Soy Dressing

Ingredients:

¼ c soy sauce or tamari

2 tbsp tahini (can substitute equal amount of peanut/almond butter)

2 tbsp maple syrup or honey

1 tsp toasted sesame oil (optional)

¼ c olive oil

Special equipment: 1 (12- to 16-oz) jar with lid

Directions:

Place all ingredients into a jar that has a well-fitting lid, close or screw on the lid, and shake the jar until the ingredients are well mixed. Add water to thin the dressing as desired.

 Basic Vinaigrette

Ingredients:

¼ c red wine vinegar, white wine vinegar, or balsamic vinegar

2 tbsp red onion, diced (optional)

2 tsp dried parsley, chives, or oregano (If using fresh herbs, increase the amount to 1 tbsp.)

1 tbsp honey

1 tbsp Dijon mustard

¼ c olive oil

Special equipment: 1 (12- to 16-oz) jar with lid

Directions:

Place all ingredients into a jar that has a well-fitting lid, close or screw on the lid, and shake the jar until the ingredients are well mixed.

American Academy of Pediatrics

DEDICATED TO THE HEALTH OF ALL CHILDREN®

Single copies of these recipes may be made for noncommercial, educational purposes. The information contained herein should not be used as a substitute for the medical care and advice of a pediatric health care professional.

The American Academy of Pediatrics is an organization of 67,000 primary care pediatricians, pediatric medical subspecialists, and pediatric surgical specialists dedicated to the health, safety, and well-being of all infants, children, adolescents, and young adults.

American Academy of Pediatrics website—www.HealthyChildren.org © 2023 American Academy of Pediatrics. All rights reserved.

Creamy Green Herb Avocado Dressing

Ingredients:

2 c fresh green herbs (parsley, chives, dill, or cilantro)

2 garlic cloves

1 avocado, pitted and skin removed

½ c low-fat plain Greek yogurt

½ lime, juiced

¼ c olive oil

½ tsp salt

Special equipment: blender or food processor

Directions:

Place all ingredients into a blender or food processor, secure the lid, and pulse the ingredients until well blended. Add water to thin the dressing as desired (or keep it as is and use it as a dip).

If a blender or food processor is not available, chop the green herbs and garlic until very fine and set aside. Remove the flesh of the avocado and place it into a bowl. With a fork, mash the avocado into a thick puree, then add the yogurt and mix the two well. Pour the lime juice into the bowl with the avocado and yogurt and mix these ingredients well. Slowly add the olive oil to the avocado-yogurt–lime juice mixture, stirring continuously to incorporate the olive oil. Add the chopped herbs and garlic to the bowl. Add water to thin the dressing as desired (or keep it as is and use it as a dip).

 Lemon Garlic Parsley Dressing

Ingredients:

¼ c fresh parsley, chopped

2 garlic cloves, chopped

¼ c lemon juice

½ tsp salt

½ c olive oil

Special equipment: 1 (12- to 16-oz) jar with lid

Directions:

Place all ingredients into a jar that has a well-fitting lid, close or screw on the lid, and shake the jar until the ingredients are well mixed.

American Academy of Pediatrics

DEDICATED TO THE HEALTH OF ALL CHILDREN®

Chapter 3

Recipes to Ensure Sufficient, High-Quality Vegan or Vegetarian Protein Intake

 Plant-Based Burgers: Mix-and-Match Legume and Grain

Serving size: 4

Ingredients:

1 c cooked grains (brown rice, quinoa, or bulgur)

1 c beans (black beans, pinto beans, or cannellini beans) or chickpeas (If using canned beans or chickpeas, drain liquid.)

1 egg

2 tsp dried spices, mixed (such as onion powder, garlic powder, paprika, ground cumin, and ground coriander)

½ c old-fashioned rolled oats (can substitute plain or seasoned bread crumbs)

2 to 3 tbsp olive oil

Directions:

Mix grains and beans in a medium-sized bowl. Mash the mixture with a potato masher or fork until the beans are well mashed. Add the egg, spices, and oats or bread crumbs and mix the ingredients well. Form 4 equal-sized patties.

Warm the olive oil in a medium-sized pan over medium heat. Place the patties into the pan and cook for 5 minutes. Flip the patties and cook for another 4 to 5 minutes.

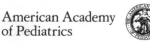

Basic Tofu

Firm tofu is ideal for this recipe because it holds its shape well when baking or panfrying.

Serving size: 4

Ingredients:

1 (16-oz) package firm tofu

Flour or cornstarch

Olive oil

Directions:

Tofu preparation methods:

Squeezing out as much liquid as possible from the tofu allows for a crispier texture and more absorption of flavors if marinating the tofu. Following are 2 options to dry out the tofu:

Method 1: Line a plate with a clean kitchen towel or paper towels and place the block of tofu onto the towel(s). Cover the tofu with another kitchen towel or paper towel, then gently push down on the tofu. Place the plate into the refrigerator for 5 to 6 hours with a heavy object on top (such as a can of beans) to help press the water out of the tofu.

Method 2: If short on preparation time, press as much water out of the tofu as possible by wrapping the tofu in a clean kitchen towel and pushing down on the tofu. Squeeze the water out of the towel. Repeat the step of wrapping and pushing down on the tofu if necessary, taking care not to break the tofu.

Tofu cooking methods:

Cut the tofu into ½-inch cubes. Coat the tofu cubes with flour or cornstarch, shaking off excess powder. Then the tofu can be cooked either in the oven or on the stove, as follows:

Oven: Preheat oven to 400 °F. Place the tofu in a single layer onto a baking sheet. Drizzle the tofu with 1 to 2 tbsp of olive oil. Bake for 10 to 15 minutes, then turn tofu cubes over and bake for another 10 minutes, until the cubes are browned and crispy.

Stove: Pour 2 to 3 tbsp of olive oil into a medium-sized pan over medium heat. Place tofu cubes in a single layer into the pan and cook for 8 to 10 minutes. Flip tofu cubes over and cook for another 6 to 8 minutes, until cubes are browned and crispy.

Tofu marination method:

Marinating the tofu for a few hours or up to overnight in the refrigerator before cooking is a great way to infuse flavor. Tofu can be marinated in a favorite sauce or combination of dried/fresh herbs and olive oil.

American Academy of Pediatrics

DEDICATED TO THE HEALTH OF ALL CHILDREN®

To marinate tofu, press the tofu to squeeze out the liquid as previously instructed (refer to Method 1 or 2), then cut the tofu into the desired shape (cubes or planks) and place it into a rimmed dish. Pour the marinade over the tofu, then cover and place tofu into the refrigerator for a few hours or up to overnight. Cook the tofu by using either previously described method (refer to Oven or Stove).

The following combinations can be served with a grain to make this meal a more complete protein (refer to the Carbohydrates section later in these recipes for grain examples).

 Pizza Tofu

Serving size: 4

Ingredients:

1 tsp garlic powder

1 tsp onion powder

1 tsp dried oregano

½ tsp salt

2 tbsp tomato paste

2 tbsp olive oil

1 (16-oz) package firm tofu

2 tbsp grated or shredded Parmesan cheese

Whole grain pasta (optional)

Directions:

Combine the garlic powder, onion powder, oregano, salt, tomato paste, and olive oil in a shallow bowl. Follow instructions for drying out the tofu (refer to Method 1 or 2), then follow instructions for marinating the tofu.

Choose a method for cooking the tofu (refer to Oven or Stove). After flipping the tofu during either method, sprinkle the Parmesan cheese on top and continue cooking as directed. Serve with a side of marinara sauce for dipping.

Tip: To make a complete protein, serve with whole grain pasta and pizza toppings (such as chopped olives, chopped green bell pepper, and mushrooms) for a fun pizza-pasta twist.

Tofu Taco "Meat"

Serving size: 4

Ingredients:

1 tsp garlic powder

1 tsp onion powder

1 tsp ground cumin

1 tsp dried oregano

1 tsp smoked or regular paprika, not sweet

1 tsp salt

1 (16-oz) package firm tofu

2 tbsp olive oil

Directions:

Combine the garlic powder, onion powder, cumin, oregano, paprika, and salt in a medium-sized bowl. Follow instructions for drying out the tofu (refer to Method 1 or 2). Instead of cutting the tofu, crumble the tofu by breaking it into small pieces (to resemble ground meat), then place it into the bowl with the seasoning mixture. Mix the seasoning and tofu together until well combined.

Add the olive oil to a medium-sized pan, and place the pan over medium heat. Add the tofu crumbles to the pan and cook for about 10 minutes, stirring occasionally.

Tip: To make a complete protein, try making a "burrito bowl" by serving with brown rice, chopped lettuce, beans, and salsa.

American Academy of Pediatrics

DEDICATED TO THE HEALTH OF ALL CHILDREN®

Single copies of these recipes may be made for noncommercial, educational purposes. The information contained herein should not be used as a substitute for the medical care and advice of a pediatric health care professional.

The American Academy of Pediatrics is an organization of 67,000 primary care pediatricians, pediatric medical subspecialists, and pediatric surgical specialists dedicated to the health, safety, and well-being of all infants, children, adolescents, and young adults.

American Academy of Pediatrics website—www.HealthyChildren.org   © 2023 American Academy of Pediatrics. All rights reserved.

Basic Lentil Soup

Serving size: 4 to 6

Ingredients:

2 tbsp olive oil

1 onion, chopped

2 carrots, chopped

2 celery stalks, chopped

2 garlic cloves, chopped

1 c green lentils

1 tsp salt

4 c water or broth

Directions:

Warm the olive oil in a soup pot over medium heat. Add the chopped onion, carrots, celery, and garlic to the pot and cook for 4 to 5 minutes, stirring occasionally. Add the lentils, salt, and water or broth. Turn heat to medium-high and bring mixture to a boil, then reduce heat to low. Cook for 40 to 45 minutes, until the lentils are soft. Add more broth or water to achieve the desired consistency.

Lentil soup variations:

- Lentil miso soup (+ brown rice)
- Lentil curry soup (+ chickpeas)
- Lentil tortilla soup (+ quinoa)

For lentil miso soup: Stir in 2 tbsp of miso paste once the lentils are cooked, then add 2 c of baby spinach or 2 to 3 bunches of baby bok choy (whole, cut in half lengthwise, or chopped) and cook for an additional 5 minutes. Serve with brown rice. Optional: Top soup with 1 tsp of toasted sesame oil and 1 tbsp of chopped green onion.

For lentil curry soup: Add 2 tbsp of curry powder or curry paste and 1 c of ½-inch cubed butternut squash or sweet potatoes. Once the lentils are cooked, add 1 can of chickpeas (drained) and stir. Top soup with chopped fresh cilantro. Optional: Substitute 1 can of coconut milk for 1 c of the cooking water.

For lentil tortilla soup: Add 1 can of diced tomatoes, 1 tsp of ground cumin, 1 tsp of dried oregano, and 1 tsp of paprika when adding the lentils and water. Serve with ¼ c of quinoa on top. Top soup with tortillas strips, cilantro, and a squeeze of lime.

American Academy of Pediatrics

DEDICATED TO THE HEALTH OF ALL CHILDREN®

Single copies of these recipes may be made for noncommercial, educational purposes. The information contained herein should not be used as a substitute for the medical care and advice of a pediatric health care professional.

The American Academy of Pediatrics is an organization of 67,000 primary care pediatricians, pediatric medical subspecialists, and pediatric surgical specialists dedicated to the health, safety, and well-being of all infants, children, adolescents, and young adults.

American Academy of Pediatrics website—www.HealthyChildren.org © 2023 American Academy of Pediatrics. All rights reserved.

Crispy Edamame

Serving size: 4 to 6

Ingredients:

1 lb edamame (frozen or fresh), shelled

2 tbsp olive oil

2 tsp seasoning (Possible combinations follow.)

Try these seasoning combinations.

- BBQ: smoked paprika + onion powder + garlic powder + ground cumin
- Ranch: dried dill weed + onion powder + garlic powder
- Asian: sesame seeds + garlic powder + ground ginger
- Latin: dried oregano + ground cumin + paprika + garlic powder

Directions:

Preheat oven to 400 °F. If the edamame is frozen, thaw and dry the edamame. (The drier the edamame is, the crunchier the final product will be.) Place the edamame onto a baking sheet, drizzle it with the olive oil, add the desired seasoning, and mix the ingredients well. Spread the edamame in a single layer. Bake for about 10 minutes. Remove the edamame from the oven and stir, then place the sheet back into the oven for another 5 to 10 minutes, until the edamame is crispy.

American Academy of Pediatrics
of Pediatrics

DEDICATED TO THE HEALTH OF ALL CHILDREN®

Single copies of these recipes may be made for noncommercial, educational purposes. The information contained herein should not be used as a substitute for the medical care and advice of a pediatric health care professional.

The American Academy of Pediatrics is an organization of 67,000 primary care pediatricians, pediatric medical subspecialists, and pediatric surgical specialists dedicated to the health, safety, and well-being of all infants, children, adolescents, and young adults.

American Academy of Pediatrics website—www.HealthyChildren.org   © 2023 American Academy of Pediatrics. All rights reserved.

Chapter 7

Recipes to Make Water More Appealing

 Fruit- and Herb-Infused Water Combinations

For 12 fl oz of water:

- Strawberry + kiwifruit: ¼ c chopped strawberries and kiwifruit
- Cucumber + basil: ¼ c chopped cucumber and 1 basil leaf
- Lemon + orange: 1 slice/wedge orange and 1 slice/wedge lemon
- Pineapple + mint: ¼ c chopped pineapple and 2 mint leaves
- Lime + cantaloupe: 1 slice/wedge lime and ¼ c chopped cantaloupe
- Blueberry + apple: ¼ c whole blueberries and chopped apples

 Flavored Sparkling Water

Ingredients:

2 c assorted fruits (such as strawberries, blueberries, and peaches)

Special equipment: blender, ice cube tray

Directions:

Puree fruits in a blender until well blended, and pour mixture into ice cube trays. Place trays into freezer. Once frozen, place 1 to 2 ice cubes into a cup and pour sparkling water over the cubes. Another option for citrus fruits that also reduces food waste is to remove the zest, slice the zest into small slivers, and place 4 to 5 slivers into each ice cube tray. Pour water into each ice cube tray until about halfway full, then place trays into freezer. Once frozen, place 1 to 2 ice cubes into a cup and pour sparkling water over the cubes.

 Fruity Ice Cubes

Ingredients:

¼ to ½ c fruit and/or herbs (such as strawberries, blueberries, peaches, and mint leaves)

Directions:

Cut a variety of fruits into small pieces (about ¼-inch thick), and place 3 to 4 pieces into each ice cube well. Add mint leaves or other herbs if desired. Pour water to cover fruit (and herbs, if using), then place trays into freezer.

American Academy of Pediatrics

DEDICATED TO THE HEALTH OF ALL CHILDREN®

Single copies of these recipes may be made for noncommercial, educational purposes. The information contained herein should not be used as a substitute for the medical care and advice of a pediatric health care professional.

The American Academy of Pediatrics is an organization of 67,000 primary care pediatricians, pediatric medical subspecialists, and pediatric surgical specialists dedicated to the health, safety, and well-being of all infants, children, adolescents, and young adults.

American Academy of Pediatrics website—www.HealthyChildren.org   © 2023 American Academy of Pediatrics. All rights reserved.

Chapter 10

Recipes for Healthful Meals Based on the Special Supplemental Nutrition Program for Women, Infants, and Children Food Package

Breakfast

 Caramelized Banana Cinnamon Oatmeal

Serving size: 4

Ingredients:

2 ripe bananas

1 tbsp olive oil

2 tbsp maple syrup or honey, divided

2 tsp ground cinnamon

1½ c old-fashioned rolled oats

1 c milk (any variety, including plant-based "milks")

1 c water

¼ tsp salt

Directions:

Peel the bananas and slice 1 banana into ½-inch rounds. Place a medium-sized pot over medium heat and add the olive oil to the pot. Add the banana slices to the pot. Pour in 1 tbsp of the maple syrup or honey and the cinnamon. Let the mixture sit undisturbed for 2 to 3 minutes to allow the bananas to caramelize. Stir bananas and cook for another minute or so until soft but not falling apart. Remove bananas from the pot and set aside.

To the same pot (no need to wash), add oats, milk, water, salt, and remaining tablespoon of maple syrup or honey. Bring the mixture to a boil, then lower the heat to a simmer. Slice the second banana into ¼-inch rounds and add the rounds to the pot. Cook for 10 to 15 minutes, stirring often. Scoop oatmeal into bowls and top it with caramelized bananas.

American Academy
of Pediatrics

DEDICATED TO THE HEALTH OF ALL CHILDREN®

Single copies of these recipes may be made for noncommercial, educational purposes. The information contained herein should not be used as a substitute for the medical care and advice of a pediatric health care professional.

The American Academy of Pediatrics is an organization of 67,000 primary care pediatricians, pediatric medical subspecialists, and pediatric surgical specialists dedicated to the health, safety, and well-being of all infants, children, adolescents, and young adults.

American Academy of Pediatrics website—www.HealthyChildren.org

Yogurt and Fruit Parfait With Cereal

Serving size: 4

Ingredients:

2 c low-fat plain yogurt, divided

2 c assorted fruit (such as berries, mango, pineapple, and peaches), divided

1 c cereal (low-sugar), divided

Directions:

Place ¼ c of yogurt into the bottom of a glass, for 4 glasses. Add ¼ c of fruit to each glass, then layer another ¼ c of yogurt, followed by another ¼ c of fruit, on top. Top each glass with 2 tbsp of cereal.

American Academy of Pediatrics

DEDICATED TO THE HEALTH OF ALL CHILDREN®

Lunch

 Lentil Minestrone Soup With Pasta

Serving size: 4 to 6

Ingredients:

2 tbsp olive oil

1 onion, chopped

2 carrots, chopped

2 celery stalks, chopped

2 garlic cloves, chopped

1 c green lentils

1 tsp salt

1 tsp dried oregano

1 (15-oz) can diced tomatoes

4 c water or broth

1 (15-oz) can red kidney beans, drained

1 c short whole grain pasta, cooked

Fresh basil or parsley

Grated Parmesan cheese

Directions:

Warm the olive oil in a soup pot over medium heat. Add the chopped onion, carrots, celery, and garlic to the pot and cook for 4 to 5 minutes, stirring occasionally. Add the lentils, salt, oregano, diced tomatoes, and water or broth. Increase heat to medium-high and bring mixture to a boil, then reduce heat to low. Cook for 40 to 45 minutes, until the lentils are soft. Once the lentils are cooked, add the drained red kidney beans and the cooked whole grain pasta to the pot. Add more broth or water as needed to achieve the desired consistency. Top soup with fresh basil or parsley and grated Parmesan cheese.

American Academy of Pediatrics

DEDICATED TO THE HEALTH OF ALL CHILDREN®

Single copies of these recipes may be made for noncommercial, educational purposes. The information contained herein should not be used as a substitute for the medical care and advice of a pediatric health care professional.

The American Academy of Pediatrics is an organization of 67,000 primary care pediatricians, pediatric medical subspecialists, and pediatric surgical specialists dedicated to the health, safety, and well-being of all infants, children, adolescents, and young adults.

American Academy of Pediatrics website—www.HealthyChildren.org   © 2023 American Academy of Pediatrics. All rights reserved.

Tuna Melts With Whole Grain Bread

Serving size: 4

Ingredients:

1 (5-oz) can tuna, drained

¼ c onion, chopped

1 celery stalk, chopped (about ½ c)

½ c canned cannellini beans, drained

1 tbsp low-fat mayonnaise

2 tbsp low-fat Greek yogurt

1 tbsp fresh parsley, chopped

1 dill pickle spear, chopped

4 slices whole grain bread

1 tomato, sliced

¼ c shredded cheddar cheese, divided

Directions:

Preheat oven or toaster oven to 350 °F. Mix the first 8 ingredients together in a bowl. Place 4 slices of whole grain bread onto a baking sheet. Place 3 to 4 tbsp of tuna mixture onto each slice of bread, then top mixture with a tomato slice and 1 tbsp of shredded cheese. Repeat steps with remaining 3 slices of bread. Bake for 10 to 15 minutes, until the cheese is melted and browned.

American Academy of Pediatrics

DEDICATED TO THE HEALTH OF ALL CHILDREN®

Single copies of these recipes may be made for noncommercial, educational purposes. The information contained herein should not be used as a substitute for the medical care and advice of a pediatric health care professional.

The American Academy of Pediatrics is an organization of 67,000 primary care pediatricians, pediatric medical subspecialists, and pediatric surgical specialists dedicated to the health, safety, and well-being of all infants, children, adolescents, and young adults.

American Academy of Pediatrics website—www.HealthyChildren.org   © 2023 American Academy of Pediatrics. All rights reserved.

Dinner

 Salmon Tacos With Corn and Black Bean Salsa

Serving size: 4

Ingredients:

2 tbsp olive oil

½ onion, chopped

2 (5-oz) cans salmon, drained

2 tsp taco seasoning

¼ c fresh cilantro, chopped

Corn tortillas

Corn and Black Bean Salsa (Recipe follows.)

Directions:

Warm the olive oil in a medium-sized pan over medium heat. Add the chopped onion to the pan and cook until browned, for 3 to 4 minutes. Add the drained salmon and the taco seasoning to the pan, breaking up the salmon into smaller chunks. Stir occasionally for 2 to 3 minutes, then add the chopped cilantro and turn off the heat. Divide the salmon among the tortillas and top it with the Corn and Black Bean Salsa.

 Corn and Black Bean Salsa

Serving size: 4 to 6

Ingredients:

1½ c frozen corn, thawed and drained

1 c canned black beans, drained

½ c onion, chopped

¼ c fresh cilantro, chopped

½ lime, juiced

¼ tsp ground cumin

¼ tsp salt

Directions:

Add all ingredients to a bowl and stir until well combined.

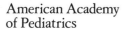

"All the Vegetables" Fried Rice

Serving size: 4 to 6

Ingredients:

3 tbsp olive oil, divided

1 small onion, chopped

3 c mixed vegetables, chopped into ¼-inch pieces

3½ c rice, cooked

¼ c soy sauce

2 eggs

Directions:

Warm 2 tbsp of the olive oil in a large-sized pan over medium heat. Add the chopped onion to the pan and stir occasionally until lightly browned. Add the vegetables and cook until the vegetables are softened, for approximately 3 to 5 minutes. (Time will vary depending on the vegetables used.) Once the vegetables are softened, add the rice and soy sauce and mix the ingredients well. Push the rice to the sides of the pan and add the remaining tablespoon of olive oil to the middle of the pan. Break the eggs directly into the pan and stir to break up their yolks. Allow the eggs to cook undisturbed for 2 to 3 minutes, then begin to mix the rice and vegetables with the eggs. Cook for another 3 to 4 minutes, until the eggs are firm.

Tips:

● This recipe is a great way to use leftover or frozen vegetables.
● Leftover rice works best in this recipe.

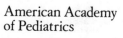

American Academy
of Pediatrics

DEDICATED TO THE HEALTH OF ALL CHILDREN®

Single copies of these recipes may be made for noncommercial, educational purposes. The information contained herein should not be used as a substitute for the medical care and advice of a pediatric health care professional.

The American Academy of Pediatrics is an organization of 67,000 primary care pediatricians, pediatric medical subspecialists, and pediatric surgical specialists dedicated to the health, safety, and well-being of all infants, children, adolescents, and young adults.

American Academy of Pediatrics website—www.HealthyChildren.org   © 2023 American Academy of Pediatrics. All rights reserved.

Recipes to Feed a Family of 4 on $31 per Day

Breakfast

 Spinach, Egg, and Cheese Breakfast Pita Pockets (About $4.00)

Serving size: 4

Ingredients:

2 tbsp olive oil

2 c baby spinach, washed and dried

4 eggs

¼ c shredded cheddar cheese

2 whole wheat pita breads

Directions:

Place a medium-sized pan over medium-low heat. Pour the olive oil into the pan. Add the baby spinach to the pan and stir occasionally for 2 minutes, until the spinach is wilted. Crack the eggs into a bowl and beat them with a fork until well mixed. Add the eggs to the pan and let the eggs sit in the pan undisturbed for 30 seconds. With a spatula, gently stir the eggs and spinach until the eggs are firm. Sprinkle the cheddar cheese on top of the egg-spinach mixture, stir the eggs until well combined, and then remove the eggs from the pan.

Cut each pita bread in half, then open each half to create a pocket. Divide the egg mixture evenly among the 4 pockets of pita bread.

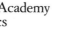 **American Academy of Pediatrics**

DEDICATED TO THE HEALTH OF ALL CHILDREN®

Single copies of these recipes may be made for noncommercial, educational purposes. The information contained herein should not be used as a substitute for the medical care and advice of a pediatric health care professional.

The American Academy of Pediatrics is an organization of 67,000 primary care pediatricians, pediatric medical subspecialists, and pediatric surgical specialists dedicated to the health, safety, and well-being of all infants, children, adolescents, and young adults. American Academy of Pediatrics website—www.HealthyChildren.org   © 2023 American Academy of Pediatrics. All rights reserved.

Lunch

 ### *Chicken Whole Wheat Pita Wraps With Creamy Ranch Bean Dip (About $13.00)*

Serving size: 4

Ingredients:

1 boneless, skinless chicken breast, uncooked

1 tsp salt

1 tsp ground black pepper

2 tbsp olive oil

2 c baby spinach, washed and dried and divided

½ large cucumber, cut into ⅛-inch slices, divided

1 c shredded cheddar cheese, divided

4 whole wheat pita breads

Creamy Ranch Bean Dip (Recipe follows.)

Directions:

To prepare chicken: Cut chicken breast in half widthwise (so chicken breast is thinner) into a total of 2 pieces. Warm a medium-sized pan on the stove at medium heat. Sprinkle each side of the chicken breast with salt and pepper. Add the olive oil to the pan. Place both chicken pieces into the pan and cook for 6 to 7 minutes. Flip the chicken and cook for another 6 to 7 minutes, until the internal temperature reaches a minimum of 165 °F. When the chicken is finished cooking, remove it from the pan, lay it flat on a cutting board, and cut it into ½-inch strips. (If you prefer to bake the chicken breast, refer to the Simple Baked Chicken Breast recipe later in these recipes.)

To prepare wraps: Spread 2 tbsp of the Creamy Ranch Bean Dip over a pita bread. Next, place ½ c of spinach to cover the entire area of the pita bread. Place ¼ c of shredded cheese into the middle of the pita bread. Place chicken strips next to the cheese. Place ¼ of the cucumber slices next to the chicken. Fold the pita bread in half to serve. Repeat steps with remaining pita breads.

 American Academy of Pediatrics

DEDICATED TO THE HEALTH OF ALL CHILDREN®

Single copies of these recipes may be made for noncommercial, educational purposes. The information contained herein should not be used as a substitute for the medical care and advice of a pediatric health care professional.

The American Academy of Pediatrics is an organization of 67,000 primary care pediatricians, pediatric medical subspecialists, and pediatric surgical specialists dedicated to the health, safety, and well-being of all infants, children, adolescents, and young adults.

American Academy of Pediatrics website—www.HealthyChildren.org   © 2023 American Academy of Pediatrics. All rights reserved.

Creamy Ranch Bean Dip

Ingredients:

1 (15-oz) can cannellini beans

½ tsp garlic powder

½ tsp onion powder

1 tsp dried dill weed

Special equipment: blender

Directions:

Place the cannellini beans, including the liquid from the can; garlic powder; onion powder; and dill weed into a blender and blend until well combined. If a blender is not available, place the beans and seasonings into a medium bowl and smash with a fork or potato masher until a thick paste forms. Add water or olive oil to thin the mixture if needed.

Adapted with permission from Muth ND. Can I eat healthy on $7 a day? American Council on Exercise blog. April 20, 2011. Accessed November 4, 2022. https://www.acefitness.org/education-and-resources/lifestyle/blog/1408/can-i-eathealthy-on-7-a-day. Copyright © 2011, American Council on Exercise. All rights reserved. Reprinted by permission.

Dinner

 Turkey and Vegetable Whole Wheat Chow Mein–style Noodles (About $12.00)

Serving size: 4

Ingredients:

2 tbsp olive oil

1 lb ground turkey

½ medium onion (white, yellow, or red), sliced

3 garlic cloves, finely chopped

2 medium carrots, peeled and cut into ¼-inch slices

2 c baby spinach

1 large red pepper, seeded and cut into ¼-inch strips

1 c green onion, chopped

¼ c soy sauce

½ c water

1 (16-oz) package whole wheat spaghetti, cooked according to package instructions

American Academy of Pediatrics

DEDICATED TO THE HEALTH OF ALL CHILDREN®

Directions:

Pour the olive oil into a large pan, and place the pan over medium heat. Add the ground turkey, sliced onion, and chopped garlic to the pan and cook for 6 to 7 minutes, stirring occasionally to break up the meat, until the meat is no longer pink. Add the remaining vegetables to the pan, followed by the soy sauce and water. Cook for approximately 4 to 5 minutes, stirring occasionally. Last, add the cooked noodles to the pan and mix all ingredients well. Cook for another 2 to 3 minutes and then serve.

Adapted with permission from Muth ND. Can I eat healthy on $7 a day? American Council on Exercise blog. April 20, 2011. Accessed November 4, 2022. https://www.acefitness.org/education-and-resources/lifestyle/blog/1408/can-i-eathealthy-on-7-a-day. Copyright © 2011, American Council on Exercise. All rights reserved. Reprinted by permission.

Snack

 Carrots and Cucumbers With Creamy Ranch Bean Dip (About $2.00)

Serving size: 4

Ingredients:

4 medium carrots

½ large cucumber

½ cup Creamy Ranch Bean Dip (Refer to Chicken Whole Wheat Pita Wraps With Creamy Ranch Bean Dip recipe earlier in these recipes.)

Directions:

Peel carrots and trim off ends. Cut each carrot lengthwise and then into sticks of desired thickness. Slice cucumbers into ¼-inch slices. Serve with Creamy Ranch Bean Dip.

American Academy of Pediatrics

DEDICATED TO THE HEALTH OF ALL CHILDREN®

Chapter 12

Mix-and-Match MyPlate-Consistent Meals

Proteins

 Simple Baked Chicken Breast

Serving size: 4

Ingredients:

4 boneless, skinless chicken breasts, uncooked

Olive oil

1 tsp salt

1 tsp ground black pepper

1 tsp additional spices/dried herbs (Possible combinations follow.)

Try some of the following seasonings to add variety by mixing these seasonings with salt and pepper before sprinkling them onto the chicken breasts:

- ½ tsp garlic powder + ½ tsp dried rosemary
- ½ tsp ground cumin + ½ tsp dried oregano
- ½ tsp onion powder + ½ tsp smoked paprika

Directions:

Preheat oven to 400 °F. Place chicken breasts onto a baking sheet. Drizzle them with olive oil and rub salt and pepper (and additional spices and dried herbs, if using) onto both sides of each chicken breast. Bake for 25 to 30 minutes, until the internal temperature reaches at least 165 °F.

Tip: Cook extra chicken to use in sandwiches, soups, salads, and wraps for the rest of the week.

American Academy of Pediatrics

DEDICATED TO THE HEALTH OF ALL CHILDREN®

Single copies of these recipes may be made for noncommercial, educational purposes. The information contained herein should not be used as a substitute for the medical care and advice of a pediatric health care professional.

The American Academy of Pediatrics is an organization of 67,000 primary care pediatricians, pediatric medical subspecialists, and pediatric surgical specialists dedicated to the health, safety, and well-being of all infants, children, adolescents, and young adults.

American Academy of Pediatrics website—www.HealthyChildren.org   © 2023 American Academy of Pediatrics. All rights reserved.

Perfect Poached Fish

Poaching is a cooking technique through which food is cooked in a liquid. Poaching works great for fish because poaching retains moisture and imparts the flavor of the liquid used for cooking. This is a basic oven-poached fish recipe that can be adapted by using different liquids and herbs or different varieties of fish.

Serving size: 4

Ingredients:

4 (6-oz) fish filets (any variety, such as cod, salmon, tilapia, or halibut)

Olive oil

2 tsp salt, divided

2 tsp ground black pepper, divided

½ c liquid (such as light canned coconut milk, lemon juice, lime juice, or soy sauce), divided

2 tsp dried herbs or spices and/or 4 tbsp fresh herbs, divided (Possible combinations follow.)

Try these flavor combinations.

- Lemon juice + 4 tbsp fresh chopped parsley + 1 tsp dried thyme + 1 tsp onion powder
- Soy sauce + 4 tbsp fresh chopped chives (or can substitute with chopped green onion) + 2 tsp garlic powder
- Light canned coconut milk + 2 tsp curry powder + 4 tbsp fresh chopped cilantro
- Lime juice + 1 tsp smoked paprika + 1 tsp dried oregano + 4 tbsp fresh chopped cilantro

Directions:

Preheat oven to 350 °F. Tear a piece of foil approximately 3 times the size of the fish filet. Place one 6-oz filet into the center of the foil. Drizzle olive oil over the fish, and sprinkle the fish with ½ tsp each of salt and pepper (and additional spices herbs and spices, if using). Bring up all sides of the foil perpendicularly to the fish, as if creating 4 walls. Place 2 tbsp of the desired liquid on top of the fish. Bring 2 opposite sides of the foil together in the middle, and roll the foil down until it meets the fish. Roll each open end toward the center until it meets the fish, creating a package that completely encloses the fish. Repeat steps with remaining fish filets.

Place each package onto a baking sheet and bake for 20 to 25 minutes, until the internal temperature is at least 145 °F.

 American Academy of Pediatrics

DEDICATED TO THE HEALTH OF ALL CHILDREN®

Single copies of these recipes may be made for noncommercial, educational purposes. The information contained herein should not be used as a substitute for the medical care and advice of a pediatric health care professional.

The American Academy of Pediatrics is an organization of 67,000 primary care pediatricians, pediatric medical subspecialists, and pediatric surgical specialists dedicated to the health, safety, and well-being of all infants, children, adolescents, and young adults.

American Academy of Pediatrics website—www.HealthyChildren.org   © 2023 American Academy of Pediatrics. All rights reserved.

Easy Cooked Vegetables

 Smashed Cauliflower and Potatoes

Serving size: 4 to 6

Ingredients:

1 small head cauliflower, trimmed and cut into small florets

1 medium-sized potato, washed and cut into ½-inch cubes

¼ c low-fat plain yogurt

1 tsp salt

1 tsp ground black pepper

Directions:

Place cut cauliflower and potatoes into a large pot. Add water until the vegetables are completely submerged underwater. Bring the water to a boil, then reduce the heat to medium and cook the vegetables for 20 to 30 minutes. Once the vegetables are tender, after approximately 15 to 20 minutes, remove the pot from the heat and drain the water from the pot. Remove drained vegetables from the pot, and place the vegetables into a medium bowl. Mash vegetables with a potato masher or fork. Add yogurt, salt, and pepper and mix the ingredients well.

Adapted from Muth ND. Appendix: recipes, reinforcement planners, and workouts. In: Muth ND. *Family Fit Plan: A 30-Day Wellness Transformation.* American Academy of Pediatrics; 2020:135–214.

 Roasted Garlicky and Cheesy Broccoli

Serving size: 4 to 6

Ingredients:

1 head broccoli, trimmed and cut into florets

3 tbsp olive oil

3 garlic cloves, thinly sliced

Salt and pepper

¼ c shredded Parmesan/cheddar cheese

Directions:

Preheat oven to 425 °F. Toss the broccoli florets with the olive oil, sliced garlic, salt, and pepper. Spread the broccoli in an even layer on a baking sheet. Roast for 20 minutes. Remove the broccoli from the oven and sprinkle the cheese on top before serving.

Adapted from Muth ND. Appendix: recipes, reinforcement planners, and workouts. In: Muth ND. *Family Fit Plan: A 30-Day Wellness Transformation.* American Academy of Pediatrics; 2020:135–214.

Quick and Fresh Salads

 Avocado-Cucumber Salad

Serving size: 4 to 6

Ingredients:

2 large cucumbers

¼ c green onion, chopped

1 lime, juiced

2 tbsp olive oil

1 tsp salt

1 tsp ground black pepper

2 medium-sized avocados, cut into 1-inch cubes

Directions:

Cut cucumbers crosswise into ½-inch slices, and place them into a medium-sized mixing bowl. Add the chopped green onion, lime juice, olive oil, salt, and pepper to the bowl and stir until mixed. Add the cubed avocados to the bowl and stir until combined.

Tip: Any variety of cucumbers will work in this recipe. If using Persian, Japanese, or English cucumbers, there is no need to peel the cucumbers because these varieties are thin skinned. If using garden cucumbers, which tend to have a thicker and more bitter skin, the skin should be peeled before cutting the cucumber.

 Grated Carrot Salad With Lemon and Parsley

Serving size: 4 to 6

Ingredients:

5 large carrots, grated

¼ c fresh flat-leaf or curly parsley, chopped

½ lemon, juiced

2 tsp Dijon mustard (optional)

3 tbsp olive oil

1 tsp salt

1 tsp ground black pepper

Directions:

Place grated carrots and chopped parsley into a medium-sized mixing bowl. Add lemon juice, Dijon mustard (if using), olive oil, salt, and pepper to the bowl and mix the ingredients until well combined.

Carbohydrates

 Basic Quinoa

Serving size: 4

Ingredients:

1¾ c water or broth

1 c dry quinoa

Directions:

Bring the water or broth to a boil in a medium-sized pot. Rinse the quinoa with water and drain it well. Add the quinoa to the boiling water and reduce the heat to medium-low. Cover the pot and cook the quinoa for 20 minutes. Turn the heat off and leave the pot covered for 5 minutes, which will allow the broth/water to be absorbed completely by the quinoa. Uncover the pot and fluff the quinoa with a fork. The quinoa is done when the kernel has "popped" open and is fluffy.

Adapted from Muth ND. Appendix: recipes, reinforcement planners, and workouts. In: Muth ND. *Family Fit Plan: A 30-Day Wellness Transformation*. American Academy of Pediatrics; 2020:135–214.

 Basic Whole Wheat Couscous

Serving size: 4

Ingredients:

1½ c water or broth

1 c dry couscous

Directions:

Bring the water or broth to a boil in a medium-sized pot. Add the couscous, cover the pot, and turn off the heat. Let the couscous stand covered for 10 minutes, which will allow the broth/water to be absorbed by the couscous. After 10 minutes, uncover the pot and use a fork to fluff the couscous.

Adapted from Muth ND. Appendix: recipes, reinforcement planners, and workouts. In: Muth ND. *Family Fit Plan: A 30-Day Wellness Transformation*. American Academy of Pediatrics; 2020:135–214.

Basic Barley

Serving size: 4

Ingredients:

2 c water or broth

1 c dry barley

Directions:

Bring the water or broth to a boil in a medium-sized pot. Add the barley, then lower the heat to medium-low. Cover the pot and cook the barley for 30 minutes. Drain excess water from the barley.

Tips:

● Add any of these grains to a salad for a heartier meal.
● Substitute chicken or vegetable broth for water to infuse additional flavor into the grains.
● Cook a double or triple batch of grains and freeze cooked leftovers for an easy addition to a meal.

Adapted from Muth ND. Appendix: recipes, reinforcement planners, and workouts. In: Muth ND. *Family Fit Plan: A 30-Day Wellness Transformation.* American Academy of Pediatrics; 2020:135–214.

A Day of DASH Recipes

 Recipe 1 (Breakfast): Veggie Frittata Muffins

Serving size: 4

Ingredients:

2 tbsp olive oil

½ onion, chopped

3 c vegetables (such as kale, bell peppers, spinach, and mushrooms), chopped into ¼-inch pieces

8 eggs

⅔ c milk (cow milk or plant-based variety)

4 whole grain English muffins or 4 pieces whole grain bread (optional)

Directions:

Warm the olive oil in a medium-sized pan over medium heat. Add the chopped onion to the pan and cook for 2 to 3 minutes, stirring occasionally. Add the vegetables to the pan and cook for another 5 to 6 minutes, until all the vegetables are soft. Remove the vegetables from the heat and cool them slightly.

Crack the eggs into a bowl and add the milk. Beat the eggs and milk together until well combined. Preheat oven to 375 °F.

Coat a 12-count muffin tin with a very light layer of oil, or use muffin liners for easier cleanup. Divide the cooked vegetables among the muffin cups. Pour the egg-milk mixture into each muffin cup until each is about three-quarters full. Bake for 15 to 20 minutes.

Optional: Serve 1 frittata muffin with whole grain toast or in between halves of a whole wheat English muffin as a breakfast sandwich.

Leftover frittata muffins can be frozen and then defrosted for a future meal.

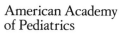

Recipe 2 (Lunch): Roasted Vegetable Grilled Cheese

Serving size: 4 to 6

Ingredients:

2 c roasted vegetables (broccoli, cauliflower, brussels sprouts, or a combination of these; refer to the Simple Roasted Vegetables recipe earlier in these recipes), divided

1 c low-fat shredded mozzarella cheese, divided

8 slices whole wheat bread, divided

4 tbsp olive oil, divided

Directions:

To assemble the sandwiches, place 4 slices of bread onto a cutting board. Place ½ c of roasted vegetables onto each slice of bread. Layer ¼ c of shredded cheese on top of the vegetables, then top each sandwich half with one of the remaining slices of bread.

Warm a medium-sized pan over medium heat, and pour 2 tbsp of the olive oil into the pan. Place 2 sandwiches into the pan and cook for 3 to 4 minutes, until the bread is golden brown. Flip the sandwiches and cook for another 3 to 4 minutes, then remove the sandwiches from the pan. Repeat these steps with the remaining 2 sandwiches.

 Recipe 3 (Snack): Almonds and Apple Slices

Serving size: 4

Ingredients:

4 apples (any variety)

½ to 1 c roasted unsalted almonds[a]

Directions:

Core and slice apples into wedges. Serve with almonds.

[a] Adult serving size of almonds: ¼ c; child serving size of almonds: ⅛ c.

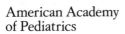**American Academy of Pediatrics**

DEDICATED TO THE HEALTH OF ALL CHILDREN®

Single copies of these recipes may be made for noncommercial, educational purposes. The information contained herein should not be used as a substitute for the medical care and advice of a pediatric health care professional.

The American Academy of Pediatrics is an organization of 67,000 primary care pediatricians, pediatric medical subspecialists, and pediatric surgical specialists dedicated to the health, safety, and well-being of all infants, children, adolescents, and young adults.

American Academy of Pediatrics website—www.HealthyChildren.org © 2023 American Academy of Pediatrics. All rights reserved.

Recipe 4 (Dinner): Chicken Black Bean Burgers With Avocado

Serving size: 4

Ingredients:

2 tbsp olive oil

1 lb ground chicken

½ (15-oz) can black beans, drained (about 1 c)

½ tsp salt

1 tsp onion powder

1 tsp garlic powder

¼ tsp smoked paprika

1 avocado, sliced into ¼-inch slices

6 whole grain hamburger buns

Directions:

Warm the olive oil in a medium-sized pan over medium heat. Mix the ground chicken, drained black beans, salt, onion powder, garlic powder, and smoked paprika in a bowl. Divide the mixture into 6 patties. Place 3 patties into the pan and cook undisturbed for 7 to 8 minutes, then flip the patties and cook for another 7 to 8 minutes, until the internal temperature reaches 165 °F. Repeat these steps with the remaining 3 patties. Place the patties onto the hamburger bun bottoms, divide the avocado slices among the patties, and top the slices with the remaining bun halves.

Burger variation:

For turkey white bean burgers: Substitute ground turkey for the chicken, cannellini beans for the black beans, pita bread for the burger bun, and dried dill weed for the paprika.

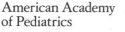

Recipe 5 (Dinner): Roasted Eggplant Casserole and Whole Wheat Pasta

Serving size: 4

Ingredients:

2 lb eggplant, cut into ½-inch rounds

4 tbsp olive oil, divided

2 tsp dried oregano

1 tsp salt

1 tsp ground black pepper

1 (24- to 25-oz) jar marinara sauce, divided

¼ c bread crumbs, plain or seasoned

¼ c grated Parmesan cheese

¼ c fresh basil leaves, chopped (optional)

Directions:

Preheat oven to 400 °F. Place the eggplant rounds in a single layer onto a baking sheet. Drizzle 2 tbsp of the olive oil over the eggplant. Sprinkle the oregano, salt, and pepper over the eggplant. Bake for 15 to 20 minutes, until the eggplant is lightly browned. Remove the baking sheet from the oven and let the eggplant cool slightly.

Spread approximately one-third of the jar of marinara sauce evenly onto the bottom of an 8 × 8–inch baking dish. Arrange 1 layer of eggplant rounds on top of the marinara sauce. Spoon another one-third of the jar of marinara sauce on top of the eggplant, then place another layer of eggplant on top of the sauce. Top with remaining sauce. Place the dish back into the oven and bake for 20 minutes.

While the eggplant is cooking, mix the remaining 2 tbsp of olive oil with the bread crumbs and Parmesan cheese. When the eggplant has been in the oven for 20 minutes, remove the dish from the oven and sprinkle the bread crumb–cheese mixture in an even layer on top of the eggplant. Place the dish back into the oven for another 10 minutes. Remove the dish from the oven once the bread crumb–cheese mixture is golden brown. Serve with whole wheat pasta. Top with chopped fresh basil (if using).

American Academy of Pediatrics

DEDICATED TO THE HEALTH OF ALL CHILDREN®

Single copies of these recipes may be made for noncommercial, educational purposes. The information contained herein should not be used as a substitute for the medical care and advice of a pediatric health care professional.

The American Academy of Pediatrics is an organization of 67,000 primary care pediatricians, pediatric medical subspecialists, and pediatric surgical specialists dedicated to the health, safety, and well-being of all infants, children, adolescents, and young adults.

American Academy of Pediatrics website—www.HealthyChildren.org   © 2023 American Academy of Pediatrics. All rights reserved.

Mediterranean-style Recipes

 Pizza Beans-and-Greens Stromboli

Serving size: 4

Ingredients:

2 tbsp olive oil

4 c leafy green vegetables (such as spinach, Swiss chard, or kale), chopped

1 tsp dried oregano

1 tsp onion powder

2 garlic cloves, finely chopped

1 (15-oz) can beans (any variety, such as cannellini, pinto, or black), drained

1 lb pizza dough, uncooked

¾ c shredded mozzarella cheese

½ c marinara sauce

Special equipment: rolling pin

Directions:

Preheat oven to 400 °F. Place a medium-sized pan over medium heat. Pour the olive oil into the pan, add the chopped green vegetables, and stir. Stir occasionally until the vegetables are wilted (about 2–3 minutes for spinach, 4–5 minutes for Swiss chard, and 7–8 minutes for kale). Add the oregano, onion powder, and chopped garlic to the pan and stir. Add the drained beans to the pan, stir until mixed evenly with the green vegetables, and turn off the heat.

To prepare the pizza dough, use a rolling pin to roll it out into a rectangle until the rectangle is approximately 10 × 12 inches (if rolling pin is not available, place flour on hands and use fingers to spread pizza dough roughly to a 10 × 12 rectangle). Spread the mozzarella cheese over the dough, leaving a 1-inch border without cheese on the sides and bottom of the rectangle and a 2-inch border without cheese at the top. Add the beans-and-greens mixture on top of the cheese. By starting at the edge closest to you, roll the dough into a 12-inch log. Once the log is rolled, pinch either end to seal the log and place the log, with the seam side facing down, onto a baking sheet. Make 2 to 3 diagonal slits on the top of the log. Bake for about 30 minutes, until the crust is golden brown. Remove the stromboli from the oven, and let it rest on the baking sheet for about 5 minutes before cutting it into slices. Cut into 2-inch slices and serve with marinara sauce.

American Academy of Pediatrics

DEDICATED TO THE HEALTH OF ALL CHILDREN®

Single copies of these recipes may be made for noncommercial, educational purposes. The information contained herein should not be used as a substitute for the medical care and advice of a pediatric health care professional.

The American Academy of Pediatrics is an organization of 67,000 primary care pediatricians, pediatric medical subspecialists, and pediatric surgical specialists dedicated to the health, safety, and well-being of all infants, children, adolescents, and young adults.

American Academy of Pediatrics website—www.HealthyChildren.org © 2023 American Academy of Pediatrics. All rights reserved.
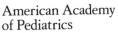

Shrimp Scampi–style Couscous Bowls With Chickpeas and Zucchini

Serving size: 4

Ingredients:

1 lb shrimp (frozen [no need to defrost] or fresh), shelled and deveined

1 (15-oz) can chickpeas, drained

3 to 4 medium-sized zucchinis, sliced into ½-inch rounds

3 tbsp olive oil

3 tbsp lemon juice

4 garlic cloves, minced

½ tsp salt

1 tsp ground black pepper

Directions:

Preheat oven to 400 °F. Place the shrimp, drained chickpeas, and sliced zucchini onto a baking sheet. Drizzle the olive oil and lemon juice over the shrimp, chickpeas, and zucchini; sprinkle the minced garlic, salt, and pepper over the top; and mix the ingredients well. Bake for 15 to 20 minutes, until shrimp is cooked through. The shrimp will be firm and its flesh white when cooked. Remove the shrimp mixture from the oven and place it on top of the couscous (refer to the Basic Whole Wheat Couscous recipe earlier in these recipes).

Crispy Fish Nuggets With Yogurt Tartar Sauce and Green Beans

Serving size: 4

Ingredients:

2 c crispy rice cereal

1 tsp garlic powder

6 tbsp olive oil, divided

1 tsp salt, divided

1 tsp ground black pepper, divided

½ c all-purpose flour

2 eggs, beaten

1½ lb white fish (such as halibut, cod, or tilapia), cut into approximately 3 × 1–inch pieces

1 lb green beans, ends trimmed

Yogurt Tartar Sauce (Recipe follows.)

Directions:

Preheat oven to 400 °F. Line a baking sheet with parchment paper or coat it with non-stick cooking spray. Place the rice cereal into a resealable bag, and crush the cereal until it becomes fine crumbs. Add the garlic powder, 4 tbsp of the olive oil, ½ tsp of the salt, and ½ tsp of the pepper into the bag with the crushed cereal, then mix the ingredients until the cereal crumbs are well coated with olive oil and seasonings.

Place the all-purpose flour into a bowl. Place beaten eggs into a separate bowl. Coat 1 piece of fish in flour, dip it into the eggs, and then place it into the bag to coat it with the crushed cereal. With the bag sealed, move the fish pieces around in the bag to coat all sides of each piece of fish. Remove the fish from the bag, and place the fish onto the baking sheet. Repeat these steps with the remaining fish pieces. Place the baking sheet into the oven and bake the fish for 8 to 10 minutes.

Meanwhile, on a separate baking sheet, place green beans in a single layer. Drizzle the remaining 2 tbsp of olive oil over the green beans, and sprinkle the green beans with the remaining ½ tsp of salt and ½ tsp of pepper.

When the time comes, remove the baking sheet of fish from the oven and gently turn over each fish piece. Place the baking sheet of fish back into the oven on the top rack, add the baking sheet of greens beans on the lower rack, and cook both for 8 to 10 minutes, until the fish is cooked through. When cooked, the fish will be firm and will flake easily with a fork.

Once the fish is cooked, remove both the fish and the green beans from the oven. Serve with the Yogurt Tartar Sauce.

Yogurt Tartar Sauce

Serving size: 4

Ingredients:

½ c plain Greek yogurt

2 tbsp mayonnaise

1 tbsp dill or sweet pickles, finely chopped

1 tsp dried dill weed

1 tsp onion powder

½ tsp salt

½ tsp ground black pepper

Directions:

Mix all ingredients in a bowl and serve with cooked fish.

American Academy of Pediatrics

DEDICATED TO THE HEALTH OF ALL CHILDREN®

Chapter 13

Recipes Featured in Table 13-3, A Sample Weekly Meal Plan

 Whole Wheat Pita Veggie Pizzas

Serving size: 4

Ingredients:

4 whole wheat pita breads

½ c marinara sauce

1 c shredded mozzarella cheese

2 c assorted vegetables (such as mushrooms, spinach, onions, peppers, and broccoli), chopped

Directions:

Preheat oven to 425 °F. Place 1 tbsp of marinara sauce onto a pita bread and spread it evenly. Place 2 tbsp of mozzarella cheese on top of the pita bread, spreading to cover the sauce. Place vegetables on top of pita pizza. Repeat with remaining pita breads and ingredients. Place pita pizzas onto a baking sheet and bake for 10 to 15 minutes, until cheese is melted.

Turkey-Spinach Meatballs With Spaghetti

Yield: 18 to 20 meatballs

Serving size: 4

Ingredients:

1 lb ground turkey

8 oz frozen spinach, defrosted and excess water squeezed out

1 tsp onion powder

1 tsp garlic powder

¼ c old-fashioned rolled oats

1 egg

2 tbsp olive oil

1 (24- to 25-oz) jar marinara sauce

1 16-oz package whole wheat spaghetti

Directions:

Place ground turkey, spinach, onion powder, garlic powder, oats, and egg into a large mixing bowl. Mix all ingredients together until well combined. Scoop 2 tbsp of mixture and roll it into a ball. Repeat with remaining mixture.

Warm the olive oil in a large pan over medium heat. Place 8 to 10 meatballs into the pan, approximately 2 inches apart. Cook the meatballs on one side for 4 to 5 minutes, then flip them to the other side and cook for another 2 to 3 minutes. Remove meatballs from the pan and set aside. Repeat steps with remaining meatballs. (Note: At this point, the meatballs are not fully cooked, but they will cook completely with the following step.)

Once all meatballs are removed from the pan, pour the marinara sauce into the previously used pan. Place all meatballs back into the pan and bring the sauce to a boil. Reduce the heat to low and cover the pan. Cook meatballs and sauce for 25 to 30 minutes.

Prepare pasta according to package directions. Serve the meatballs with the pasta.

Overnight Oats

Serving size: 4

Ingredients:

2 c old-fashioned rolled oats

2 c milk (cow milk or plant-based variety)

1 c nonfat or low-fat plain yogurt

4 tbsp honey

Toppings: nut butter, fruit, cinnamon

Directions:

Mix all ingredients except for the toppings in a large container with a lid until well combined. (Alternatively, for individual servings, place ½ c oats, ½ c milk, ¼ c yogurt, and 1 tbsp honey into a jar or container with a lid and stir. Repeat steps with remaining ingredients.)

Place the container or jars into the refrigerator overnight (at least 6–8 hours).

Serve either cold or hot. (To warm the mixture, microwave it for 1–2 minutes in a microwave-safe container). Add toppings or more milk as desired.

 Leftovers Soup

Serving size: 6 to 8

Ingredients:

2 tbsp olive oil

1 medium onion, chopped

6 to 7 c mixed vegetables (such as carrots, celery, peppers, spinach, and broccoli), chopped into small pieces

1 tsp garlic powder

2 c leftover cooked protein (such as chicken or turkey)

3 c leftover cooked pasta (or 2 c leftover cooked rice)

8 c water or broth

Place a large pot over medium heat. Add the olive oil to the pot, followed by the chopped onion. Cook onion until softened, stirring occasionally, approximately 3 to 4 minutes. Add mixed vegetables and garlic powder to the pot and stir. Stir occasionally until vegetables have softened, approximately 5 to 6 minutes. Add the protein to the pot, followed by the water or broth. Bring soup to a boil, then reduce heat to low and cook soup for 15 to 20 minutes. Add the pasta or rice to the soup and cook the mixture for another 3 to 4 minutes.

American Academy of Pediatrics

Baked Sweet Potatoes

Serving size: 4

Ingredient:

4 medium sweet potatoes

Directions:

Preheat oven to 400 °F. Use a fork to prick the outside of each sweet potato, in approximately 5 to 6 places. Place sweet potatoes onto a baking tray and bake for 40 to 45 minutes, until soft.

- "All the Vegetables" Fried Rice: Refer to recipe on page 413.
- Caramelized Banana Cinnamon Oatmeal: Refer to recipe on page 408.
- Carrots and Cucumbers With Creamy Ranch Bean Dip: Refer to recipe on page 417.
- Creamy Broccoli and Cheese Soup: Refer to recipe on page 396.
- Chicken Whole Wheat Pita Wraps With Creamy Ranch Bean Dip: Refer to recipe on pages 415 to 416.
- Frozen Yogurt Banana Pops: Refer to recipe on page 393.
- Roasted Garlicky and Cheesy Broccoli: Refer to recipe on page 420.
- Roasted Vegetable Grilled Cheese: Refer to recipe on page 425.
- Simple Baked Chicken Breast and Simple Roasted Vegetables: Refer to recipe on page 418 for chicken and recipe on page 398 for vegetables.
- Tuna Melts With Whole Grain Bread: Refer to recipe on page 411.
- Turkey and Vegetable Whole Wheat Chow Mein–style Noodles: Refer to recipe on pages 416 to 417.
- Turkey-Bean Chili With Sweet Potatoes: Refer to variation of Tofu-Bean Chili With Sweet Potatoes recipe on page 442.
- Turkey White Bean Burgers With Avocado: Refer to variation of Chicken Black Bean Burgers With Avocado recipe on page 426.
- Veggie Frittata Muffins: Refer to recipe on page 424.

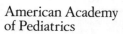

Chapter 18

Post-exercise Nutrition

 Date Nut Butter Energy Bites

Serving size: 8 to 10

Ingredients:

5 Medjool dates or any variety of dried dates

½ c almond butter or any nut butter

¾ c old-fashioned rolled oats

¼ tsp salt

1 tbsp chia seeds

¼ c mini chocolate chips or ¼ c unsweetened shredded coconut flakes (optional)

Special equipment: food processor

Directions:

Place dates and almond butter into a food processor. Pulse until well combined. Add rolled oats and pulse the ingredients until the oats are well combined. Pour this mixture into a bowl. Add salt and chia seeds and mix the ingredients well. With a tablespoon, take out 1 spoonful of date mixture and roll it into a ball. Repeat steps with remaining date mixture. Add the mini chocolate chips or shredded coconut to the mixture (if using).

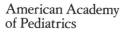

American Academy
of Pediatrics

DEDICATED TO THE HEALTH OF ALL CHILDREN®

Chapter 19

Recipes for Increasing Caloric Intake

 Avocado-Banana Smoothie

Serving size: 2 to 4

Ingredients:

1 frozen banana

1 ripe avocado

¼ c frozen spinach

½ orange, peeled and seeds removed (if any)

½ c whole milk

¼ c whole-milk plain Greek yogurt

½ c frozen fruit (such as peaches, mangoes, or pineapple)

Special equipment: blender

Directions:

Place all ingredients into a blender and blend until well combined.

American Academy of Pediatrics

DEDICATED TO THE HEALTH OF ALL CHILDREN®

Single copies of these recipes may be made for noncommercial, educational purposes. The information contained herein should not be used as a substitute for the medical care and advice of a pediatric health care professional.

The American Academy of Pediatrics is an organization of 67,000 primary care pediatricians, pediatric medical subspecialists, and pediatric surgical specialists dedicated to the health, safety, and well-being of all infants, children, adolescents, and young adults.

American Academy of Pediatrics website—www.HealthyChildren.org © 2023 American Academy of Pediatrics. All rights reserved.

One-Pot Whole Wheat Macaroni and Cheese and Peas

Serving size: 4

Ingredients:

5 c water

1 lb whole wheat short pasta (such as macaroni, fusilli, or penne)

1 c whole milk

1 (12-oz) can evaporated milk

3 c shredded cheddar cheese

1 tsp yellow mustard

1 tsp onion powder

1 tsp salt

2 c frozen peas (no need to defrost)

Directions:

Add the water and pasta to a large pot. Turn heat to high and bring water to a boil, then lower heat to medium and cook pasta for 8 to 9 minutes. At this point, most of the pasta water will be absorbed into the pasta (no need to drain remaining water). Add the whole milk and the evaporated milk to the pot, stir, and cook for another 4 to 5 minutes. Add the cheddar cheese, yellow mustard, onion powder, and salt to the pot and cook for another 2 to 3 minutes, stirring occasionally. Last, add the frozen peas, stir to combine, and cook for another 1 to 2 minutes.

American Academy
of Pediatrics

DEDICATED TO THE HEALTH OF ALL CHILDREN®

Single copies of these recipes may be made for noncommercial, educational purposes. The information contained herein should not be used as a substitute for the medical care and advice of a pediatric health care professional.

The American Academy of Pediatrics is an organization of 67,000 primary care pediatricians, pediatric medical subspecialists, and pediatric surgical specialists dedicated to the health, safety, and well-being of all infants, children, adolescents, and young adults.

American Academy of Pediatrics website—www.HealthyChildren.org   © 2023 American Academy of Pediatrics. All rights reserved.

Peanut Butter Granola With Raisins

Serving size: 6 to 8

Ingredients:

½ c smooth peanut butter

¼ c maple syrup

¼ c olive oil

½ tsp salt

2 tbsp chia seeds

3 c old-fashioned rolled oats

½ c nuts (peanuts, chopped almonds, or chopped pecans)

¾ c raisins

Directions:

Preheat oven to 325 °F. Place the peanut butter and maple syrup into a microwave-safe bowl. Microwave them for about 30 seconds, until the peanut butter is melted. Remove the peanut butter mixture from the microwave, add the olive oil to the peanut butter mixture, and mix them well. (If heating the mixture on a stove instead of in the microwave, place a medium pot over low heat. Place peanut butter, maple syrup, and olive oil into pot. Bring these ingredients to a gentle simmer while stirring continuously, until the mixture is mixed well, approximately 5 minutes.) Add the oats, salt, nuts, and chia seeds to the bowl and stir until well combined.

Pour the granola mixture onto a baking sheet and bake for 10 minutes. Remove the sheet from the oven, use a spatula to mix the granola, and place the sheet back into the oven. Bake for another 10 minutes, checking every 10 minutes to make sure the granola does not burn. Once the granola is golden brown, remove the baking sheet from the oven and let the granola cool. Once the granola is cool, add the raisins and mix the two well.

American Academy
of Pediatrics

DEDICATED TO THE HEALTH OF ALL CHILDREN®

Single copies of these recipes may be made for noncommercial, educational purposes. The information contained herein should not be used as a substitute for the medical care and advice of a pediatric health care professional.

The American Academy of Pediatrics is an organization of 67,000 primary care pediatricians, pediatric medical subspecialists, and pediatric surgical specialists dedicated to the health, safety, and well-being of all infants, children, adolescents, and young adults.

American Academy of Pediatrics website—www.HealthyChildren.org   © 2023 American Academy of Pediatrics. All rights reserved.

Chapter 20

Recipes High in Plant Stanols, Sterols, and Omega-3 Fatty Acids

 Cauliflower Cashew Alfredo Pasta

Serving size: 4

Ingredients:

5 c chicken or vegetable broth

6 c cauliflower florets, chopped (about 1 small head cauliflower)

¾ c raw cashews

5 garlic cloves, whole

2 tsp salt

2 tsp ground black pepper

2 tbsp grated Parmesan cheese or 2 tbsp nutritional yeast (vegan)

4 tbsp olive oil

1 (16-oz) package whole wheat pasta, cooked according to package instructions

Special equipment: blender

Directions:

Place the broth or water, chopped cauliflower florets, cashews, and garlic into a large saucepan or pot and bring the liquid to a boil. Once the liquid is boiling, lower the heat to medium and let the mixture simmer for 10 to 15 minutes. Drain the cauliflower, garlic, and cashews and reserve the water or broth to use later. Place the cauliflower, garlic, and cashews into the blender along with the salt, pepper, Parmesan cheese or nutritional yeast, and olive oil and blend. Add reserved water or broth as needed to thin the sauce.

Pour the sauce over the cooked pasta and toss the two to coat the pasta. If the sauce is too thick, add reserved water or broth as needed.

Tip: Although water can be used as the cooking liquid in this recipe, broth will provide more flavor.

Salmon Curry With Green Beans and Broccoli

Serving size: 4

Ingredients:

2 tbsp olive oil

¼ c onion (any color), chopped

3 garlic cloves, chopped

2 to 3 tbsp curry paste/powder (any color)

1 c water or broth (chicken or vegetable)

1 (15-oz) can coconut milk

12 oz salmon filet, cut into 3-oz pieces

3 c green beans and/or broccoli florets, cut into 3- to 4-inch pieces

3 to 4 c brown rice, cooked

Directions:

Warm the olive oil in a medium-sized pot over medium heat. Add the chopped onion and garlic to the pot and cook for 2 to 3 minutes, stirring occasionally to ensure that the garlic does not burn. Add the curry paste/powder, then add the water or broth and coconut milk. Bring curry broth to a boil, then lower heat to a simmer. Add the salmon pieces to the curry broth, cover the pot, and cook the two for 5 to 6 minutes. Add the vegetables and cover the pot again. Cook for another 4 to 5 minutes, until the vegetables are tender. Serve over cooked brown rice.

American Academy of Pediatrics

DEDICATED TO THE HEALTH OF ALL CHILDREN®

Single copies of these recipes may be made for noncommercial, educational purposes. The information contained herein should not be used as a substitute for the medical care and advice of a pediatric health care professional.

The American Academy of Pediatrics is an organization of 67,000 primary care pediatricians, pediatric medical subspecialists, and pediatric surgical specialists dedicated to the health, safety, and well-being of all infants, children, adolescents, and young adults.

American Academy of Pediatrics website—www.HealthyChildren.org

Tofu-Bean Chili With Sweet Potatoes

Serving size: 6 to 8

Ingredients:

2 tbsp olive oil

2 (14-oz) packages tofu (Refer to Tofu preparation method that follows.)

2 tsp ground cumin

2 tsp smoked paprika

2 tsp salt

2 tbsp tomato paste

1 medium onion, chopped

2 garlic cloves, chopped

2 green bell peppers, chopped

2 medium-sized sweet potatoes, peeled and chopped into ½-inch cubes

1 (28-oz) can diced tomatoes

3 c water or broth

2 (15-oz) cans black beans, drained

Directions:

Tofu preparation method:

Freezing tofu and then defrosting it before cooking mimics the ground meat texture often used in chili. To prepare the tofu, 2 days before making the chili, remove the tofu from its packaging and drain the liquid. Place the tofu into a freezer-safe container and freeze it overnight. The following day, defrost the tofu in the refrigerator and, once the tofu is thawed, squeeze out all the water, then crumble the tofu into small pieces.

Pour the olive oil into a large pot and place the pot over medium heat. Add the crumbled tofu to the pot along with the cumin, paprika, salt, and tomato paste. Cook the tofu for 4 to 5 minutes, stirring occasionally. Add the chopped onion, garlic, peppers, and sweet potatoes to the pot and cook until lightly browned, for about 3 to 4 minutes, stirring occasionally. Add the diced tomatoes, water or broth, and drained black beans to the pot and stir until combined. Bring the mixture to a boil, then reduce the heat to medium-low. Cover the pot and cook the mixture for 30 to 40 minutes, stirring occasionally and adding water or broth if needed.

Chili variation:

For turkey-bean chili: Substitute the same amount of ground turkey for the tofu.

The Dietary Reference Intake Tables

Table A-1. Recommended Dietary Allowance and Adequate Intake for Total Water and Macronutrients

Life-stage group	Total water[a] (L/d)	Carbohydrate (g/d)	Total fiber (g/d)	Fat (g/d)	Linoleic acid (g/d)	α-Linolenic acid (g/d)	Protein[b] (g/d)
Infants							
0–6 mo	0.7*	60*	ND[c]	31*	4.4*	0.5*	9.1*
6–12 mo	0.8*	95*	ND	30*	4.6*	0.5*	**11.0**
Children							
1–3 y	1.3*	**130**	19*	ND	7*	0.7*	**13**
4–8 y	1.7*	**130**	25*	ND	10*	0.9*	**19**
Males							
9–13 y	2.4*	**130**	31*	ND	12*	1.2*	**34**
14–18 y	3.3*	**130**	38*	ND	16*	1.6*	**52**
19–30 y	3.7*	**130**	38*	ND	17*	1.6*	**56**
31–50 y	3.7*	**130**	38*	ND	17*	1.6*	**56**
51–70 y	3.7*	**130**	30*	ND	14*	1.6*	**56**
>70 y	3.7*	**130**	30*	ND	14*	1.6*	**56**
Females							
9–13 y	2.1*	**130**	26*	ND	10*	1.0*	**34**
14–18 y	2.3*	**130**	26*	ND	11*	1.1*	**46**
19–30 y	2.7*	**130**	25*	ND	12*	1.1*	**46**
31–50 y	2.7*	**130**	25*	ND	12*	1.1*	**46**
51–70 y	2.7*	**130**	21*	ND	11*	1.1*	**46**
>70 y	2.7*	**130**	21*	ND	11*	1.1*	**46**
Pregnancy							
14–18 y	3.0*	**175**	28*	ND	13*	1.4*	**71**
19–30 y	3.0*	**175**	28*	ND	13*	1.4*	**71**
31–50 y	3.0*	**175**	28*	ND	13*	1.4*	**71**

Table A-1 (*continued*)

Life-stage group	Total water[a] (L/d)	Carbohydrate (g/d)	Total fiber (g/d)	Fat (g/d)	Linoleic acid (g/d)	α-Linolenic acid (g/d)	Protein[b] (g/d)
Lactation							
14–18 y	3.8*	**210**	29*	ND	13*	1.3*	**71**
19–30 y	3.8*	**210**	29*	ND	13*	1.3*	**71**
31–50 y	3.8*	**210**	29*	ND	13*	1.3*	**71**

NOTE: This table (taken from the DRI reports, see www.nap.edu) presents Recommended Dietary Allowances (RDAs) in **bold type** and Adequate Intakes (AIs) in ordinary type followed by an asterisk (*). An RDA is the average daily dietary intake level sufficient to meet the nutrient requirements of nearly all (97–98 percent) healthy individuals in a group. It is calculated from an Estimated Average Requirement (EAR). If sufficient scientific evidence is not available to establish an EAR, and thus calculate an RDA, an AI is usually developed. For healthy breastfed infants, an AI is the mean intake. The AI for other life-stage and gender groups is believed to cover the needs of all healthy individuals in the groups, but lack of data or uncertainty in the data prevents being able to specify with confidence the percentage of individuals covered by this intake.

[a] Total water includes all water contained in food, beverages, and drinking water.

[b] Based on g of protein per kg of body weight for the reference body weight, e.g., for adults 0.8 g/kg of body weight for the reference body weight.

[c] Not determined.

SOURCES: *Dietary Reference Intakes for Energy, Carbohydrate, Fiber, Fat, Fatty Acids, Cholesterol, Protein, and Amino Acids* (2002/2005) and *Dietary Reference Intakes for Water, Potassium, Sodium, Chloride, and Sulfate* (2005). The report may be accessed via www.nap.edu.

Reproduced with permission from Institute of Medicine. *Dietary Reference Intakes for Calcium and Vitamin D.* National Academies Press; 2011:1103–1115.

Table A-2. Recommended Dietary Allowance and Adequate Intake for Vitamins

Life-stage group	Vitamin A (μg/d)[a]	Vitamin C (mg/d)	Vitamin D (μg/d)[b,c]	Vitamin E (mg/d)[d]	Vitamin K (μg/d)	Thiamin (mg/d)	Ribo-flavin (mg/d)	Niacin (mg/d)[e]	Vitamin B6 (mg/d)	Folate (μg/d)[f]	Vitamin B12 (μg/d)	Panto-thenic acid (mg/d)	Biotin (μg/d)	Choline (mg/d)[g]
Infants														
0–6 mo	400*	40*	10*	4*	2.0*	0.2*	0.3*	2*	0.1*	65*	0.4*	1.7*	5*	125*
6–12 mo	500*	50*	10*	5*	2.5*	0.3*	0.4*	4*	0.3*	80*	0.5*	1.8*	6*	150*
Children														
1–3 y	300	15	15	6	30*	0.5	0.5	6	0.5	150	0.9	2*	8*	200*
4–8 y	400	25	15	7	55*	0.6	0.6	8	0.6	200	1.2	3*	12*	250*
Males														
9–13 y	600	45	15	11	60*	0.9	0.9	12	1.0	300	1.8	4*	20*	375*
14–18 y	900	75	15	15	75*	1.2	1.3	16	1.3	400	2.4	5*	25*	550*
19–30 y	900	90	15	15	120*	1.2	1.3	16	1.3	400	2.4	5*	30*	550*
31–50 y	900	90	15	15	120*	1.2	1.3	16	1.3	400	2.4	5*	30*	550*
51–70 y	900	90	15	15	120*	1.2	1.3	16	1.7	400	2.4[h]	5*	30*	550*
>70 y	900	90	20	15	120*	1.2	1.3	16	1.7	400	2.4[h]	5*	30*	550*

Females

9–13 y	600	45	15	11	60*	0.9	0.9	12	1.0	300	1.8	4*	20*	375*
14–18 y	700	65	15	15	75*	1.0	1.0	14	1.2	400[i]	2.4	5*	25*	400*
19–30 y	700	75	15	15	90*	1.1	1.1	14	1.3	400[i]	2.4	5*	30*	425*
31–50 y	700	75	15	15	90*	1.1	1.1	14	1.3	400[i]	2.4	5*	30*	425*
51–70 y	700	75	15	15	90*	1.1	1.1	14	1.5	400	2.4[h]	5*	30*	425*
>70 y	700	75	20	15	90*	1.1	1.1	14	1.5	400	2.4[h]	5*	30*	425*

Pregnancy

14–18 y	750	80	15	15	75*	1.4	1.4	18	1.9	600[i]	2.6	6*	30*	450*
19–30 y	770	85	15	15	90*	1.4	1.4	18	1.9	600[i]	2.6	6*	30*	450*
31–50 y	770	85	15	15	90*	1.4	1.4	18	1.9	600[i]	2.6	6*	30*	450*

Continued

Table A-2 *(continued)*

Life-stage group	Vitamin A (µg/d)[a]	Vitamin C (mg/d)	Vitamin D (µg/d)[b,c]	Vitamin E (mg/d)[d]	Vitamin K (µg/d)	Thiamin (mg/d)	Ribo-flavin (mg/d)	Niacin (mg/d)[e]	Vitamin B6 (mg/d)	Folate (µg/d)[f]	Vitamin B12 (µg/d)	Panto-thenic acid (mg/d)	Biotin (µg/d)	Choline (mg/d)[g]
Lactation														
14–18 y	1,200	115	15	19	75*	1.4	1.6	17	2.0	500	2.8	7*	35*	550*
19–30 y	1,300	120	15	19	90*	1.4	1.6	17	2.0	500	2.8	7*	35*	550*
31–50 y	1,300	120	15	19	90*	1.4	1.6	17	2.0	500	2.8	7*	35*	550*

NOTE: This table (taken from the DRI reports, see www.nap.edu) presents Recommended Dietary Allowances (RDAs) in **bold type** and Adequate Intakes (AIs) in ordinary type followed by an asterisk (*). An RDA is the average daily dietary intake level sufficient to meet the nutrient requirements of nearly all (97–98 percent) healthy individuals in a group. It is calculated from an Estimated Average Requirement (EAR). If sufficient scientific evidence is not available to establish an EAR, and thus calculate an RDA, an AI is usually developed. For healthy breastfed infants, an AI is the mean intake. The AI for other life-stage and gender groups is believed to cover the needs of all healthy individuals in the groups, but lack of data or uncertainty in the data prevents being able to specify with confidence the percentage of individuals covered by this intake.

[a] As retinol activity equivalents (RAEs). One RAE = 1 µg retinol, 12 µg β-carotene, 24 µg α-carotene, or 24 µg β-cryptoxanthin. The RAE for dietary provitamin A carotenoids is 2-fold greater than retinol equivalents (REs), whereas the RAE for preformed vitamin A is the same as RE.

[b] As cholecalciferol. One µg cholecalciferol = 40 IU vitamin D.

[c] Under the assumption of minimal sunlight.

[d] As α-tocopherol. α-Tocopherol includes *RRR*-α-tocopherol, the only form of α-tocopherol that occurs naturally in foods, and the *2R*-stereoisomeric forms of α-tocopherol (*RRR*-, *RSR*-, *RRS*-, and *RSS*-α-tocopherol) that occur in fortified foods and supplements. It does not include the *2S*-stereoisomeric forms of α-tocopherol (*SRR*-, *SSR*-, *SRS*-, and *SSS*-α-tocopherol), also found in fortified foods and supplements.

[e] As niacin equivalents (NEs). One mg of niacin = 60 mg of tryptophan; 0–6 months = preformed niacin (not NE).

[f] As dietary folate equivalents (DFEs). One DFE = 1 µg of food folate = 0.6 µg of folic acid from fortified food or as a supplement consumed with food = 0.5 µg of a supplement taken on an empty stomach.

[g] Although AIs have been set for choline, there are few data to assess whether a dietary supply of choline is needed at all stages of the life cycle, and it may be that the choline requirement can be met by endogenous synthesis at some of these stages.

[h] Because 10 to 30 percent of older people may malabsorb food-bound B_{12}, it is advisable for those older than 50 years to meet their RDA mainly by consuming foods fortified with B_{12} or a supplement containing B_{12}.

[i] In view of evidence linking folate intake with neural tube defects in the fetus, it is recommended that all women capable of becoming pregnant consume 400 µg from supplements or fortified foods in addition to intake of food folate from a varied diet.

[j] It is assumed that women will continue consuming 400 µg from supplements or fortified food until their pregnancy is confirmed and they enter prenatal care, which ordinarily occurs after the end of the periconceptional period—the critical time for formation of the neural tube.

SOURCES: *Dietary Reference Intakes for Calcium, Phosphorous, Magnesium, Vitamin D, and Fluoride* (1997); *Dietary Reference Intakes for Thiamin, Riboflavin, Niacin, Vitamin B_6, Folate, Vitamin B_{12}, Pantothenic Acid, Biotin, and Choline* (1998); *Dietary Reference Intakes for Vitamin C, Vitamin E, Selenium, and Carotenoids* (2000); *Dietary Reference Intakes for Vitamin A, Vitamin K, Arsenic, Boron, Chromium, Copper, Iodine, Iron, Manganese, Molybdenum, Nickel, Silicon, Vanadium, and Zinc* (2001); *Dietary Reference Intakes for Water, Potassium, Sodium, Chloride, and Sulfate* (2005); and *Dietary Reference Intakes for Calcium and Vitamin D* (2011). These reports may be accessed via www.nap.edu.

Table A-3. Recommended Daily Allowance and Adequate Intake for Minerals

Life-stage group	Calcium (mg/d)	Chromium (μg/d)	Copper (μg/d)	Fluoride (mg/d)	Iodine (μg/d)	Iron (mg/d)	Magnesium (mg/d)
Infants							
0–6 mo	200*a	0.2*	200*	0.01*	110*	0.27*	30*
7–12 mo	260*a	5.5*	220*	0.5*	130*	11	75*
Children							
1–3 y	700	11*	340	0.7*	90	7	80
4–8 y	1,000	15*	440	1*	90	10	130
Males							
9–13 y	1,300	25*	700	2*	120	8	240
14–18 y	1,300	35*	890	3*	150	11	410
19–30 y	1,000	35*	900	4*	150	8	400
31–50 y	1,000	35*	900	4*	150	8	420
51–70 y	1,000	30*	900	4*	150	8	420
>70 y	1,200	30*	900	4*	150	8	420
Females							
9–13 y	1,300	21*	700	2*	120	8	240
14–18 y	1,300	24*	890	3*	150	15	360
19–30 y	1,000	25*	900	3*	150	18	310
31–50 y	1,000	25*	900	3*	150	18	320
51–70 y	1,200	20*	900	3*	150	8	320
>70 y	1,200	20*	900	3*	150	8	320
Pregnancy							
14–18 y	1,300	29*	1,000	3*	220	27	400
19–30 y	1,000	30*	1,000	3*	220	27	350
31–50 y	1,000	30*	1,000	3*	220	27	360

anganese (mg/d)	Molybdenum (μg/d)	Phosphorus (mg/d)	Selenium (μg/d)	Zinc (mg/d)	Potassium (mg/d)	Sodium (mg/d)	Chloride (g/d)
			Infants				
0.003*	2*	100*	15*	2*	400*	110*	0.18*
0.6*	3*	275*	20*	3	860*	370*	0.57*
			Children				
1.2*	17	460	20	3	2,000*	800*	1.5*
1.5*	22	500	30	5	2,300*	1,000*	1.9*
			Males				
1.9*	34	1,250	40	8	2,500*	1,200*	2.3*
2.2*	43	1,250	55	11	3,000*	1,500*	2.3*
2.3*	45	700	55	11	3,400*	1,500*	2.3*
2.3*	45	700	55	11	3,400*	1,500*	2.3*
2.3*	45	700	55	11	3,400*	1,500*	2.0*
2.3*	45	700	55	11	3,400*	1,500*	1.8*
			Females				
1.6*	34	1,250	40	8	2,300*	1,200*	2.3*
1.6*	43	1,250	55	9	2,300*	1,500*	2.3*
1.8*	45	700	55	8	2,600*	1,500*	2.3*
1.8*	45	700	55	8	2,600*	1,500*	2.3*
1.8*	45	700	55	8	2,600*	1,500*	2.0*
1.8*	45	700	55	8	2,600*	1,500*	1.8*
			Pregnancy				
2.0*	50	1,250	60	12	2,600*	1,500*	2.3*
2.0*	50	700	60	11	2,900*	1,500*	2.3*
2.0*	50	700	60	11	2,900*	1,500*	2.3*

Continued

Table A-3 (*continued*)

Life-stage group	Calcium (mg/d)	Chromium (μg/d)	Copper (μg/d)	Fluoride (mg/d)	Iodine (μg/d)	Iron (mg/d)	Magnesium (mg/d)
Lactation							
14–18 y	1,300	44*	1,300	3*	290	10	360
19–30 y	1,000	45*	1,300	3*	290	9	310
31–50 y	1,000	45*	1,300	3*	290	9	320

Manganese (mg/d)	Molybdenum (µg/d)	Phosphorus (mg/d)	Selenium (µg/d)	Zinc (mg/d)	Potassium (mg/d)	Sodium (mg/d)	Chloride (g/d)
Lactation							
2.6*	**50**	**1,250**	**70**	**13**	2,500*	1,500*	2.3*
2.6*	**50**	**700**	**70**	**12**	2,800*	1,500*	2.3*
2.6*	**50**	**700**	**70**	**12**	2,800*	1,500*	2.3*

NOTES: This table (taken from the DRI reports, see www.nap.edu) presents Recommended Dietary Allowances (RDAs) in **bold type** and Adequate Intakes (AIs) in ordinary type followed by an asterisk (*). An RDA is the average daily dietary intake level sufficient to meet the nutrient requirements of nearly all (97–98 percent) healthy individuals in a group. It is calculated from an Estimated Average Requirement (EAR). If sufficient scientific evidence is not available to establish an EAR, and thus calculate an RDA, an AI is usually developed. For healthy breastfed infants, an AI is the mean intake. The AI for other life-stage and gender groups is believed to cover the needs of all healthy individuals in the groups, but lack of data or uncertainty in the data prevents being able to specify with confidence the percentage of individuals covered by this intake.

a Life-stage groups for infants were 0–5.9 and 6–11.9 months.

SOURCES: *Dietary Reference Intakes for Calcium, Phosphorous, Magnesium, Vitamin D, and Fluoride* (1997); *Dietary Reference Intakes for Thiamin, Riboflavin, Niacin, Vitamin B₆, Folate, Vitamin B₁₂, Pantothenic Acid, Biotin, and Choline* (1998); *Dietary Reference Intakes for Vitamin C, Vitamin E, Selenium, and Carotenoids* (2000); *Dietary Reference Intakes for Vitamin A, Vitamin K, Arsenic, Boron, Chromium, Copper, Iodine, Iron, Manganese, Molybdenum, Nickel, Silicon, Vanadium, and Zinc* (2001); *Dietary Reference Intakes for Water, Potassium, Sodium, Chloride, and* Sulfate (2005); *Dietary Reference Intakes for Calcium and Vitamin D* (2011); and *Dietary Reference Intakes for Sodium and Potassium* (2019). These reports may be accessed via www.nap.edu.

Table A-4. Tolerable Upper Intake Levels for Vitamins

Life-stage group	Vitamin A (µg/d)[a]	Vitamin C (mg/d)[a]	Vitamin D (µg/d)	Vitamin E (mg/d)[b,c]	Vitamin K	Thiamin	Ribo-flavin	Niacin (mg/d)[c]	Vitamin B$_6$ (mg/d)[c]	Folate (µg/d)[c]	Vitamin B$_{12}$	Panto-thenic acid	Biotin	Choline (g/d)	Carot-enoids[d]
Infants															
0-6 mo	600	ND[e]	25	ND	ND	ND	ND	ND	ND	ND	ND	ND	ND	ND	ND
6-12 mo	600	ND	38	ND	ND	ND	ND	ND	ND	ND	ND	ND	ND	ND	ND
Children															
1-3 y	600	400	63	200	ND	ND	ND	10	30	300	ND	ND	ND	1.0	ND
4-8 y	900	650	75	300	ND	ND	ND	15	40	400	ND	ND	ND	1.0	ND
Males															
9-13 y	1,700	1,200	100	600	ND	ND	ND	20	60	600	ND	ND	ND	2.0	ND
14-18 y	2,800	1,800	100	800	ND	ND	ND	30	80	800	ND	ND	ND	3.0	ND
19-30 y	3,000	2,000	100	1,000	ND	ND	ND	35	100	1,000	ND	ND	ND	3.5	ND
31-50 y	3,000	2,000	100	1,000	ND	ND	ND	35	100	1,000	ND	ND	ND	3.5	ND
51-70 y	3,000	2,000	100	1,000	ND	ND	ND	35	100	1,000	ND	ND	ND	3.5	ND
>70 y	3,000	2,000	100	1,000	ND	ND	ND	35	100	1,000	ND	ND	ND	3.5	ND

Females

9–13 y	1,700	1,200	100	600	ND	ND	ND	20	60	600	ND	ND	ND	2.0	ND
14–18 y	2,800	1,800	100	800	ND	ND	ND	30	80	800	ND	ND	ND	3.0	ND
19–30 y	3,000	2,000	100	1,000	ND	ND	ND	35	100	1,000	ND	ND	ND	3.5	ND
31–50 y	3,000	2,000	100	1,000	ND	ND	ND	35	100	1,000	ND	ND	ND	3.5	ND
51–70 y	3,000	2,000	100	1,000	ND	ND	ND	35	100	1,000	ND	ND	ND	3.5	ND
>70 y	3,000	2,000	100	1,000	ND	ND	ND	35	100	1,000	ND	ND	ND	3.5	ND

Pregnancy

14–18 y	2,800	1,800	100	800	ND	ND	ND	30	80	800	ND	ND	ND	3.0	ND
19–30 y	3,000	2,000	100	1,000	ND	ND	ND	35	100	1,000	ND	ND	ND	3.5	ND
31–50 y	3,000	2,000	100	1,000	ND	ND	ND	35	100	1,000	ND	ND	ND	3.5	ND

Continued

Table A-4 (continued)

Life-stage group	Vitamin A (μg/d)[a]	Vitamin C (mg/d)	Vitamin D (μg/d)	Vitamin E (mg/d)[b,c]	Vitamin K	Thiamin	Ribo-flavin	Niacin (mg/d)[c]	Vitamin B$_6$ (mg/d)	Folate (μg/d)[c]	Vitamin B$_{12}$	Panto-thenic acid	Biotin	Choline (g/d)	Carot-enoids[d]
Lactation															
14–18 y	2,800	1,800	100	800	ND	ND	ND	30	80	800	ND	ND	ND	3.0	ND
19–30 y	3,000	2,000	100	1,000	ND	ND	ND	35	100	1,000	ND	ND	ND	3.5	ND
31–50 y	3,000	2,000	100	1,000	ND	ND	ND	35	100	1,000	ND	ND	ND	3.5	ND

NOTE: A Tolerable Upper Intake Level (UL) is the highest level of daily nutrient intake that is likely to pose no risk of adverse health effects to almost all individuals in the general population. Unless otherwise specified, the UL represents total intake from food, water, and supplements. Due to a lack of suitable data, ULs could not be established for vitamin K, thiamin, riboflavin, vitamin B$_{12}$, pantothenic acid, biotin, and carotenoids. In the absence of a UL, extra caution may be warranted in consuming levels above recommended intakes. Members of the general population should be advised not to routinely exceed the UL. The UL is not meant to apply to individuals who are treated with the nutrient under medical supervision or to individuals with predisposing conditions that modify their sensitivity to the nutrient.

[a] As preformed vitamin A only.

[b] As α-tocopherol; applies to any form of supplemental α-tocopherol.

[c] The ULs for vitamin E, niacin, and folate apply to synthetic forms obtained from supplements, fortified foods, or a combination of the two.

[d] β-Carotene supplements are advised only to serve as a provitamin A source for individuals at risk of vitamin A deficiency.

[e] Not determinable due to lack of data of adverse effects in this age group and concern with regard to lack of ability to handle excess amounts. Source of intake should be from food only to prevent high levels of intake.

SOURCES: *Dietary Reference Intakes for Calcium, Phosphorous, Magnesium, Vitamin D, and Fluoride* (1997); *Dietary Reference Intakes for Thiamin, Riboflavin, Niacin, Vitamin B$_6$, Folate, Vitamin B$_{12}$, Pantothenic Acid, Biotin, and Choline* (1998); *Dietary Reference Intakes for Vitamin C, Vitamin E, Selenium, and Carotenoids* (2000); *Dietary Reference Intakes for Vitamin A, Vitamin K, Arsenic, Boron, Chromium, Copper, Iodine, Iron, Manganese, Molybdenum, Nickel, Silicon, Vanadium, and Zinc* (2001); and *Dietary Reference Intakes for Calcium and Vitamin D* (2011). These reports may be accessed via www.nap.edu.

Reproduced with permission from Institute of Medicine. *Dietary Reference Intakes for Calcium and Vitamin D.* National Academies Press; 2011:1103–1115.

Table A-5. Tolerable Upper Intake Levels for Minerals

Life-stage group	Arsenic[a]	Boron (mg/d)	Calcium (mg/d)	Chromium	Copper (µg/d)	Fluoride (mg/d)	Iodine (µg/d)
Infants							
0–6 mo	ND[f]	ND	1,000[g]	ND	ND	0.7	ND
7–12 mo	ND	ND	1,500[g]	ND	ND	0.9	ND
Children							
1–3 y	ND	3	2,500	ND	1,000	1.3	200
4–8 y	ND	6	2,500	ND	3,000	2.2	300
Males							
9–13 y	ND	11	3,000	ND	5,000	10	600
14–18 y	ND	17	3,000	ND	8,000	10	900
19–30 y	ND	20	2,500	ND	10,000	10	1,100
31–50 y	ND	20	2,500	ND	10,000	10	1,100
51–70 y	ND	20	2,000	ND	10,000	10	1,100
>70 y	ND	20	2,000	ND	10,000	10	1,100
Females							
9–13 y	ND	11	3,000	ND	5,000	10	600
14–18 y	ND	17	3,000	ND	8,000	10	900
19–30 y	ND	20	2,500	ND	10,000	10	1,100
31–50 y	ND	20	2,500	ND	10,000	10	1,100
51–70 y	ND	20	2,000	ND	10,000	10	1,100
>70 y	ND	20	2,000	ND	10,000	10	1,100
Pregnancy							
14–18 y	ND	17	3,000	ND	8,000	10	900
19–30 y	ND	20	2,500	ND	10,000	10	1,100
31–50 y	ND	20	2,500	ND	10,000	10	1,100
Lactation							
14–18 y	ND	17	3,000	ND	8,000	10	900
19–30 y	ND	20	2,500	ND	10,000	10	1,100
31–50 y	ND	20	2,500	ND	10,000	10	1,100

Continued

Table A-5 (*continued*)

Life-stage group	Iron (mg/d)	Magnesium (mg/d)[b]	Manganese (mg/d)	Molybdenum (µg/d)	Nickel (mg/d)	Phosphorus (g/d)	Potassium
Infants							
0–6 mo	40	ND	ND	ND	ND	ND	ND[h]
7–12 mo	40	ND	ND	ND	ND	ND	ND[h]
Children							
1–3 y	40	65	2	300	0.2	3	ND[h]
4–8 y	40	110	3	600	0.3	3	ND[h]
Males							
9–13 y	40	350	6	1,100	0.6	4	ND[h]
14–18 y	45	350	9	1,700	1.0	4	ND[h]
19–30 y	45	350	11	2,000	1.0	4	ND[h]
31–50 y	45	350	11	2,000	1.0	4	ND[h]
51–70 y	45	350	11	2,000	1.0	4	ND[h]
>70 y	45	350	11	2,000	1.0	3	ND[h]
Females							
9–13 y	40	350	6	1,100	0.6	4	ND[h]
14–18 y	45	350	9	1,700	1.0	4	ND[h]
19–30 y	45	350	11	2,000	1.0	4	ND[h]
31–50 y	45	350	11	2,000	1.0	4	ND[h]
51–70 y	45	350	11	2,000	1.0	4	ND[h]
>70 y	45	350	11	2,000	1.0	3	ND[h]
Pregnancy							
14–18 y	45	350	9	1,700	1.0	3.5	ND[h]
19–30 y	45	350	11	2,000	1.0	3.5	ND[h]
31–50 y	45	350	11	2,000	1.0	3.5	ND[h]
Lactation							
14–18 y	45	350	9	1,700	1.0	4	ND[h]
19–30 y	45	350	11	2,000	1.0	4	ND[h]
31–50 y	45	350	11	2,000	1.0	4	ND[h]

Selenium (μg/d)	Silicon[c]	Sulfate	Vanadium (mg/d)[d]	Zinc (mg/d)	Sodium[e]	Chloride (g/d)
Infants						
45	ND	ND	ND	4	ND[h]	ND
60	ND	ND	ND	5	ND[h]	ND
Children						
90	ND	ND	ND	7	ND[h]	2.3
150	ND	ND	ND	12	ND[h]	2.9
Males						
280	ND	ND	ND	23	ND[h]	3.4
400	ND	ND	ND	34	ND[h]	3.6
400	ND	ND	1.8	40	ND[h]	3.6
400	ND	ND	1.8	40	ND[h]	3.6
400	ND	ND	1.8	40	ND[h]	3.6
400	ND	ND	1.8	40	ND[h]	3.6
Females						
280	ND	ND	ND	23	ND[h]	3.4
400	ND	ND	ND	34	ND[h]	3.6
400	ND	ND	1.8	40	ND[h]	3.6
400	ND	ND	1.8	40	ND[h]	3.6
400	ND	ND	1.8	40	ND[h]	3.6
400	ND	ND	1.8	40	ND[h]	3.6
Pregnancy						
400	ND	ND	ND	34	ND[h]	3.6
400	ND	ND	ND	40	ND[h]	3.6
400	ND	ND	ND	40	ND[h]	3.6
Lactation						
400	ND	ND	ND	34	ND[h]	3.6
400	ND	ND	ND	40	ND[h]	3.6
400	ND	ND	ND	40	ND[h]	3.6

Continued

Table A-5 (*continued*)

NOTES: A Tolerable Upper Intake Level (UL) is the highest level of daily nutrient intake that is likely to pose no risk of adverse health effects to almost all individuals in the general population. Unless otherwise specified, the UL represents total intake from food, water, and supplements. Because of a lack of suitable data, ULs could not be established for arsenic, chromium, potassium, silicon, sulfate, or sodium. In the absence of a UL, extra caution may be warranted in consuming levels above recommended intakes. Members of the general population should be advised not to routinely exceed the UL. The UL is not meant to apply to individuals who are treated with the nutrient under medical supervision or to individuals with predisposing conditions that modify their sensitivity to the nutrient.

[a] Although the UL was not determined for arsenic, there is no justification for adding arsenic to food or supplements.

[b] The ULs for magnesium represent intake from a pharmacological agent only and do not include intake from food and water.

[c] Although silicon has not been shown to cause adverse effects in humans, there is no justification for adding silicon to supplements.

[d] Although vanadium in food has not been shown to cause adverse effects in humans, there is no justification for adding vanadium to food and vanadium supplements should be used with caution. The UL is based on adverse effects in laboratory animals, and this data could be used to set a UL for adults but not children and adolescents.

[e] The lowest level of intake for which there was sufficient strength of evidence to characterize a chronic disease risk reduction was used to derive the sodium Chronic Disease Risk Reduction Intake (CDRR) values.

[f] Not determinable owing to lack of data of adverse effects in this age group and concern with regard to lack of ability to handle excess amounts. Source of intake should be from food only to prevent high levels of intake.

[g] Life-stage groups for infants were 0–5.9 and 6–11.9 months.

[h] Not determinable owing to a lack of data of a specific toxicological adverse effect.

SOURCES: *Dietary Reference Intakes for Calcium, Phosphorous, Magnesium, Vitamin D, and Fluoride* (1997); *Dietary Reference Intakes for Thiamin, Riboflavin, Niacin, Vitamin B$_6$, Folate, Vitamin B$_{12}$, Pantothenic Acid, Biotin, and Choline* (1998); *Dietary Reference Intakes for Vitamin C, Vitamin E, Selenium, and Carotenoids* (2000); *Dietary Reference Intakes for Vitamin A, Vitamin K, Arsenic, Boron, Chromium, Copper, Iodine, Iron, Manganese, Molybdenum, Nickel, Silicon, Vanadium, and Zinc* (2001); *Dietary Reference Intakes for Water, Potassium, Sodium, Chloride, and Sulfate* (2005); *Dietary Reference Intakes for Calcium and Vitamin D* (2011); and *Dietary Reference Intakes for Sodium and Potassium* (2019). These reports may be accessed via www.nap.edu.

Reproduced with permission from National Academies of Sciences, Engineering, and Medicine. *Dietary Reference Intakes for Sodium and Potassium.* National Academies Press; 2019:565–577.

Table A-6. Estimated Energy Requirement

Age	Estimated energy requirement formula (kcal/d) (EER = total energy expenditure + energy deposition)
Infants and young children	
0–3 mo	(89 × weight [kilograms] − 100) + 175
4–6 mo	(89 × weight [kilograms] − 100) + 56
7–12 mo	(89 × weight [kilograms] − 100) + 22
13–35 mo	(89 × weight [kilograms] − 100) + 20
Children and adolescents	
Boys	
3–8 y	88.5 − (61.9 × age [years]) + PA[a] × [(26.7 × weight [kilograms]) + (903 × height [meters])] + 20
9–18 y	88.5 − (61.9 × age [years]) + PA × [(26.7 × weight [kilograms]) + (903 × height [meters])] + 25
Girls	
3–8 y	135.3 − (30.8 × age [years]) + PA × [(10 × weight [kilograms]) + (934 × height [meters])] + 20
9–18 y	135.3 − (30.8 × age [years]) + PA × [(10 × weight [kilograms]) + (903 × height [meters])] + 25

Abbreviation: EER, estimated energy requirement.

[a] PA represents patient physical activity quotient.

Adapted with permission from Otten JJ, Hellwig JP, Meyers LD, eds. *Dietary Reference Intakes: The Essential Guide to Nutrient Requirements.* National Academies Press; 2006. Accessed November 7, 2022. https://www.nap.edu/read/11537/chapter/1#iii.

Table A-7. Physical Activity Quotient for Age and Activity Level

Age	Physical activity quotient value			
	Sedentary[a]	Low active[b]	Active[c]	Very active[d]
Boys 3–18 y	1	1.13	1.26	1.42
Girls 3–18 y	1	1.16	1.31	1.56

[a] Sedentary = Typical daily living activities (eg, household tasks, walk to bus).

[b] Low active = Typical daily living plus 30–60 minutes of daily moderate activity (eg, walking at a speed of 20 minutes per mile).

[c] Active = Typical daily living plus at least 60 minutes of daily moderate activity.

[d] Very active = Typical daily living plus at least 60 minutes of daily moderate activity plus an additional 120 minutes of moderate daily activity or 60 minutes of vigorous daily activity.

Adapted with permission from Otten JJ, Hellwig JP, Meyers LD, eds. *Dietary Reference Intakes: The Essential Guide to Nutrient Requirements.* National Academies Press; 2006. Accessed November 7, 2022. https://www.nap.edu/read/11537/chapter/1#iii.

Table A-8. Acceptable Macronutrient Distribution Range by Age

Macronutrient	AMDR (as % of energy intake)		
	Children 1–3 y	Children 4–18 y	Adults
Fat	30–40	25–35	20–35
Carbohydrate	45–65	45–65	45–65
Protein	5–20	10–30	10–35

Abbreviation: AMDR, acceptable macronutrient distribution range.

Adapted with permission from Otten JJ, Hellwig JP, Meyers LD, eds. *Dietary Reference Intakes: The Essential Guide to Nutrient Requirements.* National Academies Press; 2006. Accessed November 7, 2022. https://www.nap.edu/read/11537/chapter/1#iii.

Index

Page numbers followed by *f* indicate a figure; by *t*, a table; and by *b*, a box.